The Complete Health Care Advisor

THE
COMPLETE
HEALTH
CARE
ADVISOR

HENRY BERMAN, M.D.,
DIANE BURHENNE, Ph.D.,
AND LOUISA ROSE

St. Martin's/Marek
New York

Library of Congress Cataloging in Publication Data

Berman, Henry S.
    The complete health care advisor.

    1. Medical care—Handbooks, manuals, etc.   2. Con-
sumer education—Handbooks, manuals, etc.   3. Medical
care—United States—Handbooks, manuals, etc.   4. Consumer education—United States—Handbooks, manuals, etc.
I. Burhenne, Diane P.   II. Rose, Louisa.   III. Title.
RA410.5.B46   1983   362.1   83-10928
ISBN 0-312-15765-7

Design by Kingsley Parker

First Edition

10 9 8 7 6 5 4 3 2 1

To Elsie and Melvin Berman
May and Joseph Pollack
June Rose

And in Memory of
Jack Rose, Leo Sapon and Jake Rachleff

Contents

Acknowledgments

Two of us have worked in the health care field for many years, and have learned much from our mentors and colleagues. Those who have contributed greatly to Dr. Berman's understanding of the health care system, of physician attitudes and beliefs, and of patient needs, include Drs. Irwn P. Sobel, Joan E. Morgenthau, George W. Naumburg Jr., Leo Galland, and Jack Resnick; and Mary Garfield, M.S.W.

Those who have most influenced Dr. Burhenne and helped her understand systems, the ways in which people negotiate them and how they cooperate with each other in them, include Drs. Saul M. Siegel, Grayce M. Sills, James D. Lomax, Aurelia L. Levi, and Doreen Seidler-Feller as well as Drs. Gerald Perlman and David Glassman (of the W.B.C.).

All of us thank the many people who helped to make this book as complete, accurate, and up-to-date as possible. They include Drs. Carl Baum, Bill Burr, Murry Cohen, Paul Goldiner, Pascal J. Imperato, Cam McIntyre, John Moyer, Craig Olson, Jim Shaw, Joseph Stokes III, and Alan Tower. Also Genrose J. Alfano, R.N., Mary Butler, R.N., Nancy Davidson, C.N.M., Sharon Fairchild, Chuck Fortner, R.Ph., Joanne Halstead, C.R.N., Robert W. Harley, C.L.U., Barry Jones, Margaret Pope, C.N.M., Alissa Rose and Gale Rothstein.

Special thanks to Dorothy Ruzicki, Ph.D., for her assistance with the Resource Directory and Bibliography; to Shirley Polykoff, for the book's title; to Maureen Kovac and Jean Kindem for help when we needed it; to our agent, Jane Gelfman, for her enthusiasm for the project and her encouragement; and to our editor, Joyce Engelson, for her advice and support.

Introduction

Over and over again we all hear or read about medical horror stories: uncaring doctors who avoid patients, and nurses who give the wrong medication; surgeons who perform unnecessary and dangerous operations and obstetricians who, with their love of technology, prevent women from having a positive childbirth experience; drugs that turn out to have side effects worse than the diseases they are designed to treat, and tests that make people sicker than the diseases they are used to diagnose. Because these situations happen so frequently, many people, justifiably, have become suspicious of our whole health care system.

To protect and educate yourself, you may turn to some of the innumerable books and articles that are now available. But as you try to make your way through this mass of material, how do you know what to believe?—the book that tells you that a certain new drug will cure your problem, or one that says that the power to cure can be found only within yourself?—an article that describes the wonders of fetal monitoring, or one that tells you the safest place for a healthy mother to have a baby is at home? We feel that too often opinion (home births are safer than hospital births) is presented as fact, and, furthermore, that not enough of the articles and books emphasize that the needs of individuals differ greatly.

For example, one popular and useful book, very oriented to educating consumers, unequivocally recommends *The Merck Manual* (a reference work intended for medical professionals) as a book to bring with you to a desert island. In our judgment, while some people might find security in reading it, others—those inclined to imagine the worst at all times—would find this choice of reading material terribly anxiety-producing. They would look up "headache" (pp. 1294–95 of the 1983 edition), read that it is "a common manifestation of acute systemic or intracranial infection, intracranial tumor, head injuries, severe hypertension, cerebral hypoxia, and many diseases of the eye, nose, throat, teeth, and ear," and abandon their island retreat in a panic to find a doctor. Those who do not panic go on to read that "such conditions account for only a few patients who consult a physician because of headache. The remainder usually suffer from muscle tension headache, migraine, or head pain for which no structural cause can be found." Of course, that still would not have reassured those who would be sure they were among the "few." (In our annotated Bibliography, we suggest a way to use *The Merck Manual* that we believe is helpful and list books on a variety of topics that have complete information presented with you, the consumer, in mind.)

Because medical technology is changing so rapidly, any book that claims to describe the "latest" theory or treatment is in danger of being out-of-date by the time it appears in print. Just during the time we spent working on this book, for example, a number of very promising developments occurred, including:

- the release of Accutane®, offering the prospect of an effective treatment for severe cystic acne
- governmental approval to treat certain patients, who previously required back surgery, with an injection of chymopapain
- further advances in computer applications to diagnosis, such as multi-planar reconstruction (MPR), for diagnosing a herniated disk without resorting to a potentially risky myelogram; and light-scanning, a technique to screen for breast cancer that uses no radiation

Unfortunately, along with the promising advances, the other side of the new technology has reared its ugly head: the front page of our local newspaper just featured newly discovered adverse effects of a recently developed pain killer, Zomax®.

By the time you are reading this, any of the advances we've just described may have become standard treatments or tests, or they may have gone the way of gastric freezing for treatment of ulcers (a passing fad two decades ago); Zomax may have been banned or found "not guilty." The only certainty is that there will have been a number of other possible breakthroughs, and, inevitably, other bad news.

Thus, the purpose of this book is not to answer every question you may have about diagnosing or treating a problem: these answers change each month. Rather, it is to help you understand how a diagnosis is made and how to evaluate a proposed test or treatment. Neither do we list the "best" doctors or hospitals in the country—such lists are not generally useful even at the time they are compiled, let alone a year or two later. We do, however, suggest techniques for choosing a well-credentialed doctor or respected hospital that is right for you and for your problem.

Gaining an understanding of these issues does not come easy; rather than making it simple for you to gather such information, our health care system (or non-system, as it might better be called) seems to put every possible obstacle in your way.

We intend this book as a guide through this confusing, and potentially dangerous, obstacle course—populated with people in special uniforms (white coats) speaking an unintelligible language ("semi-quantitative immunologic testing by routine hemagglutination inhibition methods is adequate only when the titers are >2,000 I.U./L of urine"). By explaining many of the secret rules and mysterious customs of this strange world, we hope to make it easier for you to complete the obstacle course, and to win a prize: high quality personalized medical care at a price you can afford, with less anxiety. In addition to giving you this information, known by insiders but seldom by anyone else, we also try to help you understand what you yourself—not your mother or husband or co-worker—need and want.

Two of us are health professionals; all three of us, like you, are patients. Most of our case histories are drawn from our own or our colleagues' experiences; we feel that by including many such examples, you will have a more vivid picture of what problems doctors and patients encounter, and, which approaches work and which fail.

Perhaps this book will help you to avoid the plight of the patient described in Chapter Two, lying in her bed in a world-renowned medical center, never knowing which doctor to turn to with her desperate questions; or the young woman in Chapter Eleven, who died from a reaction to a test she may not have needed. There is much less chance you will have bad experiences like these if you are well informed about choosing your medical care.

Despite its problems, American medicine at its best is absolutely tops. There are knowledgeable, humane doctors who care deeply about their patients, who continue to improve their skills through ongoing education, and who work within their profession to increase physician responsiveness and responsibility. (We tell you about one of those doctors, a department chairman of a medical school who became a student again in order to find out what was wrong with medical education today.)

There are surgeons who operate only when they feel there is no alternative, and who are continually looking for simpler, less invasive procedures; nurses who want to involve themselves with their patients' total care; pharmacists who take great pains to ensure that the drugs they dispense will, if at all possible, cause no adverse reaction.

We feel that it is because such good medical care is available that a book like this is so necessary. With so many excellent doctors and hospitals, it is essential that you learn how to stay out of the hands of an unskilled physician or the bed of a poorly run hospital. A hundred years ago it didn't much matter; doctors and hospitals did very little to help patients. As a matter of fact, in those times, most people were better off avoiding both. But now—when many formerly untreatable problems are completely curable, or, better still, preventable—your decisions are vitally important.

THE
COMPLETE
HEALTH
CARE
ADVISOR

CHAPTER ONE

YOUR DOCTOR IS HUMAN— BUT YOU ARE EVEN MORE HUMAN

T he titles of some of the articles appearing in medical journals these days have a new ring to them. Unlike such page turners as "Hypercalcemia Associated with Resorbable Hemostatic Compresses" or "Failure of Serum Ferritin Levels to Predict Bone-marrow Iron Content after Intravenous Iron-dextran Therapy," these new titles look like subjects any thoughtful person might be interested in: "The Nature of Suffering and the Goals of Medicine," "God and the Doctor," and "The Effects of Stress on Physicians and Their Medical Practice."

The science of medicine has advanced greatly. That which was once incredible is now possible, sometimes even routine. Imperfect and rudimentary as our present knowledge may seem, we have made enormous advances in a very brief time. Until 1833, for example, no one knew exactly what the stomach did. In that year, Dr. William Beaumont published his now famous treatise, *Experiments and Observations on the Gastric Juices and the Physiology of Digestion.* Beaumont's discoveries were made possible by an odd piece of luck. His patient, Alexis St. Martin, had a gunshot wound that failed to heal completely, leaving an opening in the abdominal wall through which the digestive process could be studied.

Nowadays, doctors can probe what lies beneath the skin with x-rays and radioisotopes and ultrasound. They can transplant organs, reattach severed hands, graft skin, begin life in petri dishes, and restore sight to the blind. With an injection or two, they can ward off fatal and crippling diseases like diphtheria, tetanus, and pertussis (whooping cough). The great scourges such as leprosy and tuberculosis and cholera can be cured. Malaria can be prevented. A traveler in time who journeyed to the present from the eighteenth century might reasonably believe that our modern physicians possessed magical powers.

1

With these advances has come a feeling of discontent. Doctors are not as happy being doctors. Patients are not so pleased to be their patients. And everybody is left wondering what has gone wrong. We feel that at the heart of the problem is the relationship between doctor and patient, the role each partner in that relationship assumes, and the responsibility each has.

Before we discuss practical strategies for finding, choosing, and dealing with doctors, we would like to offer you some insight into the medical mind. Both the role that a doctor must fill and the way he or she is trained to occupy it have a great deal to do with how the one you choose sees your problems, what his or her goals are in treating you, and how those goals enhance or conflict with your own needs and expectations.

THE ROLE OF THE DOCTOR

The role of the doctor is in some ways no different from what it always was . . . from the patient's point of view. Most of us seek out a doctor because we feel sick or are afraid we might be harboring some disease, and we don't know what to do. If you have a painful splinter, you know exactly what is wrong. You find a tweezers or a needle and take care of the problem. If you have a pain in your stomach that you fear is a sign of disease, you see a doctor. You go because you want the doctor to use his or her special knowledge and abilities to make you well or to reassure you that the pain is meaningless and transient.

If you were a primitive person, you would behave in a fairly similar fashion. For example, among the Sanpoil,[1] a northwestern American Indian tribe, diseases were divided into two groups: those that had natural and those that had supernatural causes. If your affliction belonged to the first group, you might use an herbal remedy and most likely visit the sweat lodge. Self-care would suffice. If, however, you had an illness caused by the invasion of an unfriendly spirit, you would employ a shaman to diagnose and treat your sickness. Your doctor would smoke some tobacco for inspiration. He would then begin touching you and singing, trying to find the source of your sickness. Once he had located the spirit that was causing your problem, he would extract it and immerse it in water. His efforts would be helped along by a group of your fellows who would sing and beat time with sticks.

This may seem quaintly amusing, this laying on of hands, singing, beating of sticks, and extracting spirits. (Possibly our own 1980s medicine may be similarly described in centuries to come.)

The real secret of the shaman, according to Lewis Thomas in *The Youngest Science,* is the power that resides in the laying on of hands, and this is the link between shaman and physician. "Some people don't like being handled by others, but not, or almost never sick people. They need to be touched, and part of the dismay in being very sick is the lack of close human contact. Ordinary people, even close friends, even family members, tend to stay away from the very sick, touching them as infrequently as possible for fear of interfering, or catching the illness, or just for fear of bad luck. The doctor's oldest skill in trade was to place his hands on the patient."[2]

It is becoming increasingly clear that a medical system that separates mind and body, that fails to enlist the healing powers that lie within the person being treated, and that does not involve a healing relationship, will not satisfy or even help a large number of people.

Experienced doctors, shamans, mothers who kiss a bruised knee to make the hurt go away, all understand the power of what medical studies term "the placebo effect." A treatment of no known scientific value, touching, a sugar pill, or the beating of drums becomes a focal point for mobilizing belief and positive healing energy and can therefore alleviate symptoms or sometimes actually cure.

WHY DO DOCTORS SEEM SO POWERFUL: THE SOURCES OF MEDICAL AUTHORITY

A fascinating discussion of the basis for the unusual authority physicians have possessed throughout history was published in *The New England Journal of Medicine:* "God and the Doctor," by Humphrey Osmond. Osmond identifies three different types of authority:

1. Sapiental	derived from knowledge or expertise	
2. Moral	derived from the perception that what M.D.s do is both good for the individual and socially right	
3. Charismatic	derived from a tradition in which religion and medicine were intertwined and from the need, in matters of life and death, to reinforce knowledge with the power drawn from the doctor's original priestly role	

Osmond goes on to remark that it is this charismatic element that accounts for the fact that doctors are not expected to be entirely reasonable; in fact, they may be rewarded at times for being arbitrary. "Life and death are arbitrary," writes Osmond, "and so, it is appropriate for doctors also to have this quality. Extreme rationality and consistency would only raise doubts in the patient's mind, since he knows that medicine deals with powerful and mysterious forces that are not completely amenable to reason."[3]

This kind of talk may seem contrary to the present trend toward increased consumer understanding of, and participation in, health care decisions. As you read on you will come to chapters on self-care and on becoming more informed through your own research. The fact remains that there are times when all the informed consumerism in the world cannot help or heal.

The four-year-old daughter of a doctor asked him a difficult question. "Do you think I know everything just because I'm your father?" he asked. "No, Daddy," she answered, "because you're a doctor."

People, of course, vary in their perception of this phenomenon. If you have never been extremely ill or had someone close to you who was, you may not have encountered your own need for the charismatic and magical authority that Osmond is describing, a characteristic not really so much of the doctor, but of the doctor's role. The need to believe in this authority may not arise until one is concerned with matters of life and death. You should understand that these powers do exist and that some day you may have to deal with them.

In his article, Osmond goes on to quote an amusing example of how serious illness caused one of the more authoritative men in history to encounter the power of the doctor. The two actors in this account are the seriously ill Bismarck, autocratic architect of modern Germany, and his physician, Dr. Schweninger.

> At their first meeting, Bismarck said roughly, "I don't like being asked questions." Schweninger replied, "Then get a vet. He doesn't question patients." The battle was won in a single round. Bismarck ate and drank less and kept more regular hours. When Schweninger was present, he even kept his temper. He underwent a slimming diet which consisted exclusively of herring ... it did the trick. Bismarck's weight went down from 18 to 14 stone, he slept long and peacefully, his eyes became clear, his skin fresh and almost youthful.[4]

WHERE DOCTORS COME FROM: WHAT MEDICAL SCHOOLS DO AND DON'T TEACH

To begin with, medical students are not blank slates. They are college graduates who have already developed a system of values and beliefs. Perhaps part of the inability of medical schools to create ethical, caring doctors can be traced to the process by which they select their students. Far too much attention is paid to high grades and test scores and far too little to human values, ethical attitudes, and interpersonal skills.

Perhaps the best perspective on the problems of medical education today has been offered by a man who retired from a powerful position in an important university medical center to become a medical student once again. Ludwig W. Eichna, M.D., former Chairman of Medicine at SUNY, Downstate Medical Center, Brooklyn, left his position in 1974, became a full-time medical student at the Medical Center in

1975, and completed the full program in 1979. His observations and criticisms can be found in a remarkable article published in *The New England Journal of Medicine* several years ago.[5]

What he discovered about the state of professional training answers all those questions people pose about doctors. Why don't they listen to me? Why do I feel stupid talking to a doctor? Why is too much surgery done? Why don't they think of the consequences before recommending a treatment?

Following is our brief summary of some of the principles Dr. Eichna feels should govern medical education as contrasted with what the schools really do.

"The focus and first priority of medical school education is the patient."
In practice, says Dr. Eichna, the pressure of special interest groups—students, faculty, governmental bodies—distorts the teaching. Students are often not fully qualified either in personality or commitment. Rather than learning to think and solve problems, students spend most of their time amassing facts and learning manual and technical skills. "The patient is too often a secondary consideration."

"The profession of medicine is a science, humanly conducted."
At a time when so many advances have been made in biological science, students are antiscience and antiintellectual. Eichna believes that there is a dangerous downgrading of the science of medicine.

"Learning medicine requires a proper balance between apprenticeship (practical) training and formal teaching in lectures and seminars."
"That balance does not now exist," he says. "Practical training far outweighs formal teaching." Eichna then describes a typical scene in which the students are gathered around the chart rack in the hall. The resident asks for "the numbers" (meaning the test results). "They are produced and reviewed; more tests are ordered. The patient may not even be visited or examined or may be seen only perfunctorily. Not often does one hear, 'How is the patient?' "

"The profession of medicine demands at all levels, specifically including that of medical students, the highest ethical conduct."
"It is a great disappointment to encounter the routine violation of this principle and the teaching of bad medical ethics throughout all four years of medical school" writes Dr. Eichna. "One teaches ethics by living it, by expressing it in daily actions ... the patient comes first." He observes that patients, rather than being viewed compassionately as sick people, are seen as objects that exist for the student's development. "Teaching does not deal with them as people, nor is any teaching directed toward the obligation that students have toward patients and the ways of fulfilling it."

Perhaps an understanding of the deficiencies of medical education will clarify for you the importance of finding a physician who has not succumbed to some of the attitudes described in Eichna's article. And perhaps, having found such a person, you may be more prepared to forgive him or her for being less than perfect. Indeed, if this is what a doctor's training is like, you might almost be pleasantly surprised to find someone who is thoughtful, caring, and concerned.

THE ROLE OF THE PATIENT

In addition to the depersonalization and technical emphasis we have described, there is another facet of the hospital-based training doctors undergo that colors their subsequent attitudes. In hospitals, they take care of very sick, very helpless people, who are always referred to as "patients." The word itself, with its connotation of passive suffering and endurance, prepares doctors for a relationship in which they will call the shots.

The noted sociologist Talcott Parsons, who identified a special "sick role," formulated the ways in which someone in that role was expected to behave. Parsons noted that occupying the sick role confers both benefits and obligations. Sick people do not have to be responsible in the same way as those who are well, and they are not expected to take care of themselves. They must, however, want to get well, find technically competent help, and cooperate with the helper. They must, in order to occupy the sick role, display visible signs of being sick.[6]

Stages of Adaptation to Illness	
Denial / Resistance	Person refuses help, attributes symptoms to trivial problem
Entrance into Sick Role	Person becomes a patient, seeks professional help; possible anger if illness is serious
Acknowledgment	Accepts dispensation from normal duties, accepts and follows treatment; dependency on doctor may develop
Recovery / Rehabilitation	May be difficult if "secondary gains" of sick role hard to give up

A number of observers have categorized the stages people go through when they fall ill. It is difficult to remain completely rational when confronted with a threat to your sense of wholeness and integrity. You may become angry at the doctor who gives you the bad news, or angry at yourself; you may look for another doctor who will give you a diagnosis you like better; you may develop strong feelings of dependence on your doctor. If you do have a serious medical problem you may have to restructure your priorities in life. There may also be a reorganization of roles within your family. Even the recovery stage has its wayward moments. People whose previous lives have been unsatisfactory may not want to relinquish the freedom from responsibility they may have found in the sick role.

THE NEED TO BE A GOOD PATIENT

Once in this role, fear of the doctor's disapproval prevents many people from asking for what they want. Doctors have names for patients who do not behave properly in the sick role or who do not qualify for it. They call them hypochondriacs and chronic complainers or, in medical slang, crocks. Recently, articles have begun appearing in the journals on what to do with "hateful" patients, the people who are nasty, abusive, hopelessly self-destructive or manipulative, who cause such annoyance that doctors begin to think of ways to avoid or unload them. Such patients receive poor care, so it is crucial not to be thought of as one.

Although it may seem intolerable to you that any physician would try to avoid a patient, it can happen. As you read this book, we think you will begin to understand why. What is more important, you will learn how to choose a doctor who will not react negatively to what you need, and you will discover how to make what you feel are legitimate demands without being labeled "troublesome" or "hateful."

CHANGING ATTITUDES
TOWARD PHYSICIANS AND ILLNESS

Humphrey Osmond also discussed the sick role and pointed out the difference in the perspective of earlier generations from those of us born in the last fifty years. "We grew up with a respect for illness and a wary recognition that we must honor physicians 'for the uses ye may have of them.' We knew that there was much that even the best doctor could not do, just as battle-experienced soldiers know that there are times when the best units fail and all that can be done is to fight a stubborn retreat."[7]

Today, it is not uncommon for both patient and physician to have had no personal or family experience with serious illness. Thus, "if a sick person happens to be ignorant of the rights and duties of the sick role, his or her communications are liable to be inept and to evoke aberrant responses from doctors and nurses." If you are fortunate enough not to have experienced serious illness, perhaps this book will help educate you about the "rights and duties of the sick role," so that your communications are not "inept," and you will not evoke "aberrant responses" from doctors and nurses.

We come to a doctor with a definite if unexamined set of expectations: that he or she will be highly skilled and knowledgeable about illness, will hold the personal information we give in confidence, and will always act in our best interests. In addition, we expect doctors to act, talk, and dress in certain ways. A doctor clad in the latest fashion craze or old blue jeans would seem somehow wrong to most people. We are critical of a doctor who does not seem to know enough or who acts cold or uncaring.

Most doctors feel that their goals are clear-cut: to make a diagnosis and cure the disease. They very much want to succeed, to name and conquer the illness or injury that afflicts you. If they cannot accomplish either of their goals, they may become frustrated or anxious. To combat these feelings, physicians who lack self-awareness may do a number of things such as order too many tests, withdraw, get angry if you ask a lot of questions, prescribe drugs that are not indicated, and even do unnecessary surgery.

We have talked a lot about roles and about the rules of interaction. Doctors seem so powerful and so in control that it may take an effort of the imagination to think of them as fellow human beings with all the usual responses, an effort especially difficult to make when you the patient are sick. By recognizing that your doctor is human, you will be more apt to get good and helpful reactions.

Some resent the thought of their physicians as people who face the human problems described above, but their need to see the doctor as godlike doesn't help matters. In fact, the pressure for perfection increases the stress.

If you feel that you have poor relationships with doctors, and you notice that they exhibit some of the reactions described below, you might examine your own behavior or expectations to see if either could be part of the problem. After all, physicians want to help you; it makes them feel good. If you are getting "go away" signs from the physician, it might be because you are making it impossible for him or her to help you.

PROOF THAT DOCTORS ARE HUMAN: FACTORS CAUSING STRESS IN DOCTORS

What causes stress in physicians, leading them to be less effective and even impaired? A recent article by Jack D. McCue, M.D., published in *The New England Journal of Medicine*,[8] described the following factors:

1. Working with intensely emotional aspects of life governed by strong cultural codes for behavior: these include suffering, fear, sexuality, and death—all areas in which physicians have little or no training.

2. Handling "problem" patients—that is, the "clinger," "demander," "help-rejecter," and "denier," all of whom elicit anger, avoidance, fear, and despair in the physician.

3.   The need for certainty when current medical knowledge allows only approximation—a state that makes both patient and doctor anxious, and tempts them to, in McCue's words, "collude in oversimplification and lies."

How do doctors react? Often not too well. McCue describes some of the consequences of stress.

1.   Emotional withdrawal, including retreat from family life, and putting all their energy into medicine to ensure that their efforts are above criticism—therefore, any failures must be attributed to misfortune.

2.   Social isolation—avoiding non-physicians, partly to avoid having their financial success observed by their patients.

3.   Denial of professional problems: for example, ordering unnecessary lab tests to hedge against fears and uncertainty.

4.   Irony: the "black humor" that sounds so nasty to nonprofessionals is coping behavior on the part of the physician.

BUT YOU ARE EVEN MORE HUMAN

But you are even more human; that is, you have come to the doctor in need of help. You may be feeling anxious, confused, uncomfortable, embarrassed, ignorant, and perhaps even angry that you have something wrong with you. It is the professional responsibility of the doctor to make you feel cared for by treating you with respect, listening to your concerns, answering your questions fully and clearly, diagnosing and treating your problem to the extent of his or her capabilities, and referring you to another specialist if necessary.

A good and concerned doctor will attempt to ease your anxiety, clear up any confusion you may have, and make you feel comfortable in discussing personal matters. Not only will you be a happier patient if these things are done, you will probably be a better one, far more able to participate in whatever treatment is necessary once you understand and agree to it.

Doctors know that patients are often nervous, sometimes downright fearful. If they become annoyed because you forgot to give them important information or withheld it due to embarrassment, this may be humanly understandable, but they are not really helping you.

THE IMPORTANCE OF THE HUMAN PART OF MEDICINE

For many centuries, people in and out of the medical profession have understood the importance of the human qualities that make doctors healers. Some physicians even feel that those people who have a trusting relationship with their doctor may be healthier than those who do not. Furthermore, we know of other phenomena, such as those described by Norman Cousins (in his book *Anatomy of an Illness*) in which the power of people's belief in the *vis medicatrix naturae* (the healing powers that reside in their own bodies) may help them survive even an "incurable" disease.[9]

Above all, the key to continuing good health, and to speedier recovery when you are sick, may be the "human-ness" of *both* you and your doctor, and in your healing interrelationship. Because all of us must expect that at some point we will have to place our lives or the life of a family member in the hands of a physician, condemnation of the entire species is in the long term self-defeating. And the opposite tendency, to trust every doctor completely, and never to question a diagnosis or treatment, is too dangerous. This book will try to show you the path between these extremes—the path to high quality, affordable, personalized medical care.

WHAT DO YOU REALLY WANT FROM A DOCTOR?

There are many underlying needs that people bring with them to the doctor's office along with the explicit request for medical information and treatment. If you have a certain amount of insight you may recognize your own. Perhaps you would like the doctor to be a superparent who will take care of you. You may imagine your ideal doctor to be the quintessential teacher who will give you the tools with which to make critical decisions. Maybe you wish for an impossibly intimate friend in whom anything can be confided, a friend who will always have your interest, and only your interest at heart, and who can be trusted to know when to step in and tell you what to do, and when not to; when to share doubt and uncertainty, and when not to; when to tell you all the possibilities, and when to reassure you. Or, you may be someone who wants the superbly trained technician who will give you the precisely correct output as a function of your carefully determined input.

If you have these kinds of needs, you are bound for disappointment, for no doctor, no matter how kind or willing or brilliant, can play any of these roles perfectly. What you can do, if you are aware of these feelings, is to use them to guide you in a certain direction.

WHAT QUALITIES MATTER MOST TO YOU?

A man with a bothersome elbow problem asked for a referral and was sent to a very experienced orthopedist, a busy doctor who had six exam rooms lined up, with a patient ready in each. He would see each patient, dictate the note from the room, and go on to the next. Very efficient, the better to benefit more patients from his vast storehouse of information—and not bad for his pocketbook, of course.

He made a diagnosis and gave a recommendation; the treat-ment helped somewhat, but symptoms persisted. This man, how-ever, was reluctant to make another appointment with the orthopedist. Why? After all, the doctor was extremely knowl-edgeable and had a fine reputation. The impersonal efficiency of this setup had bothered this patient. Said he, "I'd rather see someone who knows less but cares more."

There are those who would have the opposite reaction. From time to time, lists appear of the ninety-seven best doctors in New York City or the best twenty doctors in the country; they are always selected on the basis of their academic credentials. People flock to doctors whose names appear on these lists—or attempt to flock, since these doctors are generally busy heads of hospital departments and often do not practice much out-patient medicine. Given a doctor who is basically knowledgeable and well trained, do you want the one who knows the most or cares the most? You can seldom get both. The super-scientist, reading journal after journal, attending course after course, living and breathing medicine—a veritable Arrowsmith—usually has less well-developed interpersonal skills. Not always, but almost always.

There is a joke making the rounds of medical conferences about a rich and powerful man who dies and goes to heaven. While impa-tiently waiting his turn at the end of a long line before the pearly gates, he notices a tall man with a white beard and a white coat go right to the front of the line and walk in. Annoyed yet impressed, he asks, "Who is that?" The man in front of him answers, "Oh, that's God. He's just playing doctor."

Many are the doctors who have been accused of playing God. It is, for some, an occupational hazard. They have learned that patients who don't want to make decisions about their health are vastly relieved by having someone else, the expert, shoulder the burden of choice.

A teenager with a painful boil on her thigh went to see her doctor. After examining her carefully, the doctor explained that the problem could be treated in one of two ways: with an-tibiotics and hot soaks, which would probably cause it to drain in a few days and then heal, or by cutting it with a scalpel and letting it drain immediately. Medically, the options appeared about equal. The choice really depended on whether the pa-tient preferred to get the thing over with or whether she was anxious to avoid the scalpel and willing to take care of the boil at home. "It's your choice," said the doctor. The patient looked stricken. "What should I do?" she asked. Once more the doctor carefully explained her choices. Again the patient turned to him and said, "But what should I do?"

The present trend in medical consumerism, which is to view the patient as an equal partner in care, overlooks the dependency needs that many people bring to the doctor's office or the hospital bed. When people are sick or are afraid that something is wrong with them, they often regress.

What are your own reactions and wishes when you need medical attention? Do you want a doctor who will tell you what to do, or a doctor who expects you to make your own decisions? Or do you want a kind of combination approach: a doctor who will outline options but steer you in the direction that he or she feels is best for you?

Some people want to know all the probable outcomes of a course of treatment, but they may not want to know all the *possible* outcomes. For example, a patient needs a certain kind of x-ray that carries a risk. Should the doctor mention that there is a 1 in 40,000 chance of dying? Some people want that piece of information, some don't.

Everyone wants reassurance, but we don't all find it in the same way. Ask yourself how you react when someone says, "Don't worry." Are you relieved or do you hear a nagging little voice in your brain that whispers, "Don't worry about *what?*" One person is vastly consoled by a simple word of reassurance; another will only be reassured after the doctor lists every possible diagnosis and explains why all the serious ones can be eliminated.

WHAT KIND OF DOCTOR DO YOU NEED?

The following questions are designed to help you to select a physician whose style is right for you, by clarifying some of your attitudes toward physicians and some of your perceptions of yourself as a patient.

Check off each statement as either true or false *for you*. Some have to do with doctors; others are about life in general.

	True	False
1. If I take care of myself, I can avoid illness.	☐	☐
2. The more tests a doctor does, the more reassured I am.	☐	☐
3. When I think I'm sick, I can't stop worrying until my doctor tells me I'm OK.	☐	☐
4. I'm a soft touch for anyone who treats me nicely.	☐	☐
5. When my doctor doesn't return my call promptly, I start to wonder whether s/he really cares about me.	☐	☐
6. I need to know exactly what's wrong with me and what the doctor is doing.	☐	☐
7. I don't care what someone's personality is like as long as s/he gets the job done.	☐	☐

True False

8. I believe that there's a scientific solution for almost every problem. ☐ ☐

9. I almost always follow the advice of people who are more intelligent than I. ☐ ☐

10. When I'm down, kind words or even just a smile help. ☐ ☐

11. I like to be the boss in most things I do. ☐ ☐

12. Getting sick is just bad luck. ☐ ☐

13. If my doctor doesn't listen to and respond to all of my concerns, I feel shortchanged. ☐ ☐

14. When my boss tells me what to do, I don't question it. I figure s/he probably knows best. ☐ ☐

15. I only call the doctor when nothing else works. ☐ ☐

16. I generally go along with people's suggestions because I don't like to make a fuss. ☐ ☐

17. I don't read my medical insurance policies; when I need to use them, someone will help me figure them out. ☐ ☐

18. When I go to the doctor, just talking to him/her frequently makes me feel better. ☐ ☐

19. When my doctor gives me pills, I'm usually not concerned about what they are, since s/he only gives me things that are good for me. ☐ ☐

20. I don't care what my doctor does, as long as I feel better. ☐ ☐

21. Liking someone is the most important thing in a relationship. ☐ ☐

22. Because my doctor is extremely intelligent and able to figure out what is wrong with me, I feel I am in good hands. ☐ ☐

23. I'm the only one responsible for my health. ☐ ☐

24. I always accept my doctor's recommendations even if I don't like them. ☐ ☐

25. I never seem to get all the help I need with things. ☐ ☐

26. I get upset when someone tries to tell me how to do something after I've started a project. ☐ ☐

27. Just because someone is an expert in one field doesn't mean he or she is knowledgeable in another. ☐ ☐

28. Knowing that my doctor is really concerned about me helps me overlook his/her personality quirks. ☐ ☐

29. I like to make my own decisions. ☐ ☐

True False

30. When my doctor remembers something I told him/her that doesn't relate just to my medical condition, I know I'm with the right doctor. ☐ ☐

31. I can't say "no." ☐ ☐
32. If I'm seriously ill, I don't want to know what's wrong; I just want the doctor to cure it. ☐ ☐
33. I like to work alone because nothing gets done in groups. ☐ ☐
34. My doctor always knows what's best for me. ☐ ☐
35. If people care about me, I know they'll do "right" by me. ☐ ☐
36. When someone yells at me, I feel horrible. ☐ ☐
37. It makes me feel secure when my doctor gives me a lengthy explanation of my illness, even though I don't always understand what s/he says. ☐ ☐
38. I always call professional people by their titles to show respect. ☐ ☐
39. I almost always try to treat myself before I call the doctor. ☐ ☐
40. Most people seem to know more than I do. ☐ ☐

Scoring:
The above questions examine doctors and patients along four dimensions. The emotionally-oriented, technically-oriented dimensions (EMOTIONAL, TECHNICAL) relate to two physician qualities. The other-reliant, self-reliant dimensions (OTHER, SELF) relate to how much you want to be involved in your own health care. Score your responses by dimension by giving yourself one point for each "TRUE" response (the numbers next to the listed qualities are the numbers of the statements as they appear in the questionnaire):

TOTAL

Questions: 4, 5, 10, 13, 18   _____ = EMOTIONAL
           21, 28, 30, 35, 36
Questions: 2, 7, 8, 9, 14, 20   _____ = TECHNICAL
           22, 34, 37, 40
Questions: 3, 12, 16, 17, 19   _____ = OTHER
           24, 25, 31, 32, 38
Questions: 1, 6, 11, 15, 23   _____ = SELF
           26, 27, 29, 33, 39

Now add the following scores together (each category can only have a maximum of 20 points):

TOTAL
1. EMOTIONAL (__ points) + OTHER (__ points) = _____
2. EMOTIONAL (__ points) + SELF (__ points) = _____
3. TECHNICAL (__ points) + OTHER (__ points) = _____
4. TECHNICAL (__ points) + SELF (__ points) = _____

Interpretation:
Now review your scores. Which is your highest? Your highest score should give you a fairly good indication of which of the physician qualities noted is more important to you and which of the two types of patient qualities you feel more nearly represents you.

Highest Score
1. OTHER-RELIANT—   PREFERS EMOTIONALLY-ORI-ENTED M.D.: You are probably the type of person who feels that it is crucial that your physician makes you feel cared about and understood. Demonstration of technical information might not be your major concern since you feel you are not an expert in medical matters. You may feel best with a doctor who inspires confidence through caring, not through discussing medical details. You would tend to want the physician to make most of your medical decisions since you feel that a physician who shows real concern will act in your best interests.

2. SELF-RELIANT—   PREFERS EMOTIONALLY-ORI-ENTED M.D.: You would probably prefer a physician who demonstrates caring and concern by his or her attentive, sympathetic attitude rather than one who just discusses medical facts with you. What might be important to you, however, is that the physician's concern extends to your need to make many decisions for yourself. You would probably be more comfortable with a physician who works with you to make your own choices, guiding you and not just telling you what to do.

3. OTHER-RELIANT—   PREFERS TECHNICALLY-ORI-ENTED M.D.: You might prefer a physician who demonstrates his or her expertise through discussing a great deal of technical information with you. You probably feel comfortable following the advice of authorities and aren't particularly interested in making your own medical decisions. Since you believe that only medical experts should make medical decisions, you would probably feel secure with a physician who overtly demonstrates medical knowledge.

4. SELF-RELIANT—   PREFERS TECHNICALLY-ORI-ENTED M.D.: You would appreciate a physician who overtly demonstrates his or her expertise by a technical approach, sharing all of the medical details with you. You're probably the type of person who pre-

fers to make your own medical decisions but only after you have all the necessary information in detail. You would feel best with the physician who gives you all of the data and then lets you do the deciding.

If you find a physician whose style meshes with your expectations, you will have an easier and a pleasanter relationship. You will also give information more freely, helping the doctor to diagnose and treat you more effectively. Chances are, too, that you will follow treatment plans more willingly and report problems more promptly. The reason to put real effort into finding a doctor with the approach you favor is that you will most likely end up with better medical care.

CHAPTER TWO

PRIMARY CARE: WHY YOU NEED IT AND HOW TO GET IT

Mrs. B. is recovering from cancer surgery. She was operated on at a famous medical center by a gynecologist specializing in oncology. The gynecologist then referred her for follow-up treatment to a specialist in radiation therapy. She feels terribly sick. When she goes to the office of the radiologist, she tells him so. She receives another treatment anyway and collapses.

She is admitted to the hospital with renal shutdown, a condition in which the kidneys, which purify the blood of wastes and toxins, fail to function. A nephrologist (a specialist in the treatment of kidney disease) is called in. The nephrologist brings in a nephrology Fellow (a doctor taking advanced training in this subspecialty).

In the meantime, Mrs. B. develops high blood pressure. A cardiologist joins the crew of specialists (gynecologist, radiologist, nephrologist) at her bedside. Mrs. B.'s daughter comes to visit daily. "Who is taking care of me?" is her mother's recurring question.

Mrs. B. becomes desperately ill and needs dialysis. The nephrologist is called, but he is not available. He is giving a lecture. The nephrology Fellow is found but arrives too late. Mrs. B. is dead.

Mrs. B. died at a major hospital and was treated by doctors with fine medical reputations. This case is an extreme example of what can happen when Mrs. B.'s question—"Who is taking care of me?"—goes unanswered. She had highly trained specialists for almost every part of her body, and these doctors had valuable knowledge and skills to offer; but by definition, specialists are not trained to take care of the whole person nor do they view that as their role.

17

Far too many people go to a series of specialists as symptoms arise, or wait until they are sick and need an appointment on the spot before they begin looking for a good primary care doctor. In this chapter, we are going to give you some specific reasons why you need to identify that person now, not only to help you deal with a serious illness like Mrs. B.'s, but also to help you cope more easily and inexpensively with the common medical problems and concerns that are bound to arise.

We will list the types of physicians who are trained to provide general care, and describe not only the kinds of credentials these physicians should have but also the significance of those credentials.

A true primary care doctor, at least in the sense that we use the term, is someone who has studied not only the functions and diseases of the separate parts of your body but also the interrelationship of those parts. In addition, he or she will be concerned with the way you live your life, with your family situation, and with your work. Your primary care doctor will know what an important role emotions play in maintaining health and how the stresses and strains of life manifest themselves both physically and mentally.

The child with recurrent stomach aches that keep her out of school may not need elaborate and invasive lab tests. She may have a condition called "school phobia." The only way the doctor can make this diagnosis is by taking a careful history and understanding the role these stomach aches play in the family situation.

The man with the nagging cough who works in an asbestos factory is different from the man with a cough who works in a bank. The teenager who is depressed may exhibit a whole range of physical symptoms, but unless the underlying depression is dealt with, the aches and pains will continue.

Your primary care doctor is the first person to turn to with medical problems and questions. He or she will refer you to a specialist if you need one, discuss the specialist's findings with you, help you get a second or third opinion if you want one, and then explain and help you analyze the often confusing information you have been given, so that you can make a decision. If you are having financial problems, this is someone who can help you find ways to get care at the least possible expense.

> Dr. N., a family medicine practitioner, is making his hospital rounds. One of his patients, a tired young mother, is preparing to take her second baby home. He tells her how well the baby is doing, asks her how she feels, and, in the course of the conversation, learns that her husband has just lost his job. He then assures her that she will be able to call and ask questions when she needs advice—no need to pay for an office visit. He also informs her of a program that will enable her to get immunizations for her new baby free of charge.

PRIMARY CARE SAVES YOU MONEY

When you feel perfectly healthy, you may be understandably reluctant to spend any money on a visit to the doctor. If you get sick and the expenses start piling up, you may be looking for ways to cut costs. We feel strongly that the most economical course is to establish a relationship with a doctor *before* you get sick and to use your primary care giver to control your medical costs. Here is a list of reasons why this advice will save you money.

1. Primary care doctors tend to have lower fees than specialists, and can treat a wide range of problems. A headache treated by a neurologist is a far more expensive headache than one treated by a general internist or family practitioner. (If your headaches require further evaluation you can always be referred.)
2. You are much less likely to have an unnecessary operation. Should surgery be a possibility, your physician will know which surgeons are conservative and will be able to help you decide whether recommended surgery is really advisable or necessary for you.
3. Primary care doctors can reduce your reliance on expensive specialists. You may go to a specialist for a consultation but return to your primary care doctor for actual treatment. You will have the advantage of the specialist's diagnostic expertise without having to pay for costly follow-up visits.

For people with cancer, this approach may save repeated visits to distant medical centers for treatments that could be given locally. After those nationally famous cancer experts have made the diagnosis, they are available to your personal physician by phone for further advice.
4. You will save money on tests and x-rays. An experienced generalist knows what most people have, most of the time, and will order only those tests that are truly warranted. A specialist who has invested in costly diagnostic equipment is sometimes tempted to use it, even when it is not strictly necessary.

Your primary care doctor will have your complete medical history, which will contain the results of those tests and x-rays. Keeping the information in one place can save you the expense, discomfort, and added risk of having duplicate tests. (Such duplications often happen to people who make the rounds of specialists on their own.)

Probably the major reason a good generalist saves you money is that he or she is much less likely to go on what physicians refer to as a "zebra hunt." In the course of learning to make diagnoses, medical students are taught that "when you hear hoofbeats, think of horses, not zebras." This rule tends to be forgotten by those who specialize in a narrow area of medicine and who, in fact, spend much of their specialty training discussing rare diseases. If you take your headache to the neurologist, he or she is far more apt to think of aneurysms and tumors than of stress or eyestrain as causes.

MEDICAL PEACE OF MIND

Beyond purely financial and practical considerations is the sense of security you will have once you do have a physician you know and to whom you can turn with all your health problems. There are a number of ways in which your primary care doctor can keep down both your medical costs and your level of anxiety:

- by giving telephone advice and reassurance
- by helping you get the most from your insurance coverage
- by finding the right specialists and hospitals
- by identifying alternatives to a hospital stay if you want outpatient surgery
- by seeing that you do not stay in the hospital longer than necessary
- by helping you avoid having unnecessary, expensive, and sometimes painful tests when you don't really need them

WHO ARE THE PRIMARY CARE GIVERS?

There are several types of physicians who give primary care to children, to teenagers, and to adults. Don't be confused by some of the titles, such as specialist in family medicine or specialist in adolescent medicine. These physicians are indeed "specialists" in that they have completed advanced training programs, but their course of study has taught them about all the problems their patients may have. Our list contains only generalists, those physicians who are equipped to take care of a very wide range of what might ail you.

General Internist
An internist (not to be confused with *intern,* a doctor who has just finished medical school and is now receiving hospital-based training) is trained to take care of the medical problems of adults: in the physician's vocabulary the word "medical" refers essentially to treatments that do not involve surgery.

To find a true general internist may take some exploration and questioning because the field of internal medicine is really a composite of a number of different body systems and each system or organ has its own medical subspecialty: allergists take care of allergies; cardiologists treat diseases of the heart; pulmonary disease specialists handle diseases of the lung; nephrologists specialize in kidney problems; and so on through the "ologies," such as hematology/oncology, gastroenterology, rheumatology, and immunology/infectious disease.

Many internists who are trained in a subspecialty also practice general medicine; there is some danger that these highly specialized physicians may be somewhat bored by your run-of-the-mill sore throat, or migraine headache, or virus.

A good primary care giver must be interested in the routine problems that most people have—and beyond that, in the people who have them.

> Dr. G., a general internist, has seen large numbers of women with recurrent urinary tract infections (UTIs) and has decided to study this very common problem, one that has failed to generate much academic interest among either gynecologists or urologists. He reads everything he can find on the subject and then conducts a study on his own patients. Based on what he learns, he is able to recommend measures that help women avoid recurrences of this condition—and even publishes a paper on the subject in a prestigious journal.

Urinary tract infections are a good example of the kind of problem that may cross the arbitrary boundaries of professional specialization. Most women assume that the problem calls for a gynecologist or possibly a urologist, but these specialists are trained primarily in surgery, not in the medical management of disease.

Primary Care Internist

An internist who has had specific training to qualify as a true generalist is a *primary care* internist. These doctors are taught to deal with the whole patient, a concept that may sound trite or obvious unless you are aware of how fragmented hospital-based training can be. Patients are often referred to as "the kidney in room 109" or "the cardiac arrest on four." Primary care internists, in addition to their *medical* training, may also spend time learning about such surgical specialties as gynecology and orthopedics.

Family Practitioner

You may also see the term "specialist in family medicine" used to refer to this type of physician. The field has arisen out of the old and serviceable concept of the general practitioner (G.P.), the old-fashioned family doctor who took care of all your medical problems, regardless of your age or sex. Family practitioners fill a need that has never disappeared, but they do so with far more training than their predecessors. Since this is a new field and possibly unfamiliar to you, it bears some explanation.

In the early part of this century, most physicians knew a little bit about everything but not a lot about anything. There were relatively few specialists; the doctor who wanted to become one served an apprenticeship with an established specialist. This training became formalized as the century wore on and developed into hospital-based programs known as residencies. More and more physicians took specialty training; those who did not were called general practitioners.

In a city, general practitioners would usually take care of minor problems of patients of all ages. In small towns or rural settings, they would also deliver babies, set broken bones, and do minor, and sometimes even major, surgery such as removing a gall bladder or doing a hysterectomy.

As time went by, the explosion of medical knowledge caused a proliferation of specialists; the practice of general medicine was not as prestigious, certainly not from the physicians' point of view, as one of the new specialty or subspecialty fields. Medical care became more and more fragmented.

The end result of the trend toward increased specialization was a lack of properly educated generalists. The training of general practitioners was too limited and did not equip them to give care to people with serious problems. What was needed was a new field in which doctors would become specialists in general medicine.

In 1969, the field of family medicine became a recognized specialty. To qualify, a physician was required to take a three-year residency program (the same length as is required for internal medicine or pediatrics). Instead of learning about one age group or one organ system, family practice residents learn about all age groups and all the problems that might affect them, with a particular emphasis on understanding family dynamics and psychosocial problems, and an underlying philosophy that doctors must understand and deal with their patients as human beings.

At first, experienced general practitioners were given an opportunity to become board-certified (the term is explained on pp. 29–30) in family medicine by taking continuing medical education courses, passing a rigorous exam, and proving that they were competent to handle the wide variety of problems they faced in this role. During the 1970s, many G.P.s met these requirements and became board-certified family physicians. Since 1979, however, the only route to becoming a board-certified family practitioner has been to complete a residency program. To retain their board status, family physicians must meet recertification requirements every seven years.

Family practitioners can take care of every member of your family. They can take care of babies, do gynecology, treat medical problems of adults, and perform minor surgical procedures. (Many even practice obstetrics.) They feel that their knowledge of what is going on in a family as a whole enhances their ability to treat the individual members.

Pediatrician

This is the primary care physician for children. Traditionally, pediatricians have been trained to treat the medical problems of children from birth to puberty.

Most people seem to understand and use primary care more effectively for their children than for themselves. The parent who goes to a gastroenterologist for his or her own stomach ache will call on the child's pediatrician for everything from rashes to ear infections to problems with bed-wetting and school adjustment.

For most parents, a pediatrician with an interest in child development and behavior is invaluable. A large percentage of questions and concerns are not strictly medical. Why won't my child eat puréed vegetables and does it matter? How can I get her to take naps? Is he droopy and withdrawn because of the new baby?

There are a number of pediatricians who have taken extra training and developed skills in dealing with these behavioral areas. You can certainly ask directly if the pediatrician has some background in this area: the latest catch-phrase for such counseling is "anticipatory guidance."

Specialist in Adolescent Medicine

Usually this is a pediatrician, but sometimes it is an internist or family practitioner who has taken extra training in the medical, developmental, and emotional problems of adolescence. Like the pediatrician, the adolescent specialist is a primary care doctor for a given age group. Right now, there are thirty-five formal training programs for this specialty in major hospitals around the country.

A physician in this field should be both medically and personally skillful in handling a wide range of problems and concerns: everything from eating disorders such as anorexia nervosa or bulimia, to acne, to painful periods (dysmenorrhea). A trained adolescent specialist is also familiar with problems of substance abuse (alcohol, cigarettes, drugs) and should be comfortable in dealing with family/school, social, and personal problems.

Many specialists in adolescent medicine also do general pediatrics; some, usually those associated with an adolescent clinic, care exclusively for teen-agers. At this time, there are no boards, but physicians with significant training and experience in the field will generally be members of the Society for Adolescent Medicine and/or will belong to the adolescent section of the American Academy of Pediatrics.

Physicians experienced in treating this age group establish a confidential relationship with their patients and will explain to parents how vital the issue of trust is in giving good medical care.

SPECIAL CONSIDERATIONS FOR WOMEN

Although being a man is no guarantee of receiving high quality health care, being a woman seems to make the goal even more difficult to achieve. Articles and books written by both health care professionals and feminist activists describe the history of abuse women have suffered at the hands of the medical profession, and the problems women still face today. Most physicians are men. Men control most medical schools, hospitals, and other health care institutions. Women are more likely to have their problems diagnosed as "neurotic" or "hysterical," and as a result they are given far more prescriptions for sedatives and tranquilizers. Women are also subjected to more unnecessary surgery than men.

We feel that the guidelines we propose as the basis for finding good health care are the same for both sexes. Because of a tradition of discrimination, however, women may have to work harder at finding doctors who will treat their concerns with respect and make them feel cared for.

Until fairly recently, women have been unable to enjoy the advantages of real primary care medicine because most general physicians left the care of the reproductive organs to gynecologists. Fortunately, the women's movement has brought about a greater awareness and interest in women's health problems; many doctors have reconsidered the wisdom of having women divide up their bodies and their care. For example, a woman with annoying frequency of urination may have a vaginal infection, a urinary tract infection, or a stress-related problem. A good generalist can sort things out for her, referring her to an appropriate specialist only if necessary, and spare her confusion and extra expense.

An important question for a woman to ask when looking for a primary care doctor is "Do you do routine gynecology?" Family practitioners are all trained to do this, and so are the new breed of primary care internists. Specialists in adolescent medicine who have taken fellowships have been trained to do pelvic exams and are usually especially up-to-date on the subject of birth control.

Many women don't realize that gynecology is primarily a surgical specialty and that the height of the gynecologist's skill is to perform such operations as hysterectomies (removal of uterus) and oophorectomies (removal of ovaries).

Most gynecologists are not well versed in matters such as the behavioral aspects of various birth control methods or the most recently recommended treatments for those minor problems that are major annoyances to women: vaginal infections. Despite their medical knowledge of the sexual organs, gynecologists are not necessarily qualified to do sex counseling. Although some do develop a genuine interest in the more routine aspects of their field, most are more valuable as consultants who can make difficult diagnoses or treat more serious disorders.

Mrs. V. is dismayed to find herself pregnant even though she has faithfully followed all the instructions for using her diaphragm. After obtaining an abortion, she asks her gynecologist to check the way the diaphragm fits, and he assures her it is correct. He explains that there is a lower failure rate with birth control pills and suggests she consider taking them. Mrs. V. says she'll think about it.

A few months later, unable to get a prompt appointment with her gynecologist for a bout of vaginitis, she sees a gynecological nurse-practitioner at a woman's health clinic who, in the course of the exam, explains that her uterus is tilted and suggests that she use an arc-spring diaphragm. When she does, she is immediately aware of the difference in fit. Why didn't her highly trained gynecologist know?

In the interests of comprehensive care, women would do best to find a good general internist or family practitioner who does routine gynecology. If the best or only primary care doctors around are all men, a woman who feels more relaxed and less embarrassed getting gynecological care from another woman would have a problem.

One solution would be to use a woman gynecologist. Another would be to find a gynecological nurse-practitioner who, because she specializes in the routine aspects of gynecology, may be extremely helpful when it comes to questions of birth control, vaginal infections and irritations, and menstrual problems. (These professionals work in women's health clinics, in gynecologists' offices, and sometimes in prepaid health plans.)

Women who rarely or never see a primary care doctor should find a thorough gynecologist who in addition to doing a pelvic exam always does a breast exam and a blood pressure check.

PRIMARY CARE FROM NONPHYSICIANS

What about the nonphysicians who give medical care? Who are they and what kinds of problems do they treat? For information on the full range of practitioners other than physicians, we would recommend reading a comprehensive book on non-traditional medicine. But there are two kinds of professionals we will mention here: osteopaths and chiropractors.

Osteopath

A doctor of osteopathy (D.O.) has graduated from college and a four-year school of osteopathic medicine and has often gone on to take a hospital-based residency. The training these days is very much equivalent to an M.D.'s training. Unlike most physicians, osteopaths are trained to do spinal manipulations for back and neckaches. Some osteopaths have trained in the same hospital programs and specialized in the same fields as have M.D.s. If you are considering using an osteopath for your primary care doctor, you would want to have the same information on credentials that you would with any doctor: school, residency, boards, and hospital affiliation (all discussed later in this chapter. Although there are some hospitals run by osteopaths, the best trained D.O.s generally have privileges at the same hospitals that M.D.s use.

Chiropractor

The field of chiropractic is based on the theory that almost all medical problems emanate from abnormalities of the spine. Chiropractors are usually but not always college graduates. They have attended a four-year chiropractic school. In the course of their education, they are introduced to all fields of medicine, primarily to help them know when to refer a patient they are seeing to a physician. Some states allow chiropractors, despite their shorter, less extensive course of training, to do almost anything a physician does. Other states restrict their practice to spinal manipulation for the relief of musculo-skeletal problems.

We feel strongly that people should rely on a good physician (or a well-educated osteopath) for medical care. Should you need manipulation for some type of muscular problem, your doctor may refer you to a chiropractor or physical therapist for that treatment.

WHAT TYPE OF DOCTOR SHOULD YOU CHOOSE?

Now that we have listed the various kinds of generalists, you still have the problem of deciding which type to use. For some people the choice may be limited. If you live in a rural area far from any major city, there may be only one doctor. Easy. You may, however, have to decide when to leave town and doctor for another opinion or for treatment that is available only in a larger place.

If you live in a small town that is a suburb of a larger city, you will have to decide whether you want the convenience of a local doctor or greater choice of physicians and a longer drive. Some suburbs are infamous in medical circles for the poor quality of their doctors and hospitals. Smart medical consumers in these places head for the city when possible.

To complicate matters, though, there are skillful doctors with impeccable credentials who just love living in the country. You will never be able to judge the quality of a doctor by his or her zip code.

If you like the idea of having everyone in the family see the same doctor—and if everyone in your family likes the idea—a family practitioner offers great advantages. You may be able to schedule things a bit more conveniently when both parent and child need routine appointments.

You may be able to save money on visits if the flu you took to the doctor's office for a diagnosis begins to make its way through the rest of your family. A telephone call may be all that is necessary to confirm the fact. When medical problems or stresses affect the health and well-being of father or mother, the family practitioner may be able to help everyone else cope.

If cost is the major factor in your choice, you may have more opportunities to save money by using a family practitioner; but since fees vary greatly depending on what part of the country you live in, you should get some specific fees quoted before you make a decision on that basis.

Sometimes, though, having the family practitioner see every family member is not the answer. An adolescent struggling with problems of separation may want his or her own doctor. Spouses may really prefer to have different doctors.

In many cities, family practitioners are not able to obtain admitting privileges at major hospitals, where specialists hold all the political cards; therefore, in the case of serious illness, you or your child would have to be admitted by another doctor—either an internist or a pediatrician.

In general, we recommend either a family practitioner or general internist for adults, an F.P., or pediatrician, for children, and, if possible, a specialist in adolescent medicine or a physician with a real interest in, and knowledge of, this area for teenagers.

TRAINING AND CREDENTIALS: WHAT THE DOCUMENTS REALLY MEAN

The latest writings on how to be a savvy medical consumer have you researching a physician's credentials: medical school, residency, board status, and hospital affiliation. This sounds good until you, the lay person, have to decide what it all means. You can garner some of the information in the library—and we will tell you what reference books to consult. (See the Resource Directory for this chapter.)

You can ask the doctor about credentials directly unless you feel uncomfortable questioning the figure in the white coat, surrounded by imposing framed certificates. The root of this discomfort may lie in the realization that, to understand the full significance of the answers, you almost have to become a doctor yourself. Was Dr. Y. trained in surgery at such and such a famous hospital in 1969? You are impressed by the hospital name. Dr. Y.'s colleagues are somewhat less impressed. They know that at that time, the training offered there, in that particular field, was less than outstanding.

Certain paper credentials are important. They establish a minimum level of competence and training, but none of these documents will give any indication of the human qualities of a physician or of his or her skill in the art of medicine.

THE MEANING OF MEDICAL SCHOOL

Ask the deans of U.S. medical schools to list the ten best medical schools in the country and they will come up with fairly similar lists—

names like Harvard, Yale, Johns Hopkins, and Columbia. These places are renowned for their famous researchers, and attract large grants and donations. The deans' criteria for naming them the best, though, are not necessarily those factors that are of the most importance to you.

As we noted in the first chapter, many physicians and physician-educators are now beginning to question the way that medical schools select their students and the way those students are trained. Until recently, there has been a heavy emphasis on science background; college students planning to attend medical school have spent far more time in chemistry, biology, and other science courses than in the humanities. The outcome of this process is very well described in a remarkable book, *Gentle Vengeance*, by Charles LeBaron, a Harvard Medical School student (see Bibliography).

Furthermore, admissions committees of medical schools have generally placed a strong emphasis on grades. Unfortunately, whether or not a doctor is caring and sensitive to patient needs does not correlate with academic performance. From the patients' point of view, the medical school a doctor attended is not of paramount importance. To physicians, however, this is a significant credential because graduates of the better medical schools find it easier to be accepted into good training programs and onto the staffs of good hospitals. Within the medical profession, U.S. and Canadian schools are generally considered tops; those of England and South Africa, approximately their equal.

What does it mean if a doctor has attended a foreign medical school? We suggest you focus not on this fact but on what further credentials the doctor in question has obtained. There are fine physicians who are graduates of foreign medical schools—or of those schools in the United States that are regarded as less strong. You can identify such physicians by the quality of the residency training programs they subsequently completed, and by the fact that they are now on the staffs of good hospitals.

The one situation in which a medical school credential might be of special significance is in finding the right consultant in a highly scientific and research-oriented field. Top grades in a top school would indicate excellent scientific ability. We hope, though, that should you need a researcher as a consultant, you would have a primary care doctor guide you in making your selection.

INTERNSHIP AND RESIDENCY

In the last year of medical school, students must decide what specialized area of medicine they want to study; they then apply for acceptance into a hospital training program in that field.

Internship is the first year of postgraduate training, and these days it often serves as the first year of residency, the next step in specialty training.

Fledgling doctors are usually thrown into a hectic schedule of patient care with no orientation or training in how to communicate with patients or deal with the human side of sickness. They begin to refer to the people they care for by their diseased organs: "the liver in room 114." Interns and residents spend most of their time seeing very sick patients in a hospital setting. This sort of education, which emphasizes the technical side of hospital medicine, does little to prepare doctors for the world that most of them will inhabit—the world of office practice.

The point of this critique of training is to make you aware of what the certificates do and do not certify. Doctors are taught a great deal about diseases and not very much about the people who have them. How much time residents spend working in the "clinic" (the part of the hospital that cares for ambulatory patients) may be far more important in preparing them for private practice than all the discussions of rare diseases and enzyme interactions.

In the medical world, certain residency programs are considered highly desirable. They are based in large and famous teaching hospitals and are conducted by doctors primarily renowned for their research contributions. Again, as with medical school, the most famous programs, which emphasize complicated diagnoses and rare diseases, do not necessarily produce the best primary care doctors.

You do, however, want to be sure that the physician you choose has completed his or her residency program. Generally, the programs run by U.S. or Canadian hospitals are the most highly regarded.

FELLOWSHIP TRAINING

Physicians who have completed medical school, internship, and residency may decide to learn more about a given subspecialty area. For example, an internist who becomes especially interested in heart disease would enter an accredited training program and upon completion would be entitled to call him- or herself a cardiologist. Fellowships are organized and offered by hospitals and take one or two years to complete.

BOARD STATUS

Here is a useful credential to understand. Boards are examinations (written and, in some cases, oral) given by qualified physicians in a specific field to determine whether the applicant has assimilated a certain body of knowledge.

In order to be eligible to take the boards, a physician must have completed a residency that has been approved by the board in that field. In certain fields, such as obstetrics and gynecology (OBGYN), candidates cannot take the exam until they have performed a certain number of surgical procedures. In others, pediatrics for example, they must have two years of practice experience after completing residency. Internal medicine and family medicine candidates, on the other hand, may take board examinations immediately after completing residency.

If you have a choice of doctors, we would urge you to select someone who is board-certified or at least board-eligible. (See Resource Directory for information on how to determine a doctor's board status.)

There are various reasons why board-eligible physicians may not have taken and passed their boards. They may be studying for the test; they may be avoiding it; or they may have failed it one or more times.

There is often no difference in skill and knowledge between the board-eligible and the board-certified physician. There is probably a much greater difference between those who are board-eligible and those who are not. On the other hand, a specialist who has taken and passed the board exams is someone who is sensitive to the importance of reassuring the public—to the extent it is possible—that he or she is well trained.

Double-boarded physicians. These are doctors who have completed the training and passed the boards either of two separate fields such as pediatrics and psychiatry or of a specialty and a subspecialty such as general surgery and cardiac surgery. (Subspecialty is a word that has proved confusing to some people who take it to mean that a subspecialist knows less than a specialist. Perhaps superspecialist would be a better term for those who spend extra time studying a small area of a larger field; for example, cardiologists are subspecialists in the field of internal medicine.)

There are some situations where the physician trained in two separate fields might be especially desirable. If you have a chronically ill child with a severe behavior problem, you might have more coordinated care from a doctor trained in both pediatrics and psychiatry. In most cases, "double-boards" will be of more importance in selecting consultants than in finding someone for primary care.

HOSPITAL AFFILIATION

Hospital affiliation is a very important guideline. Good physicians will not want to put their patients in second-rate hospitals; good hospitals will be selective and demanding in choosing their physicians. Chapter Five has a discussion of the different types of hospitals and some of the signs of a good hospital. If you are new to a community, your company benefits manager might be one logical source of information. If you meet a nurse, an ambulance attendant or a fire-fighter, he or she may have an informed opinion.

In most places, the citizenry seems to agree that certain hospitals are far more desirable than others. Of course, at times the lay people agree that one hospital is the best, while the doctors all know that a less famous hospital actually gives better care. In the words of one prominent physician, "When my patients are sick, I admit them to the university hospital. That's what they want. When I myself am sick, I go to ———— hospital."

The number of hospital affiliations a doctor maintains is a function of the size of the city and how much time the hospital demands in exchange for admitting privileges. (Often, to be a member of the staff, a doctor must put considerable unpaid time into teaching or working in the hospital's clinic.) In smaller cities, qualified doctors may be able to admit patients to any of the hospitals in town; in big cities like New York, doctors are usually associated with only one or at most two hospitals.

Many doctors use one hospital for most of their patients and admit only occasional cases to the other hospitals where they have privileges. If it is important to you to go to a particular hospital, you will want to know which one the doctor you are considering regularly uses.

There are various reasons why a doctor might choose a given hospital: it is the most medically prestigious; it has a reputation for good patient care; it is convenient to the doctor's office; it has convenient parking (for the doctor); it is easy to get a patient admitted there; it has residents to handle urgent problems so that the doctor won't be called away during office hours.

But be cautious: hospital affiliation taken by itself is not an ironclad guarantee that you have found the right doctor or even that the doctor is perfectly competent. Even some of the most famous institutions in the country have given privileges to the occasional misfit.

MEDICAL SOCIETIES

Medical societies organize conferences, publish journals, and generally provide an educational forum for their membership. Doctors commonly join the county medical society, the state medical society and the American Medical Association (AMA) for political and social reasons, so that membership in these groups is not a useful guideline for you in choosing or knowing more about a doctor.

Membership in other types of medical societies, however, may be an important clue to a doctor's special areas of interest. If a physician is a member of an organization such as the Psychosomatic Medicine Society, he or she is interested in the behavioral aspects of your medical problems. (We would like to note that when doctors use the term *psychosomatic*, they are referring to the interconnections between human emotions and physical health. They do not mean that the medical problem is in any way not a real one.)

Do not be put off by the odd names of some of the societies. The doctor who displays a certificate of the Manipulative Medicine Society will not use devious means to get you to swallow your penicillin tablets. He or she will have learned techniques to relieve backaches and muscle spasms.

Some societies have fairly strict requirements for membership. For example, the American Academy of Pediatrics or the American College of Physicians (for internists) is restricted to those who are board-certified. Some organizations require that physicians publish articles in their field before becoming members.

FACULTY APPOINTMENTS

A faculty appointment to a medical school is another credential worth discussing. In some situations, however, the appointment follows from the hospital affiliation. For example, every physician who is on the staff of The Mount Sinai Hospital in New York City or of Beth Israel (an affiliated hospital) has a faculty appointment to The Mount Sinai School of Medicine. Without credentials needed to obtain a faculty appointment, no doctor is allowed to be on the staff of either hospital.

The kind of faculty appointment that is especially important to you, the patient, is the one given to a physician who is actively involved with the teaching of clinical skills to medical students, interns, or residents. In some programs, the student or resident actually spends time in the physician's office. If the doctor you are considering is involved in this kind of training, here is a sure sign that you have found a highly regarded clinical practitioner, a fact that might persuade you it is worth having an extra person in the room during your examination.

WORD OF MOUTH

By now you may be convinced, as we are, that formal credentials tell only part of the story. You can use the lack of proper credentials to strike a doctor off your list of possible choices, and you can be assured by the presence of certain credentials that a doctor has been well trained. Nevertheless, you still do not have the vaguest idea of what kind of human being you are about to encounter. For this information, you must turn to the people you know and ask for advice. When you do this, you need to ask not only for the names of doctors they like but also why they like them and what qualities they value.

Because it is so difficult for the nonmedical person to judge medical expertise, many people have taken to looking for all sorts of other clues as to the probable stature of a physician. One person may proudly tell you that Dr. Impressive's waiting room is always crowded and that you will have to wait an hour or more to be seen. This is the successful-restaurant approach: if everyone else wants to eat here and is waiting to get in, it must be good. It is a poor basis upon which to choose a doctor.

Furthermore, you don't know how many days of the week the doctor sees patients and how many hours the office is bursting at the seams. Young doctors just opening a practice are often advised to schedule patients close together so that the office will seem busy and full.

Using this type of logic, a new and inexperienced administrator for a large group practice was upset that the waiting rooms never seemed full. He had been trained in a system that paid no attention to patient convenience and had, therefore, concluded that the practice was not doing well. What he failed to grasp was that scheduling was skillfully handled; the doctors had decided to value the patients' time as well as their own.

In a similar fashion, people may be impressed by a doctor's rich and famous patients, expensive address, even by a brusque manner. They take these things as signs of financial success, which they then equate with clinical skill. Unless you enjoy long waits or require expensively furnished waiting rooms, we suggest you ignore recommendations based on such factors.

You should also be somewhat wary about the recommendation from a friend who sees "the world's best doctor" for a complicated medical problem. Your friend may be seeing someone who is primarily a specialist when what you need is a generalist.

The most valuable things you will learn about doctors from their patients are firsthand observations of the physician's behavior and human qualities: "Dr. M. always gives me plenty of time," or "Dr. S. is very gentle and explains everything." In using this sort of information you can try to take into account the kinds of needs and expectations you have. For example, if you too want a doctor who explains everything, Dr. S. may be just your ticket. If you're more comfortable with the old-fashioned "let me worry about it" type of doctor, you might find young Dr. S. unreassuring. This would have nothing to do with that doctor's knowledge or skill but everything to do with how happy you are when you leave his or her office.

In fact, if a doctor possesses the right paper credentials, your friend's hearty recommendation may be the best credential of all. When you make an appointment you will be asked where you got the doctor's name, so be sure that your friend pays bills on time and does not make unreasonable demands; otherwise, you may not be greeted warmly or given an early appointment.

If You Are Planning to Move

If you already have a primary care physician, he or she will be your best resource in finding a suitable doctor in your new community. At a minimum, your present physician can supply you with the names of physicians with good credentials and, if you are lucky, he or she may even be able to refer you to a friend or acquaintance. If a member of your family has a serious chronic problem such as lupus or cystic fibrosis, your present physician should be sure to identify a doctor who would be a suitable replacement.

Be sure to arrange to have your medical records sent to the new physician. To save time, you may want to take them with you; however, laws vary from state to state concerning your right to have your own records.

What do you do if you suddenly become ill while on a trip or in a town you have just moved to and haven't the foggiest idea of what doctor to call? Because you do not have the time to find a doctor through the process we have described, your best bet would probably be to go to the emergency room of the largest hospital in town. After you have been treated, ask for names of physicians associated with the hospital who are well qualified to follow up the care the ER provided.

ACCESS, COST, AND QUALITY

When health planners discuss medical care, they generally break it down into these three areas. Of the three, quality is the most difficult for anyone, whether physician or nonphysician, to describe. We have already discussed paper credentials as well as the human qualities that are important in a doctor. Still, the world's most brilliant and most caring physician may not do you much good if you can't get an appointment when you need it.

Access
The importance of access depends on your state of health and the level of anxiety you experience when you feel you need to talk to or visit the doctor. Access can be broken down into the following components:

- office location
- office hours
- appointment availability
- after-hours availability.

Waiting time in the office might be a factor, although we would tend to put it under cost (hidden—and to you) or quality (of service, not of care). The more often you need to see a doctor, the more urgent your medical problems, and the less mobile you are, the more important is ease of access. If, for instance, you had a child who suffered from frequent, severe asthma attacks, you would find it important to have an

M.D. not only nearby but also easily reachable after hours or well covered by a colleague who was readily available.

If you are seldom sick and therefore see your doctor primarily for screening tests and routine physicals, access is not as important, but availability might be an issue. Suppose your hectic work schedule keeps you running all day. The fact you could make an evening or Saturday appointment would be a real boon to you and a deciding factor when it came to picking a doctor.

If you commute some distance to work, you may wonder whether to have a doctor near where you work or where you live. If you are generally healthy, it is convenient to have a doctor near your job; if you have serious health problems, you may find it an advantage to have a doctor near your home.

How long you must wait to get a routine appointment is generally a less important issue. It would be a rare physician indeed who was not able to find time for his or her very sick patients. If you are a new patient, though, you may have trouble getting an appointment on short notice unless you are being referred by another doctor for an urgent problem.

Somewhere in between the routine and the urgent falls the kind of problem that you may want to take care of immediately even though it is not medically necessary. If you are in pain or are very uncomfortable—or if you are extremely worried—you may want to see your doctor right away. In many cases, the telephone can fill the gap. Once you have established yourself as a patient, you will be able to call in for telephone advice, whether you are suffering from a bee sting or wondering if your child's fever and sore throat are caused by something more than the usual virus.

When you call, unless the doctor is free at that moment, you can expect to wait some amount of time for your call to be returned. This policy protects you when you are the one in the doctor's office and need undivided attention. Ask if there is a regular time to call in. Many doctors, especially pediatricians, reserve an hour during the day for returning calls and answering questions.

After-hours availability. It is midnight and all is not well. That slightly queasy feeling you had all evening has developed into severe abdominal pain. Is it something you ate? Could it be appendicitis?

A phone call to your doctor may save you a trip to an emergency room. Should the trip be necessary, he or she will recommend an ER and either meet you there or consult over the telephone with the emergency room doctor who has examined you.

It is unreasonable to expect doctors to be available twenty-four hours a day, seven days a week. You should, however, make sure there is a good coverage system—perhaps two or three other doctors in the same specialty who share after-hours "call" and are on the staff of the same hospital.

Cost

Before deciding on a doctor, ask the office what the charges are for various types of visits: for a complete exam, for a follow-up visit, for shots for children, and for any other kind of visit you know you would need. All other things being equal, by all means choose the doctor who charges less; if anything, this would indicate someone who cares about the needs of his or her patients.

In comparing costs, take into account the fact that some doctors do more, and therefore charge more, per visit; but the total cost to you will be less. Suppose, for example, you are trying to pick out a doctor for your newborn and cost is an important factor. One pediatrician will see the baby at one, two, four, and six months (the number of visits that are considered medically necessary), and charge $40 per visit. This doctor gives two immunizations at each visit at no extra charge, and thus bills $160 for the first six months.

Another doctor schedules a monthly visit and gives an immunization at each visit. The office visit costs half as much: $20. But there is an additional $10 fee for the immunization. The total for six months of well-baby care from this doctor will come to $180 for the first six months.

Fees vary according to the length of the visit. A brief exam, a shot, and a quick "how are things going" will cost less than a visit to a pediatrician who takes the time to find out how the new baby is affecting your life, your spouse's life, your job, and your other children. This doctor will have to charge more per visit.

For many people, the extra few dollars is money well spent. New parents may be able to nip problems in the bud by being made more aware of them at an early stage. If, for example, a young mother is having stress-related symptoms because she is doing too much, the pediatrician or family physician may be able to help her to focus on ways of managing her responsibilities more effectively.

Finally, you should not assume that a younger and less well-established doctor will have lower fees. We know of highly regarded older physicians who actually charge less than some of their young colleagues. Unlike the young baseball player from the minors whose salary is less than five percent of Steve Garvey's or the twenty-five-year-old tenor who does not expect to equal Pavarotti's income, new young doctors often feel that they must charge as much as their older colleagues in order to be taken seriously.

(For a detailed discussion of health insurance coverage, see Chapter Twelve.)

FIRST IMPRESSIONS

Within the first visit or two, you should be able to decide if this doctor is right for you. You will have impressions of the efficiency and courtesy of the office staff, the attention paid to your convenience, and most important, the way the doctor treats you as a person.

> The office floor is covered with a costly Chinese rug; the very good chairs are real leather. The prints on the wall are tasteful and expensively framed. On the tables are current copies of *Architectural Digest* and *Art in America*. The office windows frame striking views of lake and trees. The wait is somewhat long, but the staff is pleasant. After the doctor has done a thorough examination, the patient, a thirty-five-year-old woman who describes herself as anxious, has a question. Somewhat embarrassed at its triviality, she brings up a complaint that has been troubling her: an occasional difficulty in swallowing food.
>
> The doctor asks a few questions and then, fixing her with an amused and kindly look, explains that she is experiencing something he terms "globus hystericus" (that proverbial lump in the throat), a psychological difficulty. Nothing real here. No problem. The visit is over. (The bill is $130, which includes an electrocardiogram.)

For some patients, this doctor would be perfect. The expense of the office decor and the bill are reassuring: this doctor is expensive because he is good. The doctor's kindly and amused manner in diagnosing a psychological complaint would have relieved many patients' anxieties.

This woman, however, decided not to return to this physician. She wasn't really sure why. His credentials were impeccable; he was affiliated with a hospital noted for good patient care; and he came highly recommended by another doctor. Something about the style of the experience, all that gloss, was somewhat off-putting.

Several years later, still experiencing the same occasional problem, she checked a medical reference book and learned that her symptoms were not those of "globus hystericus," (although it appeared likely that any problem she had was minor.)

In analyzing her negative reactions, we would note several contributing factors.

· She was put off by the expensive furnishings
· Her anxiety was not allayed by being told that her problem was psychological. In fact, she felt patronized
· She thought the bill somewhat high
· Her perception was that she was being asked to be impressed by style rather than substance

Was this really the wrong doctor for her? It so happened that she lived in a fairly large city. What if she came from a small town where no other doctor had such good recommendations and credentials? In his favor, we note the following factors:

- The doctor did not order a large number of tests. He did the electrocardiogram because the woman reported episodes of chest pain and was anxious about their cause
- He could have done an expensive work-up for her swallowing problem. Had he done so, she might have received unnecessary surgery
- Even though his explanation was probably wrong, he had upheld that cardinal rule of medicine: first do no harm
- From his point of view, his expensively decorated office might reflect pride in his occupation and a desire to please his clientele

The first impression his patient received, however, from both his style and his manner, was that she could not "trust" this doctor. In her case, she had other equally well-recommended doctors to choose from, so she did not have to decide whether or not to suspend judgment.

It is difficult for you, the lay person, to make an assessment of a doctor, especially if you are worried about a symptom or are feeling unwell. To help you, we reproduce the following very thorough check list from a book we highly recommend called *Beyond the Medical Mystique: How to Choose and Use Your Doctor,* by Marvin S. Belsky, M.D. and Leonard Gross (see Bibliography).

PATIENT'S CHECK LIST

First Phone Call
Does medical assistant give her name when answering phone?
Is she warm, concerned?
Do you feel rushed?
Are your questions answered?
Does she ask what's wrong with you, and if it's urgent?
Does she put you through to the doctor if asked?
Does she give you traveling instructions?
Does she answer your questions about the doctor's fee schedule, hospital affiliation, availability?

First Visit
Is office cheerful, comfortable?
Are you greeted pleasantly?
Does the medical assistant inquire about your condition?
Does she inform you of the approximate delay, if there's to be one?
Is your chart made out promptly in an area of confidentiality?
Are the desks of the medical assistants neat?
Are the medical assistants friendly, reassuring?

Are there appropriate reading materials, including magazines of general interest as well as health magazines?

Is there a "no smoking" sign, indicating overall concern for patients' health?

Is the waiting room crowded?

First Encounter with Doctor

Does the doctor welcome you or does he ignore your entrance, continuing to peruse his work or talk on the phone?

Does his consulting room meet the same criteria as the waiting room?

Is the doctor's desk neat?

Are you given close attention, or does the doctor interrupt to take calls, respond to his assistants?

Are you oriented by the doctor about the nature of examination?

Do you feel rushed when talking to him?

Does he take a thorough history?

Does he show an interest in you outside of your presenting symptom?

Is he a good listener?

Does he seem to empathize with you?

Does he share his own background and interests?

Does he use jargon?

Does he smoke?

Is he obese?

Does he answer your questions freely regarding his medical training, hospital affiliation, emergency protocol, fee schedule?

Examination Room

Is the purpose of the tests explained by the medical assistant?

Are the tests done with apparent skill and concern?

Is the equipment modern or shopworn?

Does the medical assistant welcome and answer your questions?

Is the examination room clean, neat, modern?

Are delays in the examination room explained, or are you lost and forgotten?

Are there magazines in the pre-examination rooms?

The Examination

Does it proceed without interruption?

Does the doctor offer information about procedures?

Does he answer questions to your satisfaction?

Does he proceed systematically and thoroughly?

Does he accept suggestions?

The Evaluation

Does the doctor summarize his findings, note the data gathered, and explain his conclusions?

Does he put you at ease, or do you feel rushed?

Does he preach, talk down, give orders, speak quickly?

Does he encourage questions?

Does he use jargon?

Does he encourage you to call him in a few days, or whenever you feel the need?

Does he consistently and intensively follow up on the data gathered?

If you use this very thorough list to organize your impressions, you will come away with a more objective and accurate first impression than the woman in our example was able to gather. You do not want a doctor whose office is sloppy, poorly equipped, and staffed by rude people. You may, depending on your personality, forgive a doctor whose magazines are old or who talks too quickly, if you feel he or she is really trying to explain something to you.

MUST YOU FIND THE PERFECT DOCTOR?

Can you? Theoreticians have painted a wonderful portrait of the perfect healer, someone so knowledgeable and dedicated, so kind, so caring, so respectful of our right to information yet so sensitive to our need for protection that we are guaranteed a response exactly calibrated to our emotional state. There are doctors who come very, very close to filling this description, and we hope you will be able to find one. But the fact that you cannot find exactly the right emotional fit between you and your physician does not mean that you have the wrong person or that there is something wrong with you.

If you find a well-trained, pleasant, and conscientious doctor, you may have to work a bit at creating the kind of medical relationship you want. If you do not have the luxury of being immediately understood, you may have to explain your needs—for information, for reassurance, for another look at your problem, or for an outside consultation if you want one. How to succeed in this enterprise is the subject of our next chapter.

CHAPTER THREE

HOW TO DEAL WITH YOUR DOCTOR

Perhaps someday, when doctors are far more skillful in the human side of medicine, a chapter like this will be unnecessary. After all, why should patients have to prepare themselves for office visits by taking notes, walk on eggs when mentioning the possibility of a referral, or maneuver delicately to be seen on time for a scheduled appointment. Obviously, they shouldn't.

Having read our opening chapter, though, you should now have a fairly good idea of the ways in which doctors are selected and educated. They do not enter a cohesive training program, one in which patient care is the goal governing a carefully planned sequence of medical school courses and postgraduate training. Instead, they are fed into a system with mixed purposes. A great deal of what happens in medical schools and hospitals has to do with the needs of those institutions, for turf, for grants, for staff—or because that's just the way things have always been done.

Not only do they receive little instruction in the human side but doctors in training actually undergo negative learning. They are taught, for example, to pursue diagnosis and exhaust all possible forms of treatment without examining how necessary or desirable this is from the individual patient's point of view. They learn to identify the hospital patients they see by their diseases rather than by their names.

Fortunately, there is a countertrend to the increase in specialization. Many young doctors, those who want to see a return to more human values in medicine and who are interested in the personhood of their patients, are entering fields like primary care internal medicine and family practice. Older and more experienced generalists have learned from their own observations, if not from their training, the importance of applying human warmth and concern as well as the last word in medical technology. There are some wonderful doctors out there— *41* knowledgeable, concerned human beings—and we hope you will find one of these to be your personal physician.

No matter what their social skills, most doctors are conscientious and really want to help their patients. This chapter is your guide to tapping that helpful streak.

It is extremely difficult for most people to confront a doctor with a complaint, a demand, or a direct expression of dissatisfaction with the care they are receiving. (In general, even doctors are unable to confront other doctors.) But if you understand such matters as how doctors organize their practice, their goals in treating patients, and what their "sore spots" are, you will have an easier time getting what you need.

HOW YOUR EXPECTATIONS MESH
WITH THOSE OF YOUR PHYSICIAN

Do you want a doctor who will give you an immediate appointment, see you on time, give you uninterrupted attention, and spend as long as you want answering your questions . . . and who is immediately available by telephone? If so, you must find a doctor in "solo" practice, meaning that you are the sole patient.

Doctors are always doing a bit of a balancing act, trying to meet everybody's needs. If they take a long time answering each patient's questions, they risk running so far behind schedule that they anger the others who are waiting for their turns. They can decide to see fewer patients a day; but then it takes longer to get an appointment, and their patients will pay a higher fee. If they take calls as they come in, they are constantly diverted from the patient who is sitting in front of them, full of confusion and anxiety. If they have the receptionist tell everyone who calls and wants to be seen today to "come right over," they will be playing havoc with their own and everyone else's schedule.

Some people, those whose appointment calendars are bursting at the seams or who resent long waits in waiting rooms, prefer the doctor who will not say "come right over," unless the problem is really urgent or there has been a last-minute cancellation. Others would rather put in their time in the doctor's outer chambers, knowing they can be seen any day they really want to.

Similarly, there are those who find themselves distracted and annoyed when their doctor takes phone calls during an examination. They want the doctor's uninterrupted attention. Those of a different temperament may not particularly mind and are pleased with the trade-off: that they can call in and talk to the doctor when they choose. Trade-off is the key here. You can't have it both ways.

If you like and trust your doctor but are upset with his or her administrative style, you can certainly discuss it. You can ask if there is a way or time to schedule an appointment so that you do not have to wait more than fifteen minutes. Perhaps, for example, you can get the first appointment of the day.

If you feel your doctor's attention is constantly diverted by phone calls or questions from the office staff, you can explain that you have difficulty organizing your thoughts and remembering information if your visit is full of these interruptions. If you and the doctor are able to find solutions to these problems, so much the better. If not, you will have to decide how much these things matter to you.

It is important to decide on the bottom line. It is unlikely that you will find a doctor who will do everything the way you wish. If you have a caring, knowledgeable doctor, you may decide that although you are not enchanted with his or her administrative skills, these are of lesser importance to you. You may have to wait for a semiurgent appointment longer than you want to, but when you finally see the doctor, you may find that you can take as much time as you need to ask questions and discuss your concerns.

HOW TO TALK TO YOUR DOCTOR

There are some ways of dealing with doctors that are guaranteed to drive them up a wall; there are others that will ensure that you enlist their full cooperation.

RULE ONE:
TELL THE DOCTOR YOUR PROBLEM, NOT YOUR SOLUTION

For example, say, "I have a painful sore throat, a fever, and spots on my tonsils," instead of "I want a prescription for penicillin." The doctor will usually examine you, do a throat culture, and wait to prescribe penicillin pending the outcome of the culture. He or she may suggest aspirin for the pain, rest, and plenty of fluids.

If you aren't entirely happy with this procedure, you should ask why the doctor is recommending each component (throat culture, taking aspirin, drinking fluids, rest, etc.).

What if the doctor answers your questions carefully, but you still aren't satisfied?

RULE TWO:
AVOID PUTTING YOUR DOCTOR ON THE DEFENSIVE

Ask "Is it possible penicillin will help?" rather than, "Why aren't you giving me penicillin?" You should get a helpful answer. What if you remain unconvinced and still want that penicillin? Say, "I really would feel safer if I could have some penicillin." If the doctor will not accede to your request, he or she should give very clear reasons why not. In general, good doctors answer all questions carefully and don't get upset when you disagree; because they are sure of their knowledge, they remain unintimidated.

The last thing you want is to get into a power struggle with your doctor. Whoever wins, your treatment suffers. If you get a prescription for penicillin against the doctor's better judgment, you are taking a powerful drug and spending your money for no good reason. If the doctor tells you that you can't have it but doesn't explain why, you will feel resentful and uncooperative.

RULE THREE:
GIVE THE DOCTOR ALL THE INFORMATION

People may, due to embarrassment, withhold information that would help in making a diagnosis and planning treatment. Your doctor is required to hold all information you give in the strictest confidence. If you are a heavy drinker, a homosexual, a pack-a-day smoker, whatever it is that makes you fear the doctor's disapproval, you are risking the quality of your medical care if you fail to present all the relevant information.

TALKING TO YOUR DOCTOR ABOUT TESTS

Most tests done in a doctor's office—blood tests, cultures, EKG, urinalysis—are harmless: your only questions would concern whether they are worth the cost. Of course, if the tests are necessary to diagnose a serious problem, cost is not a consideration. But if they are done primarily because that is the doctor's "routine," you may spend a hundred dollars or more for no real benefit. (The usefulness of screening, as opposed to diagnostic, tests and the problem of false positives are discussed in detail in Chapter Eleven.) Ask your doctor:

Why is the test being done?
What is the cost?
Are there any associated risks? (For example, a liver biopsy may cause serious bleeding; an exercise stress test can cause a heart attack.)
(If the test is costly or risky) Can my problem be treated without doing the test?

WAITING FOR THE LAB REPORT

"I'll have the results of these tests in a few days," says the physician, tucking away a vial of blood. "The office will call you if anything is abnormal." How do you spend the next few days? Do you put the whole thing out of your mind or do you chew your nails and keep reminding yourself that no news is good news?

It's fairly common for physicians to have the staff call only those patients who have abnormal results. It saves time. If that makes you anxious, you can ask to be called no matter what the results or you can ask when you should call in to find out. The doctor's office should be cooperative even if this is not the usual policy.

AVOIDING X-RAYS YOU DON'T NEED

X-rays are another matter: you must make every effort to minimize their use, since radiation poses a cumulative risk. Always be sure the x-ray is really needed for the diagnosis and treatment of your problem. Always tell a new doctor about any x-rays you have already had to evaluate the problem under discussion. He or she may be able to review the earlier films, thereby reducing or eliminating the need for more studies.

In particular, avoid routine chest films (which are of little or no value) and question the use of skull films after a head injury. What is important is what has happened to the brain, not the skull, and x-rays are rarely helpful in making this assessment.

If you did not lose consciousness and if your physical examination was normal, you do not need a skull x-ray. In fact, one study found that most skull films of children are taken either because of parental demand or so that the doctor can practice "defensive medicine" (the avoidance of malpractice suits[1]).

Pregnant women should be especially careful to avoid x-rays, and both sexes should have their gonads shielded with a lead apron unless the x-ray is being done of that area.

(For further reading on the subject, see the Bibliography.)

HOW TO ASK FOR AN OUTSIDE CONSULTATION

First discuss your concerns about your treatment in detail; it may be that your doctor will come up with a new approach that sounds good to you. Otherwise, the logical thing is to seek another opinion.

If you feel that your present doctor is basically competent, you are probably better off asking him or her to select a consultant. Your doctor can make informed choices, discuss your case with the consultant, arrange for you to have an appointment on an urgent basis if it seems necessary, and send copies of your medical records and test results. It is very much to your advantage to have the consultant start where your primary care doctor left off instead of having to go over the same ground, repeat tests, and wait for results.

Remember, your doctor feels bad that you are not getting better— rather helpless, too. When powerful people feel helpless, they may take it out on the nearest weaker person—and that would be you. But, if you let the doctor choose the consultant, he or she will feel more in control and will use his or her energy to arrange for the best possible consultation.

This approach assumes that you still respect your doctor but are not happy about how this particular problem is being treated. If you are completely dissatisfied, you are better off going through the process of finding a new primary care doctor and having the new person arrange for a consultation if necessary.

WHY YOU DON'T WANT ONE OF THE TOP TEN DOCTORS IN THE COUNTRY

You may have a doctor in mind, someone you think would be the right person to go to for your problem. Proceed the same way you would in the matter of asking for penicillin. After your doctor mentions a name, ask why that person is being recommended. You could then say, "I've heard that Dr. Z. is a real expert in this sort of problem. What do you think?" Practicing physicians know that the doctors with the biggest names are not necessarily the best at diagnosing and treating patients.

Every so often, a magazine article or a book appears that identifies the "best" physicians in your city or in the country. Inevitably, the list includes the names of doctors who are famous researchers or heads of departments in major teaching hospitals, who never, or almost never, actually see patients. Calls to these big names will lead to a referral to one of their associates or to a Fellow they are training.

Unless you have an extremely rare disease that no one can diagnose, we would never recommend a doctor who is primarily a research scientist. Your goal should be to find an expert clinician who is skilled in dealing with medical problems as they occur in real people rather than test tubes and who knows how to find answers to questions he or she cannot answer.

THE ETIQUETTE OF REFERRALS

In general, you should assume that the consultant will make recommendations to the referring doctor, who will implement them with you. Sometimes, especially in hospitals, the consultant won't even give you information directly but will instead send a report to your own physician.

Suppose you decide you really prefer working with the consultant and want him or her to become your doctor? If the consultant is a specialist, we would advise against this. You need a primary care doctor. (We discussed the reasons why in the previous chapter.)

If the consultant is also a primary care doctor, you will ruffle the fewest feathers if you wait a while. If your present doctor is looking worse and worse and the consultant better and better, of course you can change doctors, but if you try to switch after the first visit, consultants may become uncomfortable and hem and haw. You probably make them feel the same way they felt in high school at the thought of dating their best friend's steady. At issue is the touchy matter of stealing patients. The consultant knows that doctors whose colleagues suspect them of doing this don't get any more referrals.

What do you do if the second opinion is different from the first opinion? You may be justifiably confused and decide you want a third opinion. By all means ask for one. There is always the hope that while the opinions are coming in, you will get better. Ask your primary care physician to help you make sense of the various recommendations.

If there seems to be a lot of medical doubt and differences of opinion, do nothing. No surgery, no high-powered medications. Should you get worse, the proper treatment plan will become more obvious. If you get a little better, you may not need anyone else's opinion.

WHAT IF YOUR DOCTOR HAS MADE A MISTAKE?

What do you do if you learn that your doctor has missed a diagnosis or given you the wrong treatment?

> A woman comes to see her physician because of a deep cat bite on her finger. In order to prevent infection, he prescribes an antibiotic. Instead of healing, the wound becomes so badly infected that only an admission to the hospital and intravenous antibiotics save her finger. In the hospital, she learns that her physician had prescribed the wrong antibiotic, unaware that it was not effective for a cat bite.

Her doctor is an excellent physician with good credentials, respected both before and after this error by his colleagues, who all know that at some point every one of them will make mistakes. They devoutly hope and pray that whatever errors they make will not harm their patients. That is why it is so difficult for physicians to police other physicians.

If you feel that your doctor's mistake is understandable, and you are otherwise satisfied that he or she is competent, you need not feel you are making a mistake by not going off to find a new doctor.

> Don't be too hard on your doctor for making a single mistake, especially if no lasting harm has been done.
> Pay close attention to how the doctor acts after discovering the error. This is indicative of his or her abilities and ethics.
> Stick with the doctor who frankly admits an error and is upset and apologetic. This is someone who learns from mistakes.

If, however, the doctor's reaction is defensive and self-justifying, you might very well consider a change.

A second error, no matter how concerned your doctor is, may well indicate that this is not someone to trust with your life.

HOW TO GET WHAT YOU WANT— AND WHAT YOU SHOULD WANT

There are certain situations in which patients and doctors often lock horns. From the patient's point of view the doctor is inhuman, selfish, uncaring. From the doctor's, the patient is childish, unreasonable, and demanding. An example of such a situation is the House Call. Patients who have heard of, or remember, the good old days are often heard to ask . . .

WHY DON'T DOCTORS MAKE HOUSE CALLS ANYMORE?

Reason number one: they are human. They don't want to leave an office full of patients, get up at some odd hour, or travel an unreasonable distance to see a relatively minor problem. If you live near their home or office and you request a house call at the beginning or end of the working day, you might get one. Otherwise it is extremely unlikely.

Reason number two: During the day, they must leave a waiting room full of patients to attend to you. This is fine if you are the patient getting the house call. If, however, you are the person who had to wait an extra hour or two, you will not be so appreciative.

Reason number three: Patients will not pay for or cannot afford the cost of this service. Let us assume the doctor sees three patients an hour, charging perhaps $30 or more per visit. Counting traveling time, a house call may take an hour or more of the doctor's day. Are you ready to pay $100 for a house call?

> A joke making the medical rounds recently concerns a psychiatrist whose toilet is stopped up. He calls the plumber in the middle of the night. The plumber makes the "house call" and hands the psychiatrist a bill for $80. The psychiatrist is visibly upset and exclaims, "$80! But I'm a psychiatrist and I only charge $70." The plumber nods sympathetically and replies, "Yes, when I was a psychiatrist I also charged only $70."

The joke reflects a certain bitterness on the part of physicians toward people who are more willing to pay large sums of money to electricians and TV repairers than to doctors, who, after all, perform a somewhat more vital service.

Reason number four. The more urgent the need for a house call, the more likely it is that it will not be enough. Someone sick enough to need immediate attention will probably need an x-ray, an EKG, or a blood, or urine test. When you request a house call, if the doctor says, "I'll meet you at the emergency room," it is because, having heard the reason for the request, the doctor knows that your problem cannot be taken care of in your home.

> A physician received a call one night from the husband of one of his regular patients. The man explained that he had just made love to his wife, who then seemed to have collapsed; he couldn't wake her up. The husband was requesting a house call, but the doctor told him to carry his wife to the car and meet him in the emergency room. It turned out she had ruptured an ovarian cyst, was bleeding internally, and was in shock; she needed immediate transfusion and surgery. If the doctor had made a house call, the patient would almost definitely have died.

Incidentally, notice that if the husband had waited for an ambulance to arrive, she might also have died. Ambulances are often a poor choice of transportation for a critical emergency when minutes matter. (More about this in Chapter Six.)

Reason number five: The best treatment for your problem is sitting in your medicine cabinet. You may be calling for relief from severe pain from a problem that is not itself that urgent: a bad sore throat, earache, or headache. The reason your doctor will tell you "take two aspirin and call me in the morning" is that, as several studies have shown, aspirin (or acetaminophen) is as effective for relieving pain as oral prescription medications. (See Chapter Ten for further discussion of these two remedies.)

As for treating the cause of the pain—the ear infection or the strep throat—an antibiotic takes 24 to 48 hours before it has killed enough bacteria to affect the pain. There is little to be gained by being seen at midnight instead of at 9:00 A.M.

WHEN DOCTORS DO MAKE HOUSE CALLS

The kind of house call that does make sense is one that is scheduled for a person who should not leave home: a patient who was discharged from the hospital and needs sutures removed, or a very infirm patient with a chronic disease. If the doctor knows what the problem is ahead of time, and has the proper equipment, he or she may be able to fit a home visit into the day's schedule.

WHY DID YOU CALL ME *NOW?*

A second area of frequent miscommunication involves the after-hours call. People fall into one of two groups: the larger group contains those who feel that they cannot bother the doctor after working, or waking, hours and that they must suffer; the second group waits out the day, hoping that the problem will disappear, and then, anxiety increasing by the hour, finally calls.

You don't call a doctor in the middle of the night unless you are truly worried. You are upset about whatever symptom or pain you are experiencing, and you are upset that you are going to disturb the doctor. Often, one of the first questions you will be asked is, "Why did you call me now?" This is a question that sets off a whole chain reaction of misunderstanding, for people often interpret this to mean "Why did you bother me now?"

Doctors who ask this question are usually trying to get information. What they want to know is "What has happened that has caused you to become concerned enough to call me now?"

To avoid confusion, we suggest you take two or three minutes before dialing to work out what you are going to say. You want to be able to give enough information so that the doctor can help you. Think about the question of why you are calling *now*.

> Has there been some change that is causing you to worry? For example, your child has had a slight fever all day, which you considered unimportant. The fever has suddenly shot up to 103° F.

> The longer your headache persists, the more you are afraid you have something dangerously wrong. You are not in unbearable pain, but your fear is now in the red zone. You don't know whether to head for the nearest brain surgeon or try to go back to sleep.

> You have been using home remedies and rest to treat your child's sore throat. Your spouse comes home, criticizes you for allowing the problem to go untreated for so long, and insists that you call the doctor.

After you have determined the reason for your call, assemble any information you need, and if you are feeling tense, jot down a few notes.

For example: no fever in morning . . . fever of 99° F by mouth in afternoon . . . child wakeful, irritable . . . took temperature ten minutes ago and was 103° F . . . have given aspirin in such and such a dose . . . last dose given at seven o'clock. Am afraid of meningitis, convulsions, brain damage, etc.

Part of the reason you should have a relationship with a physician is to be able to get medical help when you really need it. Reassurance is part of that help, but in order for the doctor to give that reassurance, you need to express what is really worrying you, even if in the saying it seems foolish.

CALL SOONER, NOT LATER

If you or your child begins to develop worrisome symptoms, there are a number of advantages to calling your doctor early in the course of the illness:

1. You will be anxious for a shorter period of time.
2. If you call during the day, you may be able to have an immediate appointment.
3. If you call early in the evening you will not wake the doctor.
4. You may get a recommendation for a home-care treatment.

We tend to be sympathetic with physicians who become annoyed with patients who call at 2:00 A.M. to ask about relatively minor symptoms that began twelve hours earlier. We also feel that any concerned physician will be responsive to someone who calls at a reasonable hour to discuss almost any problem.

ARE YOU THE RIGHT PERSON
TO MAKE THE CALL?

Quite often, the worries or criticism of another person may cause you to make an after-hours call. Typically, one parent is concerned about a child and gets the other parent to make the call. Sometimes one spouse is not feeling well and the other one makes the call.

The problem this creates is that the doctor is talking to the wrong person. For example, you might not be all that concerned about your child's fever, but spurred on by your worried mate, you call, discuss it, and accept the doctor's reassurance. When you hang up the phone, your spouse says, "Did you mention the fact that the boy next door had a fever last week and ended up with pneumonia?"

Now you are in a dilemma. Do you call again with this information and annoy the doctor, or do you refuse to do this and anger your spouse?

More commonly, a husband calls to discuss his wife's illness, a mother calls to discuss her teen-ager's illness, or an adult child calls about the illness of an elderly parent. People who are retarded, senile, mentally ill, or mute obviously cannot be expected to do the calling. Neither can young children. Otherwise, it is very important to have the person who is the patient speak to the doctor. Why?

Only the patient can answer the doctor's questions thoroughly.
Only the patient can decide whether the doctor's recommendations are acceptable.

MAKING THE CALL

Having decided that you do need advice and that you are the one to make the call, and having made notes if necessary, you call the doctor's number and get the answering service.

> Explain that you are a regular patient, that you are not feeling well, and that you need to speak to the doctor.
> State that your problem cannot wait until the office opens.
> Be prepared for the possibility that your own doctor is not available and is covered by another doctor.

When the doctor calls back, you want to make sure that you get all the help you need. Your goal is to appeal to the doctor's helpful side. If the hour is very late and your call is prompted by large doses of anxiety, this first step is very important.

1. Start by being somewhat apologetic. It is best to begin your conversation by acknowledging that you are calling late or after regular hours. The later the call, the more important this part is.

We suggest an opening such as, "I hate to call you at this hour, doctor, but . . ." By prefacing your call this way, you will make it clear that you are appreciative, a quality doctors dearly love in their patients.

2. Get to the point quickly. First, explain why you are calling now. If it is because you just saw a TV show that you think described the dread disease your child has, say it. If the pharmacy closes in an hour, so you want to find out now if you are going to need some medicine, say it. If your friend died of similar symptoms, say so.

The sooner the doctor understands exactly why you have called, the sooner he or she will be able to respond to your needs. And if you were moved to call because of your spouse's concerns, don't be embarrassed to say that; the doctor should ask to talk to your spouse, which is the best solution anyway.

3. Be prepared to accept telephone advice. That is probably what you are going to get. And don't say, "How can you tell what's wrong over the telephone?" At least seventy percent of all medical diagnoses are made from listening to what the patient says and asking further questions. For simple illnesses, the percentage is even higher.

If you have confidence in your doctor, if he or she asks careful questions and seems appropriately concerned, you can safely accept telephone advice—especially if it includes follow-up instructions, such as "Call me if it gets worse," or "Make an appointment to see me in two days if you still have the fever."

4. If you want a house call, say why. As we have explained, it is unlikely you will get one, but when the doctor hears your concerns, he or she may be able to help you understand why a house call is not necessary.

5. Don't get angry if your doctor says, "Take two aspirin and call me in the morning." Although this may seem like an unfeeling cliché, what your doctor means is, "Don't worry. The problem can wait till morning. Get a good night's sleep now and let me hear from you."

6. Don't feel you must tolerate rudeness or inattention. If the doctor seems uninterested in your problem, angry to be disturbed, or does not call back within fifteen minutes for a problem you feel is very urgent or within an hour for a somewhat less urgent problem: mention your concerns—if not on the spot, then at the time of your next visit. There will be times when you need medical help after hours, and you must have someone who will be accessible and responsive.

7. If you call after hours often—unless you are acutely ill each time—be prepared to have the doctor become increasingly annoyed with you. If your doctor feels that you could have called sooner or waited until the next day, he or she may feel put upon. Actually, people who call after hours for medically trivial reasons often have an emotional need to find out whether the doctor will "always" be there.

8. Be prepared to get a call back from your doctor's associate. If you do not like the associate, you can tell your own doctor why you were dissatisfied. Doctors take night and weekend calls in rotation with one or more colleagues in the same field. Doctors who are always available may seem wonderful to you but not to their families.

THREE THINGS YOU CAN DO
TO ENRAGE YOUR DOCTOR

1. Accept a prescription for a two-week course of medication. Take a few pills sporadically and forget the rest. Tell the doctor the medication didn't work.

2. See your doctor for a problem and then consult another doctor. Return to your doctor for further treatment without sharing the information that you have consulted another doctor.

3. See your doctor, accept a treatment, and go home. Talk to Mrs. So-and-So next door, who warns you that her uncle developed a terrible problem after following that particular recommendation. Decide not to follow the treatment but do not inform your doctor of this decision.

All the above situations involve lack of honesty and cooperation, two basic ingredients a doctor needs in order to be effective. In the first case, you may be embarrassed at having forgotten to take the pills, disturbed by unexpected side effects, or afraid of some risk. You may hate swallowing pills. By not sharing this information, though, you are interfering with the doctor's ability to find a successful way to treat your problem. In the second case, if you have sought another opinion, and have not told your doctor, you are withholding information and treating your doctor with disrespect.

The third case is similar to the second, with an added insult: instead of consulting a qualified professional, you have taken the advice of a lay person. In all of these situations you are not fulfilling your part of the bargain, and you will pay for your failure by getting poorer medical care. (See the discussion of the sick role in Chapter One.)

THREE THINGS DOCTORS CAN DO TO ENRAGE YOU

1.   Keep you waiting for an hour with no explanation. When you are finally seen, offer no apology for the delay.
2.   Inform you that though you are suffering from chronic pain, there is nothing physically wrong and the problem is "all in your mind."
3.   Tell you that it would be a waste of valuable time to answer your questions.

The issues here are respect and caring. The doctor who schedules patients with no regard for the value of their time, the doctor who dismisses a patient's request for help with the pat phrase, "It's all in your mind" (without explaining the mind-body connection and offering further help or advice on what to do about the problem), and the doctor who dismisses a patient's legitimate questions as being a waste of his or her time will arouse hostile feelings that destroy the trust that is necessary for the doctor to be effective.

WHEN TO CHANGE DOCTORS

At the end of the previous chapter, we cautioned you not to have unrealistic expectations of your physician. Still, should you be unhappy with your present doctor, you need not resign yourself to an unpleasant medical relationship.

If you question the correctness of a diagnosis or treatment, your first step should be to discuss your concerns frankly with your present doctor. No reputable doctor will object to your wish to have another opinion, if that's what you want, and in fact, will help you find an appropriate consultant. If a doctor criticizes you for wanting another doctor's opinion, you should strongly consider switching.

You might also want to switch if you are dissatisfied with the way the doctor takes care of you. If seeing the doctor makes you more, rather than less, anxious or if you feel you are being treated with a lack of concern or respect, you will quite understandably want to make a change. Since it will cost you time and money to do so, we advise you to discuss what is bothering you with your present doctor.

You might say, for example, "I feel that you brush aside my questions," or "I felt more and more anxious when you did not return my call for such a long time." Although, as we explained earlier, physicians are not selected for their interpersonal skills and are not well trained in the "human" side of medicine, as a group they very much want to help people get well. You may be surprised by the positive response you get.

If you remain unsurprised, if your complaints go unheeded or are turned into criticisms of you ("you are not trying to get well," or "you are unable to understand medical terminology"), it is time to seek a new physician.

Why Do Doctors Talk Medicalese?

Although sometimes it is because of obliviousness—they assume everyone uses words like "myocardial infarction" (heart attack) and "hypertension" (high blood pressure)—at other times medicalese hides ignorance. We offer the following examples:

The *thyroid* is a gland in the neck; smaller glands adjacent to the thyroid regulate calcium and phosphorus metabolism, and are called the *parathyroid* glands. A condition in which these glands are under-active is known as *hypoparathyroidism*. If the cause of this under-activity is not known, the condition is described as *idiopathic hypoparathyroidism* ("idiopathic" means "cause unknown"). Those people with a poorly understood inherited disorder in which it appears that the parathyroid is under-active because bone and kidney are unresponsive to the action of the parathyroid glands, are said to have *pseudohypoparathyroidism;* one of the signs is certain bone deformities. Those people with similar abnormalities of bone, but without the other symptoms of pseudohypoparathyroidism are diagnosed as having—do you see it coming—*pseudopseudohypoparathyroidism.*

Acute viral hepatitis is usually caused by one of two viruses—called virus A and virus B. If it is not caused by either, but by a virus that has not yet been isolated, it is called *hepatitis non-A non-B.*

Generally, it seems that the less well understood a problem, the more elaborate the medicalese.

IF YOU HAVE TROUBLE TALKING TO DOCTORS

We have written a great deal about the education and background of doctors and about their human failings, not to be critical but to give you some perspective. Our hope is that by understanding the way doctors think, you will be better equipped to deal with them. Here and throughout the book, we stress your rights as a patient and include specific advice for the typical problems that arise in communication. But if, armed with all this knowledge, you march into the doctor's office and still find yourself lapsing into uncertainty, here are some suggestions for coping:

Plan ahead. If you have been experiencing certain symptoms, write down what they are and when you have them, e.g., "Have had a bad cough for a week, worse at night, cough medicine doesn't help."

If you have more than one problem, list each one, with its particular symptoms, separately.

Prioritize your list. It may be that you will not have enough time to get to everything, so make sure you mention first what troubles you the most.

Try rehearsing to yourself what you are going to say. The authors of *The Well Body Book*[2] suggest that you role-play not only your part of the conversation but the doctor's too. If your rendition of the doctor is critical or impatient or condescending, remember that these are your fears of what the doctor is thinking.

When you see the doctor, explain why you have a list and what it consists of. "I decided to write down a brief list of exactly what is bothering me because I find I forget to mention things." Some doctors have had bad experiences with people who come in with a huge shopping list of complaints and theories. You do not want to be seen as one of these.

Take notes on what the doctor says and repeat back precisely his or her conclusions and recommendations. Make sure you understand everything you must do.

HOW TO COME HOME WITH SOME ANSWERS

For those people who become anxious to the point of forgetting what to tell the doctor, these paper and pencil techniques may save a lot of uncertainty. To add to this approach, we are including a useful list of questions from an equally useful article by Mike Oppenheim, M.D. published by *Woman's Day*.[3] Dr. Oppenheim feels that people should expect to leave the doctor's office "with some answers to the following questions."

What is my problem?
What caused it?
What should I do about it?
When should I get better and what should I do if I don't?
Do I really need this [medication]?

In these first three chapters, we have tried to lay the groundwork for dealing with medical people. In the three chapters that follow, we will build on your understanding of the needs of doctors and patients and explain how they affect some specific and difficult situations: deciding whether to have surgery, entering a hospital, and using an emergency room.

CHAPTER FOUR

HOW TO HAVE ONLY THE SURGERY YOU NEED

There is probably no decision quite so difficult to make, so fraught with anxiety, as the decision to have surgery. Rightly so, we think, because there is a real difference between deciding to try a medical treatment and committing yourself to the surgeon's knife.

Most medical treatments have more gradual effects than surgical ones, and if there are difficulties they are completely or partially reversible. Once your gall bladder is removed, however, it is gone, never to be seen again.

Surgery also involves cutting, making a wound, creating a problem to solve a more serious one, something that surgeons have learned to accept but that their patients still regard with varying degrees of squeamishness or fear. (And, of course, it is the patients who will suffer the consequences if something goes wrong.)

THE EMOTIONAL STRESSES OF SURGERY

In addition to all the stresses generally associated with being in a hospital, the stress of surgery imposes a unique set of demands. People who have chosen surgery with expectations of relief or cure must also deal with deep-rooted fears of being "put to sleep," a state many people associate with death. Indeed, some surgical patients do fear that they will not wake up.

The surgery itself holds the threat of damage and mutilation, a violation of one's sense of bodily integrity. If the part of the body that is being operated on has symbolic significance, there may be further stress. For example, if a woman feels that her uterus is the source of her femininity, her sense of loss after a hysterectomy may lead to depression and a difficult convalescence.

Fear of surgery may be beneficial if it helps you avoid an operation you do not need and impels you to seek out the best surgeon and the safest setting for one that you do. Some of what we are going to tell you in this chapter may seem frightening. Our goal in presenting this information is not to scare you into avoiding a procedure that will save your life or spare you great pain but to help you decide whether what is being recommended will in fact do one or the other.

Far too often, the need for surgery is presented and discussed only by surgeons, most of whom by training and interest believe surgery is a good and curative thing. Sometimes it is; sometimes it isn't.

YOUR PRIMARY CARE DOCTOR
IS AN IMPORTANT HELPER

The most common mistake people make is to bypass their personal physician. Perhaps they want to save money by avoiding extra doctors' fees. Perhaps they have no idea of how helpful a doctor who is not a surgeon can be in this situation. Whatever the reason, they often neglect to use their most helpful resource.

We will give you two typical scenarios that dramatize the difficulties you may create for yourself if you don't involve your personal physician.

You have had abdominal pain on and off, and your physician has told you that one more serious episode means you need to have your gall bladder removed. The pain returns and you decide that you need surgery.

Your mother learns of this and announces that she can get the name of a wonderful surgeon. He helped her neighbor, who was in terrible pain. Everyone thinks he is the best!

You call the wonderful surgeon's office yourself and make an appointment. You are uncomfortable about what you have done, so you don't call your primary doctor to ask that your medical records be sent.

What do you say if the surgeon wants to perform tests you have already had? How do you proceed if you don't like what this surgeon tells you? Do you go to Surgeon Number Two who, you are told, saved the life of somebody's cousin? Suppose you do and Surgeon Number Two disagrees with Surgeon Number One; now what? How are you going to decide which recommendation to follow?

The best thing you could do now would be to call your own doctor, explain what you have done, and ask for advice. You are better off with a case of embarrassment than you are with unnecessary surgery or the wrong surgeon.

Another common scenario: you see the surgeon to whom you were referred by your primary care doctor. You listen carefully to an explanation of why the operation is necessary, posing occasional questions and getting brief and unsatisfying answers.

The surgeon is forceful and compelling, and you feel foolish asking questions when you know that your real motive is not desire for enlightenment but fear. After all, you reason, you are now in the hands of a surgeon recommended by your own doctor. Therefore, you suppose that you ought to accept the need for surgery without further question.

In this situation, the person who can explain to you in simple English what the surgeons are telling you in fluent surgeonese is your primary care doctor. One is reminded of the old popular song that begins, "If I ever needed you / I need you now." If ever your primary care doctor has a role in explaining alternatives and helping you make decisions, it is here.

Your own doctor can do a number of things for you, such as:

· finding the right surgeon for the problem
· finding the right surgeon for *you*
· preparing you for the consultation
· making sure that the surgeon works at the right hospital
· recommending surgeons for second and third opinions
· helping you sort out whatever differences of opinion exist
· evaluating what the surgery will accomplish
· determining whether you have other medical problems that would interfere with the success of the surgery
· offering continuity of medical care should your surgery cause medical problems to develop

Saving money by going straight to a surgeon is likely to be a poor decision for anyone, but if you have existing medical problems or are at high risk because of age or your particular history, you are clearly inviting trouble. If you have not involved your own doctor, the surgeon will call in one or more specialists if medical complications arise after surgery. The result: fragmented care and a higher bill.

WHAT DO THE RISKS MEAN TO YOU?

Everyone has heard the horror stories, the errors, complications, reactions that the victim might have been spared, the additional procedures that were done because of bungling. Let us assume, though, that you have eliminated the possibility of incompetence by securing the services of a knowledgeable and talented surgeon, one who practices at a hospital known for its fine surgical service.

No matter how skilled the practitioner or how safety-conscious the hospital, there are still inherent risks associated with surgery. Of course, there are risks associated with almost any kind of medical treatment, but many of them, as we just noted, occur gradually and can usually be reversed. In surgery, the things that go seriously wrong tend to happen fast.

If you are rushed—mangled, bleeding internally, and unconscious—from the scene of an automobile accident to the operating room where a team of specialists races against time to save your life and repair the damage, you have been spared the difficulties of making the kinds of decisions that this chapter is about. Whatever the outcome, the benefits definitely outweigh the risks.

Surgery often involves making choices. To identify what they are, you need information from the surgeon and help from your primary care physician. Some problems can be treated either with drugs or with surgery. For example, people with coronary artery insufficiency can take medication or have by-pass surgery. Even when surgery is the sole recommendation, there may be more than one procedure to choose from. For example, a woman with very early breast cancer, depending on her exact diagnosis, may have to decide whether to have a modified radical mastectomy, a simple mastectomy, or a lumpectomy.

Finally, you may be called upon to choose between surgery and no surgery. In some cases, the decision can be postponed either for months or indefinitely. As you go about gathering information, you need to consider the risks and how you feel about them.

When we suggest that you consider how you feel about taking risks, we are asking you to enter a realm of decision-making that is ignored by most of the medical profession. When doctors want to order a test or treatment, they may discuss with you the question of risk versus benefit. Usually that discussion reflects the doctors' feelings about risk-taking. Almost never will they explore with you what kinds of risks *you* are willing to take and why.

Doctors give very little conscious thought to the way in which they present risk/benefit information and how the presentation will affect a patient's decision; unconsciously they may present alternatives in a way that favors surgery. Yet, the patient who accepts a treatment when told there is a "ninety percent chance of success" might refuse it if told that it had a ten percent chance of failure.

A recent article in *The New England Journal of Medicine*[1] related the results of an experiment that crystallizes the problem people have with making risk/benefit decisions. In the experiment, a group of people were asked which of two treatments for lung cancer they would choose. (None of the subjects actually had lung cancer.) The first, a surgical procedure, had a ten percent chance of killing them immediately from the surgery itself but had a better overall chance of saving their lives than did the second treatment, radiation therapy, which would not kill them but would save fewer lives.

When told about the chances of *dying* with either treatment, many chose the radiation therapy, since that would never kill them right away. When, however, the alternatives were presented in terms of *survival*, people tended to choose surgery because it gave them a greatly increased life expectancy should they survive.

Try the experiment on yourself. Answer the next two questions "yes" or "no."

> Your physician tells you that you have a serious disease that may prove fatal. If you choose a certain treatment you have a sixty-eight percent chance of living more than one year. Do you choose it?
>
> What if the treatment proposed gives you a thirty-two percent chance of dying within the year? Would you choose it?

These were the odds given in the experiment cited above. When an operation for a disease was described in terms of life, people tended to choose that operation. When presented in terms of death, they tended to shy away. The odds, however, are the same.

Furthermore, if this study is any indication, you can expect to be very much influenced not only by the way that the doctor answers your questions about the risks of a given treatment but by your gut feelings about the nature of the treatment.

For example, one group being studied was given information about the risks of Treatment A versus Treatment B. Ten percent of patients who have Treatment A will die during the treatment, they were told, but those who survive will live an average of 6.8 years. No one will die from Treatment B, but the average life expectancy is only 4.7 years. Forty-two percent of the group considered the risks and chose Treatment B.

When another group was presented with exactly the same information except that now Treatment A was identified as surgery and B as radiation therapy, only twenty-six percent of subjects chose the latter. Evidently, people have feelings about radiation therapy that cause them to avoid it, even though the purely numerical results sound more attractive to them.

Different strokes for different folks ... but be sure that you understand what strokes you will be getting. If you would choose a procedure that you are told has a ninety percent chance of saving you but avoid one that you are told has a ten percent chance of killing you—something is wrong. You may be preventing yourself from making the decision that is right for you because you are not thinking clearly about the choices, or are confused by the numbers, or have prejudices about one of the treatments.

To make the right choice you need to try to understand how you feel about living with uncertainty and how you respond to consequences in the near, as opposed to the distant, future. Here are some questions to ask yourself when you are faced with making life and death decisions.

Am I unrealistically hoping for a miracle cure to come along?

Do I have family obligations that I must consider? (It may be of utmost importance to you to live for several more years in order to leave your family financially secure.)

Do I lose anything by waiting to make a decision?

Faced with the kind of stress this situation provokes, some people simply avoid thinking about it. They don't really decide *against* having recommended surgery; they just decide to do nothing. Doing nothing, though, is also a decision. It may or may not be the right one.

When you don't trust the physician who is recommending surgery, that is another matter; then all the numbers in the world are irrelevant. If this is the case, you should keep shopping. If necessary, go to a famous referral center such as the Cleveland Clinic or Massachussetts General Hospital.

SURGEONS LIKE TO OPERATE

By our definition, the very best surgeons are those who, in addition to being technically skillful, are also thoughtful and conservative, and who only recommend surgery when it is clearly the best treatment.

There are many surgeons who, while qualifying as technically "good," lack selective judgment and are all too willing to operate. Why? Some seem to have an underlying need for power or prestige, or to demonstrate that they have the ability to cure, the skill to defeat disease. A few do it for the money.

In our experience, however, the most obvious and universal reason surgeons are too willing to operate is because they love doing operations. They sincerely believe that in doing surgery they are saving your life or your health, and they take umbrage at any suggestion that they are mercenary. After all, even though they are generally not paid to teach resident physicians, they will get up at 2 A.M. to assist the young surgeon in the operating room (after recommending the surgery)—proof that they sincerely believe in the power of the scalpel to purify and heal. And their enthusiasm for the curative powers of their art may sway you.

Here is yet another reason why we recommend the involvement of primary care doctors. They will not be unquestioningly enthusiastic about the ability of surgeons to heal, since their training emphasizes a medical (that is, *nonsurgical*) approach.

There are surgical procedures that will work wonders for you, and there are those that will do you no good whatsoever. There are times when surgery is the best choice and times when it is not so clearly indicated.

We are going to talk very specifically about the risks of surgery. As we have already stated, our goal is not to frighten you. Rather, we hope that you will make surgical decisions with extreme care and with as much consultation as you feel you need. Many health insurance policies now pay for a second opinion; some even pay for a third. Even if you must pay the cost of a consultation yourself, you will have made a good investment if you thereby save the risk and pain of an unnecessary operation.

Some surgical procedures are safer, more routine than others, but all have inherent risks. Any problems that do occur tend to fall into three categories: the risks of anesthesia, the risks of the actual surgery, and the postoperative risks.

ANESTHESIA

A number of years ago, a professional black athlete died on the operating table because he did not get enough oxygen while under anesthesia. The anesthetist did not realize what was happening because she was inexperienced in interpreting changes in black skin tone. (She should have been checking the color of his mucous membranes to find out whether the oxygen level was adequate.)

Scary? It should be. Even a simple procedure carries serious risks. This kind of catastrophe is relatively rare, but not unheard of.

AWAKE OR ASLEEP?

For most people, local anesthesia (which numbs only a specific part of the body) is much safer than general anesthesia (which puts a patient to sleep); however, a tiny percentage will suffer a reaction to local anesthetic drugs.

General anesthesia carries greater risks and must be very carefully administered by a well-trained practitioner. Since skilled postoperative care is also necessary in order to prevent anesthesia-related problems, the quality of the hospital where you have your surgery is an important factor.

Major surgery must be done under general anesthesia, and most of the drugs used are considered safe for most people, except for the unlucky few who have what doctors term an "idiosyncratic reaction." Who will experience it cannot be determined ahead of time.

Find out whether you have a choice of local or general anesthesia. Of course, safety is your first consideration, but if you have a choice, you must also take into account your feelings. Some people are terrified of being unconscious; others of being awake and witnessing their own surgery.

WHO WILL GIVE THE ANESTHESIA?

There are two types of qualified professionals who administer anesthesia: an anesthesiologist, who is a physician, and a nurse-anesthetist. (The word anesthetist is not as precise and may refer to either.)

The patient does not choose this practitioner; some combination of the hospital and surgeon will. You can, however, ask questions beforehand about a part of your care, which is just as important, if not more so, than the surgery itself.

Will you have a board-certified anesthesiologist or a resident he or she is supervising? Or is the physician just a general practitioner, or only partially trained in anesthesiology?

Will you have a nurse-anesthetist? If so, is he or she a certified registered nurse-anesthetist (C.R.N.A.), and will he or she be supervised by an experienced anesthesiologist who is responsible for no more than two nurse-anesthetists?

Too often, the risks of anesthesia are not fully explained. They will appear minimal to you if the surgery is either life-saving or performed to prevent great pain and suffering. But knowing what they are may make you decide to try an alternative treatment if surgery is not your only, or necessarily your best, choice. Once you fully understand the risks, you may decide that cosmetic surgery, for example, is just not worth it.

An attractive young woman with a slightly crooked nose decided to have plastic surgery. The decision was made to do the procedure in the surgeon's office, and she was given injections of several different drugs to kill the pain. She had a severe unexpected reaction and died suddenly.

QUESTIONS THE ANESTHESIOLOGIST SHOULD ASK YOU

Before your surgery, the person who is going to be giving the anesthesia should meet with you to explain what will be done and to ask some important questions about your previous medical history.

1. Do you have any allergies?
2. Do you have any medical problems the anesthesiologist needs to know about, such as cardiac or respiratory disease, sickle cell anemia, diabetes?
3. Are you taking any medication?
4. Have you had anesthesia in the past?
5. If so, how recently? (Some anesthetic agents cannot be given again until a certain amount of time has passed.)

6. Have you ever had problems receiving or recovering from anesthesia?
7. Have you ever had a fever or other problem after taking any kind of anesthetic?
8. Have you ever had a reaction to a local anesthetic, such as a shot given in the dentist's office?
9. Do you have a history of abnormal bleeding?

THE RISKS OF THE SURGERY ITSELF

You can die from anesthesia for a minor procedure or for major surgery. The danger of a surgical procedure, however, is generally proportionate to the seriousness of the problem it is designed to treat. For instance, a hernia is not a grave problem. If you had to, you could live with it, but the surgery used to repair your hernia is not especially tricky or dangerous. (One notable exception to this rule is the tonsillectomy, which has serious risks associated with it. See discussion on pp. 75–77.)

Some types of surgery are hazardous either because of the organ that is being tampered with or the extensiveness of the procedure. Brain surgery, for example, is always very risky as are open-heart surgery and certain kinds of very extensive cancer surgery. The following table may give you a clearer idea of the increasing risks of not having surgery. The higher the category number, the more dangerous it is to postpone surgery. Problems listed under categories IV, V, and VI are clearly worth the risk of surgery. Below IV, the decision to have surgery is more a function of your own fears and priorities.

For most types of surgery, especially those in the lower categories, the immediate surgical risk has less to do with the procedure itself and more to do with the skill of the surgeon. Some surgeons are referred to by their colleagues as "butchers," a phrase that requires no explanation. Their patients usually survive, but with a much higher rate of postoperative complications than the patients of more skillful surgeons.

The incompetent surgeon may earn the title of "butcher" by making mechanical errors. For example, there is a procedure known as a hemigastrectomy, which translated means the removal of half of the stomach. One young resident was surprised to learn that this operation was not almost invariably fatal. At the hospital associated with his medical school he had observed seven patients undergo a hemigastrectomy. All seven died. He was shocked to learn later in his training that the overall mortality rate is less than five percent.

Another kind of error the less skillful surgeon makes is caused not by lack of skill but by lack of judgment.

In a large teaching hospital, where the students claimed the unofficial motto was the phrase "See one, do one, teach one," a

RISKS OF AVOIDING SURGERY

CATEGORY	RISKS OF NO SURGERY	PURPOSE OF SURGERY	EXAMPLES
I	None	Cosmetic	Eye muscle surgery, rhinoplasty, face-lift, cosmetic breast surgery
II	None	To relieve pain, or solve a problem	Bunionectomy, removal of ganglion, hysterectomy for prolapse, back surgery, joint reconstruction/replacement, vasectomy
III	Almost None	Same as II but also to avoid some risks	Hernia repair, tubal ligation if pregnancy would be dangerous, cryosurgery for Class II Pap, myomectomy for fibroid tumor
IV	Significant	To eliminate a condition that is threatening loss of an organ or limb—or that could be fatal	Amputation of gangrenous toe, hysterectomy for recurrent severe bleeding, surgery for carcinoma in situ of cervix, hip pinning, appendectomy
V	Almost 100%	To eliminate a serious problem that would probably be fatal without surgery	Hysterectomy for cancer of the endometrium, bowel resection for cancer, removal of brain tumor, repair of abnormal heart valve
VI	100%	To save life or limb in emergency	Repair of major blood vessels injured in accident, evacuation of subdural hematoma, removal of ruptured spleen, tracheotomy for respiratory obstruction

young woman was admitted with lower abdominal pain. On examination, she was found to have a large mass in her abdomen and was taken directly to the operating room. There the surgeon made an incision and disclosed a huge lump. It was in a place where nothing should have been and was surrounded by unusual-looking tissue. The surgeon, without further ado, set about removing it. The lump turned out to be her only kidney.

RISKS AFTER SURGERY

Postoperative problems may be the direct result of poor surgery, such as a wound infection caused by careless aseptic technique, or they may occur because the patient is in very poor health and more susceptible. Someone weakened by metastatic cancer is more apt to have serious complications even in the most competent hands. Some common problems that may occur are infections, either at the site of the incision or in the bloodstream (septicemia), pneumonia, and pulmonary embolus (a blood clot that forms in the leg, breaks away, and goes to the lung).

The actual physical dexterity of the surgeon is a very significant factor. The very best surgeons are both speedy and careful of the way they handle body tissue. In order to operate on an abdominal organ, for example, the surgeon must cut through a number of layers of skin, fat, and muscle, and must move various vital innards aside to get at the problem area.

The more carefully this is done, the less damage afterward and therefore the less chance of infection. Among physicians the phrase "respect for tissue" indicates a quality that is the hallmark of the very skillful.

Speed is important because it minimizes the time spent under anesthesia and leaves you open to infection for a shorter period of time. A recent report in *The New England Journal of Medicine*[2] found that for every hour beyond the first that it took to do an abdominal hysterectomy, there was an increase of two percent in the risk of postoperative infection.

Those who possess this combination of care and speed consistently get the best results and are the most popular and admired teachers. Residents who are training to be surgeons want to work with them. It is a good sign when the surgical residents are enthusiastic about your choice of surgeon.

LONG-TERM RISKS OF SURGERY

Then, finally, there is the risk that you will develop new problems after the surgery. For instance, someone who has a ruptured or diseased spleen removed is prone to infection with pneumococcus. Anyone who has had abdominal surgery is at a higher risk later in life for intestinal obstruction caused by adhesions. Women who have had hysterectomies often talk of not feeling well for many months post-op, even though presently there is no "medical" explanation. (The truth is that physicians do not fully understand the function and interaction of all the parts of the body.)

SURGICAL RISKS VERSUS SURGICAL BENEFITS

With all the risks and dangers we have discussed, how do you go about deciding when surgery is justified and whether the risks are worth the good things the surgery will do? If the benefit is a bumpless nose (a Category I problem on our chart), the authors of this book would not take the chance of dying for it, but you might. Give some people the choice of dying from cancer or having an operation that has a fifty percent chance of saving their lives and they respond, "Show me the way to the operating room." To others, the thought of dying from surgery is so horrifying that they forgo the operation and try all sorts of unscientific treatments such as Krebiozen® or Laetrile®.

To enable you to make an informed decision, the surgeon should tell you . . .

- the risks of the procedure and how statistically common each is
- the benefits of the procedure and what percent of the time it produces those benefits

Only you can decide whether to have surgery. Only you know how much suffering a given problem is causing and how much risk is acceptable to improve your condition. One person accepts a one percent chance of dying rather than going through life with frequent severe abdominal pain; another wouldn't take the risk.

An Example of Risk/Benefit Analysis

If you are interested in the statistical underpinnings of surgical decisions, you might find this next section helpful. It is drawn from Dr. George Crile, Jr.'s excellent book, *Surgery: Your Choices, Your Alternatives*[3] and is based on his eye-opening discussion of risk versus benefit and of how the qualifications of your surgeon must be included in your decision to have or decline surgery.

Dr. Crile discusses alternative treatments for low-lying, small- to medium-sized cancers of the rectum. One treatment is radical surgery (cutting out the cancer and nearby lymph nodes). Reported mortality rates for this procedure range from 1.8 percent to 18 percent.

The other treatments are electrocoagulation (use of an electric current to destroy the tumor) and radiation therapy, both of which have a zero mortality rate. (Nobody dies from either of these treatments.)

The justification for surgery is the possibility that the disease has spread (metastasized) to nearby lymph nodes. Yet, as Dr. Crile points out, of 100 patients with this problem, 70 have no spread to lymph nodes and will not benefit from a radical procedure. Of the 30 with spread, 24 cannot be cured by any treatment. We are left with only 6 people out of the original 100 who would benefit from radical surgery.

Furthermore, significant expense and discomfort, including a colostomy, accompany surgery. Also, most patients with this problem are in their sixties, with a life expectancy of ten to fifteen years. If they die from surgery, they die immediately, whereas if they die from cancer left in the lymph nodes, it is usually after living comfortably for five to ten years.

Let's suppose that five percent of your surgeon's patients die. Would you guess that surgery is the better choice?

Let's see what would happen to 100 people who had surgery compared with 100 who had one of the more conservative treatments.

Surgery and Electrocoagulation

Surgery

With your surgeon, 5 out of 100 people will die. Of the 95 who survive surgery, 70% (67 people) do not have metastatic disease and live 15 years each.   67 x 15 = 1005 patient-years.

Of the remaining 28, 80%, (22 people) are incurable. They live 7.5 years each.   22 x 7.5 = 165 patient-years.

The remaining 6 are cured by the surgery. Let's assume they live 15 years each.   15 x 15 = 225 patient-years.

Total patient-years for this treatment = 1260

Electrocoagulation

Electrocoagulation cures 70; they live 15 years each.   70 x 15 = 1050 patient-years.

Remaining 30 are not cured
and live 7.5 years each. $30 \times 7.5 = 225$ patient-years.

Total patient-years for this treatment $= 1275$

Given these calculations, electrocoagulation is the better choice. Mortality for surgery would have to be, at most, 3 percent to present a clear advantage, a figure attained at only a handful of major medical centers.

HOW TO TALK TO A SURGEON

The above heading may sound like an attempt at humor. It is not. Surgeons are different from other physicians, and the way they relate to patients is a result of that difference.

An ophthalmologist is talking to a fellow physician (not a surgeon) who expresses negative feelings about having to cut into a person. The ophthalmologist somewhat surprisingly agrees. "I am always terrified before doing an operation," he says. "Every so often, I've thought about cutting off my hands so that I wouldn't be tempted to operate on anyone else."

What's unusual about this surgeon is that he readily admits to these feelings; his willingness to acknowledge them is part of what makes him an excellent surgeon and an excellent physician. Whatever you feel about the nature of human aggression, it is not normal behavior to take a knife and carve up people who have done nothing to wrong or enrage you. Most surgeons have repressed their fears and their reluctance; otherwise, how could they get themselves to cut people open, remove chunks of their insides, and sew them back up again?

The result of this repression is a lack of responsiveness to the anxiety and fears and individual humanness of the patient. The more critical and dangerous the type of surgery, the more emotionally upsetting it is to the person who performs it, and therefore, the more repression is necessary. Anyone who has tried to talk to a neurosurgeon will understand this, at least in retrospect.

If you find a surgeon who is warm, understanding, willing to spend time answering all your questions, and capable of dealing with your anxiety, you are in luck. Given the nature of surgeons and surgery, it is unrealistic to expect this.

Having said all this, what do you do if you are the patient of a surgeon who is not one of the great communicators?

· Remember that you have your primary care doctor as a backup. You are seeing this surgeon for technical skill rather than caring or concern.

· Ask questions directly. Hinting that you have something on your mind will get you nowhere.
· Try to avoid challenging the surgeon's knowledge or authority. Preface questions with some statement such as "I am confused. Can you explain further?" Your goal is to call on his or her protective impulses rather than the defensive ones.

DO YOU NEED A SECOND OR THIRD OPINION?

If you have been referred to a surgeon by your primary care doctor, who thinks an operation will probably be necessary, then in a sense, the surgeon's recommendation is a second opinion. Suppose after talking to this surgeon and perhaps checking back with your own doctor, surgery seems reasonable to you, and you have no particular doubts or concerns. In this situation, there would usually be no need to ask for another opinion.

There is a difference between getting *another* opinion and getting a *second* opinion. You might want another opinion because you are not sure you have gotten the right advice, or because while you think you probably do need surgery, you did not like the style, or trust the competence, of the particular surgeon. Logically, in such situations, you would see another surgeon. If you liked that person better, you would probably switch doctors, even if the advice is the same.

Getting a second opinion is an insurance term for a more formal process. Nowadays, fortunately, most health insurance plans pay for a second opinion whenever surgery is recommended. Studies have found that fifteen to twenty percent of the time, the second physician will recommend against surgery. (See p. 80 for a list of procedures for which we particularly recommend a second opinion).

The intent of this program is not to give the patient access to a second possible operating surgeon but to a second surgical *opinion.* The insurance company will therefore stipulate that the surgeon rendering the second opinion is not allowed to perform the actual surgery. Thus, if you like the second surgeon better, you are out of luck. Had you made the appointment and paid for the visit yourself (assuming your insurance would not cover the costs of a simple office consultation), then you could easily have changed doctors.

Therefore, you should request a formal second opinion only if you like and have confidence in the skill of the first surgeon but feel the need to confirm that an operation of any kind has to be done. Explain to the surgeon that should one be necessary, he or she is your choice but that you would feel better with a second opinion. Second opinion panels are carefully chosen by insurance companies; commonly the surgeons on the list are medical school professors who seldom take new surgical patients. If what you want is another surgeon, not just another surgical opinion, you would be better off to forgo the formal second opinion route offered by your insurance company.

HOW TO HANDLE A CONSULTATION

1. Be completely honest with the second doctor. Explain your reasons for wanting another opinion.
2. Tell the second doctor what was recommended and why.
3. If you do not agree with or like that recommendation, explain why.
4. If you did not like the first surgeon, say so.

You may have heard the phrase "doctor shopper" and fear being labeled as such. The people who really anger doctors are those who go from one doctor to another without revealing that this is what they are doing. Such behavior makes doctors feel manipulated and mistrustful of the patient.

WHICH IS THE RIGHT OPINION?

A good rule of thumb is, "When in doubt, do nothing." What makes this an especially good rule for surgical issues is that many surgeons have the opposite inclination.

There is a very extensive operation called a Whipple procedure that is sometimes done for cancer of the pancreas. Although it is a very difficult piece of surgery entailing a high rate of mortality and usually offering only a meager hope for cure, there was a surgeon at a very respected hospital who liked to do this procedure so much that the residents claimed his motto was "When in doubt, Whipple it out."

There is an old medical joke that asks, "What does a gynecologist consider an indication for a hysterectomy?" The answer: "The presence of a uterus."

If you have consulted two surgeons who disagree, you may feel you need a third opinion to break the deadlock. Many insurance policies will cover the cost of a third consultation. Or, you and your primary care physican might decide that if two highly qualified people cannot agree the best thing is to do nothing.

ELECTIVE SURGERY

When the surgery in question is not being performed as a life-saving measure to cure cancer, to remove an otherwise fatal brain tumor, or to correct a serious congenital abnormality, in other words, if waiting a few weeks or months will not really change the outcome (see Categories II and III on the chart), you can safely take the advice of a reputable surgeon who tells you that surgery is not necessary. It is unlikely that you will be hurt by such a recommendation from one who is trained to solve problems by operating on them.

QUESTIONS TO ASK THE SURGEON

Do I need this surgery immediately? If so, why?
How long can the surgery be postponed?
How dangerous would it be to postpone the surgery?
Will the surgery be less successful if I wait?
Will my life be threatened if I wait?
What will the surgery accomplish?
What are the risks of the surgery itself?
What are the postoperative consequences of the surgery?
How long will it take to recover from this surgery?
What are possible complications and how common are they?
How often have you done this procedure?
What rate of success have you yourself had with this procedure?
What kind of anesthesia would I need?
What are the qualifications of the person who would administer it?
Which hospital would you use and why?
What is the surgical fee?

What do you do if, after getting as much information as you can, there seem to be as many pros as cons? The best decision for you may have to do with your own personality.

Do you like getting things over with or do you enter a swimming pool one toe at a time? For some people, action itself is of value; it seems decisive, and therapeutic. For others, "making decisions" is anxiety-producing. (We've put the phrase in quotes to remind you that doing nothing is really a decision too.)

Will you blame yourself if you make the wrong choice and the surgery does not work out well, or will you accept the results of your decision as the luck of the draw?

Bear in mind, too, that the way information is given to you may affect your decision, as the study we discussed earlier revealed. You might try writing down the risks and benefits of the surgery being proposed in terms of both survival and mortality to make sure you are not being swayed by the manner in which these facts are presented.

UNNECESSARY OPERATIONS

In an article in *Woman's Day Magazine*[4], the noted health writer Jane E. Brody pointed out that "The United States has the highest rate of surgery in the world—twice that of England, for example—and the rate goes up each year. In 1978 approximately one American in ten had an operation. This country also has the highest ratio of surgeons to population—a situation that some experts believe leads to questionable operations." We have already noted that by temperament and training, surgeons believe in surgery.

How can you, a lay person, avoid an operation you don't need? You can start by taking a close look at the way surgeons think. In order to illustrate for you the process that leads to unnecessary surgery, we are going to discuss in some detail tonsillectomy and hysterectomy—two of the operations that are most commonly overperformed. Although the specific indications for other types of surgery will, of course, differ, the kind of reasoning that surgeons use when they recommend surgery remains a constant.

TONSILLECTOMY

In the 1950s, tonsillectomies were extremely common and were frequently done as office procedures. Doctors who saw endless cases of children with infected tonsils reasoned that if the tonsils (which were thought to be functionless lumps of tissue) were removed, they could no longer become infected. Simple? There are only a few problems with this line of thinking.

First, nature was not quite so dumb as those doctors assumed. The body's first line of defense in dealing with the host of infectious agents that enter the nose and mouth are the tonsils. They become enlarged and get "infected" because they have stopped a virus or bacteria from progressing onward and downward to wreak further havoc. Removing tonsils because they become swollen is something like ordering the cavalry to stop sending scouts ahead because they get killed more often than the rest of the troops.

Even if you are prepared to lose this valuable protection, there is another problem with tonsillectomy: it carries risks that are seldom justified by any benefits. Death from tonsillectomy may result from bleeding—it often occurs a few days post-op, after the patient has been discharged and is far away from a hospital—or from postoperative airway obstruction or from lung problems caused by aspiration of blood or tissue.

Deaths from tonsillectomy are statistically rare, but because the procedure is still so common, there are a significant number. With antibiotics available to treat tonsillitis, people do not die from infected tonsils.

There are two clear and easily definable reasons to have a tonsillectomy. One is a serious kind of infection known as a peritonsillar abscess; the other is enlargement of the tonsils to the point that it becomes literally impossible to breathe. The risks of either of these conditions justify the risks of surgery.

A third indication, which is still being studied, is the frequent recurrence of tonsillitis (an inflammation of the tonsils) specifically caused by a bacterium known as Group A betahemolytic streptococcus.

Experts disagree over the number of episodes that constitute "frequent"; some say three in one year, some five, some seven. All agree, however, that these infections should be carefully documented by throat cultures.

Here is where things become murky. The word tonsillitis simply means that the tonsils have become infected with something. That something could be viral or bacterial. Many people look at a sore throat and swollen tonsils and make a pronouncement of "strep throat" without realizing that it cannot be diagnosed simply by looking at it or having it.

In a study reported in *The New England Journal of Medicine,* researchers followed sixty-five children who had histories of recurrent throat infections (twenty-six in six consecutive years) that had not been "documented." Only eleven of these children had the same kind of recurrent infections during the first year of the study. Of the remaining fifty-four children, forty-three experienced either no throat infections, or one or two. "We conclude," write the authors, "that undocumented histories of recurrent throat infection do not validly forecast subsequent experience and hence do not constitute an adequate basis for subjecting children to tonsillectomy."[5]

There are still too many doctors, however, who recommend surgery for a patient who has had a few sore throats that have never been properly evaluated. One study that looked at the incidence of tonsillectomy in twenty-two states showed that the state that did the procedure the most frequently did it about ten times as often as the state that did it the least. It can hardly be that the children of the first state needed ten times as many operations as the other children, and it is extremely unlikely that anyone in the second state was deprived of a necessary tonsillectomy.[6]

Many tonsillectomies are performed as much to treat parental anxiety as to cure the child's medical problem. Concerned about frequent sore throats and sickness, and frustrated by the feeling that nothing is being done to prevent them, many parents insist on seeing an ENT (ear, nose, and throat) specialist. Surgeons, as we have pointed out, are trained to do surgery and will only rarely recommend a "medical" approach, especially when that means treating each sore throat as it occurs. So to make the parent feel less anxious, or more effective, or less helpless, the child gets a tonsillectomy.

By understanding that the tonsils have a valuable service to perform, that their removal entails risk, and that this procedure is properly used only to treat certain very specific conditions, you can make sure that your child will avoid an unnecessary operation. If you are concerned about frequent sore throats, your best bet is to consult a primary care physician, not a surgeon. Pediatricians, in particular, seem to take great care to avoid unnecessary tonsillectomies.

HYSTERECTOMY

The incidence of this procedure has increased so rapidly that a number of studies have been done to determine just how often it is really indicated. Diana Scully, in her book *Men Who Control Women's Health,* writes that "A recent study of a second-surgical-opinion program in New York found that 43% of 384 recommended elective hysterectomies . . . were not confirmed in a second opinion."[7]

Since hysterectomy is major surgery, involving a week in the hospital, bills of $5,000 or more, major short-term risks and long-term effects, we think women need to explore every possible medical alternative before resorting to surgery. Although there are a few clear indications, such as cancer of the lining of the uterus or heavy bleeding and pain caused by large fibroid tumors, hysterectomies are too often recommended for reasons that are either vague or unsound. Close to three quarters of a million women had hysterectomies in 1975; at the present rate of increase, eventually more than one out of every two women could expect to have her uterus removed by age 65!

A number of theories have been advanced for the popularity this operation enjoys with its advocates, ranging from the historical male perception of the uterus as the seat of all female complaints to the present oversupply of surgeons. There are gynecologists who take a very conservative approach, but many others still seem to act as if the mere presence of a uterus were indication enough for a hysterectomy. ("When in doubt, take it out," a phrase all OBGYN residents are familiar with, sums up what has been a fairly typical attitude.) In the same study discussed above, the state with the highest rate of hysterectomy did the procedure seventy (!!) times as often as the state with the lowest rate.[8]

If a hysterectomy is recommended to you, proceed with caution and get more than one opinion. Here are some questions to ask:

1. Is there a medical treatment for this problem?
2. Can I try the medical treatment before resorting to surgery?
3. What is my diagnosis?
4. (If the diagnosis is "precancerous condition") What percentage of women with this condition actually develop cancer?
5. (If fibroids) How large are they, and can they be watched?

Prevention of cancer of the cervix and of the endometrium (the lining of the uterus)—two relatively common forms of cancer—is advanced as reason enough to remove a uterus. But both of these diseases can be diagnosed fairly easily and treated successfully. Cancer of the cervix develops slowly; regular Pap smears (every couple of years) will reveal changes in the cells before they become malignant. Should treatment be necessary, there are far simpler and safer ones than hysterectomy.

Endometrial cancer, which is a danger largely to postmenopausal women, can generally be diagnosed by an endometrial biopsy done on any such woman with vaginal bleeding. If the biopsy shows the presence of cancer, then a hysterectomy would be indicated.

In the past, when contraception was less reliable, and when abortion was illegal, hysterectomies were commonly done on women with vague complaints who really wanted to be sure they would not get pregnant again. This approach was never sound medically but was at least understandable, given the abortion laws. Now it is indefensible.

When gynecologists discover that a patient has fibroid tumors (benign growths in the uterus), they often recommend a hysterectomy; however, the mere presence of fibroids does not justify an operation. First of all, these tumors shrink after menopause and often disappear. If they are not causing undue pain and bleeding, your doctor can observe them to make sure that they are not growing and causing problems. Women with fibroids who wish to have children may need a procedure called a myomectomy in which the fibroids are removed but the uterus left in place.

Many gynecologists see no reason why a woman would want her uterus once she has completed child-bearing; after all, she doesn't "need" it any more. Older women are often advised to have surgery rather than medical treatment because of this underlying assumption.

Depending on the problem, a woman might very well decide that her situation warranted a hysterectomy, but all too often, she is unaware of the bias of her doctor, who presents information in such a way that surgery seems the only choice.

Oophorectomy (Removal of the Ovaries)

Whenever a hysterectomy is performed, the question of what to do about the ovaries arises. Should they be left in, or should they be removed in order to prevent ovarian cancer, a disease that is very difficult to treat and has a high mortality rate.

The question is worth asking, but too often the only person who answers it is the surgeon. Removing the nonfunctioning ovaries of a postmenopausal woman is far different from talking a woman in her late thirties or early forties into having her ovaries removed. An oophorectomy at this age will cause a "surgical menopause," which is often far more abrupt and difficult than normal menopause.

In theory, any symptoms can be effectively treated with estrogen but in practice, the synthetic stuff just doesn't do what the natural hormones do. Again, a second opinion would probably be a good idea. Many highly regarded gynecologists favor the oophorectomy because of the difficulty they have encountered treating cancer of the ovaries, but you should hear both sides of the question before choosing.

OTHER PROCEDURES TO BE ESPECIALLY WARY OF

Radical Mastectomy
Just a few years ago, almost every woman with breast cancer had a radical mastectomy, a very extensive operation with serious postoperative problems. Now the most extensive procedure, except for very unusual cases, is a modified radical mastectomy, a much less mutilating procedure, which leaves the chest muscles in place. Even this procedure is being questioned as more and more women are choosing to have a simple mastectomy (removal of breast only) or a lumpectomy (removal of tumor).

Coronary Bypass
This is the current hot procedure. Hardly a day goes by—or so it seems—when the newspaper does not contain an account of some notable who is resting comfortably after double or triple or quadruple bypass surgery.

Many thoughtful and conservative physicians, however, are troubled by this situation; what is not clear to them is the extent to which the risks of this operation outweigh the benefits, when compared with "medical management" or less invasive procedures. The studies that have come out so far suggest that only certain selected cases are best treated with bypass surgery.

Dilation and Curettage of the Uterus
This procedure can be done as a means of diagnosing the cause of abnormal bleeding or as a way of treating it. Although the procedure is considered minor surgery, all surgery has its risks. In many cases, watching and waiting, or hormonal treatment, can resolve a problem.

Elective Orthopedic Surgery
Consider such surgery carefully. Orthopedists like to "fix things." They are the carpenters of the medical profession. What you must ask them is what will happen after surgery. Will the joint that looks or feels funny but works for you now be significantly better, or are there possible consequences of the repair you would rather not live with? Will the problem stay fixed or will it possibly require further surgery?

Be sure to get another opinion before you have an operation to fix something that you could live with if you had to. And find out whether there are alternative treatments, such as manipulation, physical therapy, or exercise. Back problems in particular will often respond well to conservative treatment, poorly to surgery; neurosurgeons tend to be more skillful and conservative in handling these than orthopedists.

Cholecystectomy (Removal of the Gallbladder)
Here is another controversial procedure. This is a major operation requiring up to a week in a hospital. Many people clearly need it to save their lives or spare them great pain. But there are others, with only x-ray evidence of the presence of a gallstone, who are told they must have their gallbladders removed. To avoid an unneeded operation, our recommendation as usual is: first, be evaluated by a primary care doctor.

If you are having recurrent pains and other digestive ills and have x-ray findings that show a significant problem with your gallbladder, your primary care doctor will refer you to the right surgeon. But the simple presence of a gallstone, or some occasional indigestion, is not worth the risk of major surgery.

If you are told you need a procedure that appears on the following list, we hope that a blinking red light will flash in your mind's eye, that you will ask a lot of questions, and that you will get a consultation or a second opinion.

PROCEDURES THAT ARE OVERPERFORMED

Tonsillectomy
Hysterectomy
Oophorectomy (removal of ovaries)
Elective Cholecystectomy (gallbladder removal for asymptomatic gallstones)
Elective Orthopedic surgery
Coronary Bypass surgery
Radical Mastectomy
Dilation and Curettage (scraping out of uterine lining)
Cesarean Section (discussed in Chapter Nine)

OUT-PATIENT SURGERY

Must you go to the hospital for surgery? Several years ago, the American College of Surgeons gave its blessing to ambulatory surgery by declaring that "where feasible, surgeons should consider out-patient, or office, surgery as an alternative to operations in the hospital."[9] (The term ambulatory surgery means that rather than remaining in the hospital, you will be able to walk out the door of the facility and go home.)

The first financially successful free-standing facility, the Surgicenter, was established in Phoenix by Dr. John Ford and Dr. Wallace Reed in 1970. The idea has spread, and there are now more than 100 free-standing facilities. In the meantime, hospitals, not wishing to lose out on business, have established their own ambulatory surgery centers; a survey done by the American Hospital Association in 1980 found that 70 percent of the 2,000 hospitals questioned were offering out-patient surgery.[10]

In all likelihood, this option will be available in your community, and according to a recent article in *The New England Journal of Medicine,*[11] there are seventy-five surgical procedures that can be done on an out-patient basis. Nowadays, most health insurance plans are smart enough to pay for out-patient surgery since it saves them substantial amounts of money; some companies even pay additional sums to surgeons who operate in their own offices to cover the extra supplies that are needed.

Many subspecialists, plastic surgeons and hand surgeons in particular, have well-equipped small operating rooms in their offices. Check your insurance policy to make sure it covers an office procedure.

Your surgeon may or may not be a fan of the ambulatory approach. Breast cysts, for example, can be removed either in a hospital or in an out-patient surgery center. A recent study[12] showed that in one state only twenty-two percent of excisions of breast cysts were performed in the hospital, while in another state, eighty-two percent were done there. The gap between these figures is indicative of the difference in physicians' attitudes. Some surgeons only feel comfortable working in a hospital. If your surgeon will not consider out-patient surgery, you will have to decide whether to give up the doctor or give up the ambulatory surgery.

If you really want out-patient surgery, ask yourself:

1. Will my insurance cover it?
2. Can I save a significant amount of money?
3. Do I have a responsible adult to help me when I return home?
4. How do I feel about hospitals? Would I feel more anxious in a hospital or does the idea of going home after surgery somehow frighten me?

If your insurance does not cover out-patient surgery, you will be stuck with a large bill to pay, which makes the hospital a better choice. If you have no insurance, ambulatory surgery will save you hundreds of dollars.

In choosing ambulatory surgery, you should also consider how much care you will need after your operation. If you live alone, you might explore the possibility of having a home health aide or visiting nurse. Your doctor would be able to recommend a service that would provide someone suitable. Because health insurance most often does not cover this, you will have to decide whether you can afford the expense.

Many people find entering a hospital an anxiety-producing experience and would prefer recuperating at home in familiar surroundings. Recovery is sometimes faster, because being up and about as soon as possible can prevent complications and speed healing. In addition, you avoid some risks, such as hospital-acquired infection, which we will discuss in the next chapter.

HOW DO YOU KNOW THAT
AMBULATORY SURGERY IS SAFE?

If you trust your surgeon to operate on you, you can trust his or her recommendation to have your surgery on an out-patient basis. A good surgeon is not going to take any risks, especially in these litigious times. The opposite may not be true. Some doctors, generally those not trained as recently, are still nervous about this approach. Others may not have "operating privileges" at an ambulatory facility.

WHAT KIND OF HOSPITAL DO YOU NEED FOR SURGERY?

Generally the choice is between a medium-sized community hospital, a larger hospital involved in the training of physicians, and a major medical center. There are community hospitals that give excellent care, and there are major medical centers that are badly overrated. If you have chosen a skillful and conscientious surgeon, you can safely rely on his or her judgment. For major surgery, avoid small proprietary hospitals. Only unethical or self-deceiving surgeons would ever recommend them—possibly because they have a financial interest in such a place or cannot get privileges at larger institutions.

If you are choosing between a moderate-sized hospital (150–300 beds) that is a training site for physicians and has a good reputation in the community, and a major medical center, you might focus on the quality of the nursing care. Community hospitals commonly show much more concern for your needs as a patient, without sacrificing anything on the technical side. Often, good surgeons who have privileges at both types of institution prefer to operate at the kind of community hospital we have described. They will be the first to recommend the medical center if they think you need it.

Major medical centers, almost inevitably, give less personalized care. The world-renowned surgeon who operates there is apt to delegate much of your pre-op and post-op care to a Fellow, leaving you to rely on the ministrations of a less experienced physician—not quite your image of the super-expertise you had hoped to find.

In the next chapter, we are going to discuss the types and qualities of hospitals much more thoroughly. As you begin to read it, you will see that we have a consistent point of view. In this chapter we began by encouraging you to avoid unneeded surgery. Next, we plan to help you spend as little time as possible in the hospital.

CHAPTER FIVE

HOW TO
PLAY HOSPITAL

We might well have called the first part of this chapter "How Not to Go to the Hospital." Often people who would actually prefer to stay home assume that a given operation or illness requires a hospital admission. We will discuss alternatives to hospital care and the advantages of staying out of the hospital whenever possible.

Nevertheless, at some point in the course of a lifetime, most of us will have to spend some time in a hospital, hence the title. Although the experience will not seem like a game, a certain amount of gamesmanship is required when dealing with the cast of characters and rules you will encounter.

Our advice: read this chapter while you're hale and hearty, or at least before you enter the hospital doors. Our aim is to give you enough general information, plus some specific strategies, so that you can influence the quality of care you receive, the cost of your treatment, the length of your hospital stay, and the way you feel about what is happening to you.

Hospitals are confusing and confused institutions with goals that are sometimes incompatible. You, the patient, quite reasonably assume that hospitals are there to take care of you when you're sick. And they did start out with that purpose; however, something seems to have happened along the way.

HOW THEY BEGAN

First of all, we are talking about a very ancient institution. When religion and medicine were part of the same endeavor, the place of worship was also a shelter for the sick. In the Egypt of the Pharaohs, people brought their medical problems to the temples to be cured by doctor-priests. In the Middle Ages, hospitals were shelters for the aged, the destitute, and the homeless, as well as places for the care of those who were seriously ill. They were founded and run by religious orders whose members viewed nursing the sick as God's work. These early hospitals were well run and clean by the standards of the day. Kings and dukes and philanthropists all founded hospitals—again as charitable institutions. But as the seventeenth century rolled in, orderliness gave way to unbelievable squalor, and hospitals throughout Europe so deteriorated that, while they did identify a social need, they often filled it to the great detriment of their clientele:

> "The ward of St. Joseph's is reserved for pregnant women; honest or vicious, healthy and unhealthy, they are all together. Three or four women in this state lie in the same bed, exposed to insomnia, to contagion [from] their diseased neighbors, to the risk of injuring their children."—Jacques Tenon quoted in *The House of Healing*[1] by Mary Risley

WHO IS THE HOSPITAL DESIGNED FOR?

Nowadays you won't have to share a bed; you'll lie on clean sheets (until the reforms of the late nineteenth century, putting clean sheets on the bed for each new patient, let alone changing them for the same occupant, was in many hospitals an unheard of luxury). The people who take care of you will wash their hands and use clean instruments to examine you. The surgeons, who less than two hundred years ago took pride in operating-room coats so stiff with blood they could stand alone, now follow exact and scrupulous scrubbing rituals to prevent infection.

You will not be required to pray or give public thanks to the hospital benefactors for allowing you to be a patient, as did the inmates of certain Victorian institutions. You may, however, have the sense that you ought to behave in a grateful manner, to appreciate the fact that the hospital has managed to find you a bed and supply you with nurses.

Because you are sick and in need of care, it is no wonder that you feel dependent, less in control, anxious. But why do the rules and procedures make you feel like an object, not a person? Is it medically necessary for you to put on pajamas and lie in bed if all you are going to do is have tests? Must you have unnecessary quantities of blood drawn—as Norman Cousins describes in his book *Anatomy of an Illness*[2]—because the hospital cannot coordinate your lab work?

The major and minor indignities of hospital ways are experienced by sick people who are feeling vulnerable and who are least able to shrug off an annoyance or behave assertively.

In one famous hospital in New York City, a tense teen-ager scheduled for knee surgery is kept for hours in a waiting room so crowded that she does not have a chair to sit on, even though the admission is a scheduled one, not an emergency.

In another hospital with a reputation for good patient care, not even a medical degree and admitting privileges can save you from the unthinking routines that have developed. Recently, a staff doctor who became a patient there (he was in the midst of passing a kidney stone) was left sitting in a chair in a corridor for an hour awaiting an x-ray. It was simply more convenient to have people who needed x-rays wait together in the corridor than to make an effort to bring them to the x-ray department when the staff was prepared to do their procedure.

In neither of the two examples above was a patient's life endangered. Nor does it endanger your life to be awakened at six in the morning for a temperature check or roused from a much needed nap to be given a pill. You can survive bad hospital food and odd mealtimes as well as brusque nurses, surly aides, and unidentified young persons in white jackets who appear unannounced at your bedside to give you yet another examination.

But at a time when you need all of your energies to rest and to heal, hospital routines undermine the serene and humane atmosphere they ought to create. When Norman Cousins, who was seriously ill, decided that the hospital was working against his recovery, he signed out, checked into a hotel, engaged full-time nursing help, and began doing active things to restore his health. He was fortunate in having a doctor sympathetic to his needs and plans—and also in making a good recovery. As you may have gathered by now, the authors are less than enthusiastic about hospitals as "houses of healing."

PATIENT CARE DOESN'T ALWAYS COME FIRST

Part of the problem with hospitals, from the patients' point of view, is that patient care is not the highest or the clearest priority. In many ways, doctors are the primary customers; not surprisingly, their needs come first. In fact, the quickest way for a hospital to increase business and attract more patients is to attract more doctors.

Those doctors do not usually focus on what it is like to be a patient in the hospital; they are interested in what it is like to be a doctor there. They want to know what kinds of equipment the hospital has, how easy it is to get a patient scheduled for surgery, what referral specialists are on the staff, and how easy it will be for them to park. Some of these factors are important to you; others not at all.

In some cities, hospitals have an "open staff" arrangement: a doctor who is qualified to be on the staff of one is generally considered qualified to be on the staff of the other hospitals in town. In such a situation, patient preference may carry a lot of weight; the hospitals will compete with each other to attract patients by providing programs and services oriented to consumer needs: outreach wellness programs, birthing rooms, and same-day surgery centers.

In the larger cities, most doctors are on the staff of just one hospital, or two at the most, and patients are generally admitted wherever their doctor has "privileges." The major teaching hospitals compete with each other not so much for patients as for medical prestige: doctors famous for theoretical contributions to medicine, sophisticated new equipment, and specialized departments.

Hospitals must also serve many masters. If they are teaching hospitals, they must satisfy the medical schools with which they are affiliated. There are stringent regulations to follow. The policies governing how hospitals are paid—by Blue Cross, Medicare, and Medicaid—are positively Byzantine, and they can lead to unusual pricing practices, such as the infamous $1.00 aspirin tablet that shows up on many a hospital bill, and odd rules. For example, the hospital may require that everyone admitted have certain blood tests or x-rays regardless of whether they are medically necessary or have been recently performed. These rules carry the day, even while they increase your discomfort and inflate the cost of medical care.

When Jimmy Carter was president and was grappling with the problem of controlling medical costs, he recalled his previous experience as a member of the board of a hospital in Georgia. The board had approved the purchase of a new piece of equipment and had then taken measures to make sure the equipment would be used enough to pay for itself. At that time, he had been looking at the situation from the perspective of the hospital, not the patient. As president, he suddenly saw the problems such a point of view causes.

A hospital is a highly specialized institution that does some things marvelously well—we'd hate to have open-heart surgery anywhere else—and other things not so well. Make sure that your problem needs to be treated in a hospital, and/or that you are the kind of person who will feel more secure there. Some people see it as a safe haven; others have learned to give themselves intravenous injections in order to stay home.

Think about your own needs and attitudes first, and then discuss the possibilities with your doctor. What follows may help you avoid an unnecessary hospitalization or some of the very real dangers of a too lengthy stay.

WHY HOSPITALS ARE THE WORST PLACES TO BE IF YOU'RE NOT REALLY SICK

1. The longer you are in a hospital the more chances for error. Medications really are given to the wrong patient; people do fall out of hospital beds and fracture skulls (the beds are kept high for the conve-

nience of the doctors and nurses). You may be sent to the x-ray department for an invasive and potentially hazardous procedure that was ordered for someone else.

2. The longer you are in a hospital, the better the chance to develop a nosocomial infection (that is, an infection acquired in the hospital). Because there is such heavy use of antibiotics in hospitals, the microorganisms that flourish there are those that, having become resistant to the most common antibiotics, are often hard to treat and require drugs that can be almost as dangerous as the diseases they fight.

3. Once you are in, it is hard to get out. A little girl is admitted with a high unexplained fever. The fever, it turns out, is caused by a urinary tract infection. Despite the fact that if the diagnosis had been made in the doctor's office, she would not have been admitted, she will now stay in the hospital until there is no fever. Then, if the fever persists a day or two longer than is usual, the doctor may order a test that has as a side effect a rare but dangerous allergic reaction. Had the child been home, an extra day of fever might not have seemed so remarkable nor would it have been so simple to order a test.

4. Being a patient in a hospital is an infantalizing experience. You must take off your own clothes, put on a hospital gown that makes you feel exposed and vulnerable, have your food brought to you on someone else's schedule, get permission to use the bathroom, perhaps. Although some of the hospital rules are clearly necessary for your own health and comfort (if you had visitors until 4 A.M., it would be poor security, disturbing to your roommate, and maybe even to you), many others are convenient for the hospital but bad for you. They make you feel powerless at exactly the time you may well need to feel more in control.

5. Finally, being a hospital patient may make you think and feel that you are sicker than you are. If you are being treated at home, it may seem to you that your disease is not so serious after all—otherwise you would have to be in a hospital! This is particularly true of children with chronic diseases. Minimizing their hospital stays may help them to feel less different from other children.

Far too often, the length of time you spend in the hospital is determined by local medical custom, rather than by carefully documented studies. One organization has compared hospital stays in different parts of the country and found dramatic differences.

The Commission on Professional and Hospital Activities has identified a group of hospitals from different regions to participate in their Professional Activity Study (PAS); the results of this study are analyzed and published in a series of books. (See Resource Directory for details.) The commission has found, for example, that the average length of stay for a routine delivery is four days in the Northeast but only two days in the Northwest. The average length of stay for a hysterectomy in the Northeast is seven days, whereas in the West it is five days. In the Northeast, the average length of stay for a mastectomy is over a week, but in the West, ten percent of patients are discharged in two days.

Unless you have a particularly complicated medical problem, there is no increased risk to your health with the minimum length of stay. Indeed, by decreasing the risk of hospital-acquired infection, such a decision may improve your health.

WAYS TO SHORTEN A HOSPITAL STAY

Some caution is in order before you enthusiastically push for a shorter length of stay. First, study your health insurance policy. It may only cover certain types of care or procedures in full, or at all, if they take place in the hospital. If you would like to be discharged much sooner than the average person with your problem, you or your physician could discuss the situation with your insurance agent or benefits officer. If your shorter stay could save the insurance company a substantial amount of money, they might be willing to work out a special arrangement with you to cover out-patient tests and home nursing, for example.

Discuss your desire to spend as little time as possible in the hospital. Ask what is the minimum time that is medically necessary. If you need to convince your doctor that a shorter length of stay is feasible, call the Utilization Review Department of the hospital to get the PAS average length of stay for your condition, and discuss this information with your doctor.

Elective Surgery

Most elective admissions (hospital admissions that are planned ahead of time as opposed to emergency admissions) are for surgery; commonly patients are admitted one day ahead for tests and a general physical.

In many hospitals, arrangements can be made for the tests and physical exam to be done ahead of time and for you to be admitted the day of surgery. If you are told that it is against hospital policy, you are certainly free to question that policy. (The patient representative mentioned later in this chapter may be helpful here.)

Remember that hospitals vary in rules and procedures. If another hospital would be equally satisfactory and your doctor has privileges there, you might inquire whether it has a more flexible policy.

If you are having major surgery under general anesthesia, you should probably expect to stay overnight; but you may well be ready to go home the next day. Much will depend on how well you feel at that point and what your home situation is. If you can walk well enough to use the bathroom and if you have a responsible live-in adult at home, you are in a position to question your doctor about discharge. Be sure to raise this as a possibility before surgery.

There are some sound reasons to keep people in the hospital after an operation. For example, they may be unable to eat and require intravenous (I.V.) feeding or they may need intravenous or intramuscular (I.M.) medication. Here a skilled technician and careful observation is necessary.

There are other reasons that are quite common but perhaps not so sound, such as the need for frequent temperature or blood pressure checks, for more tests to be done, or for sutures to be removed. If you have a capable person at home, you can have him or her check temperatures or learn to do blood pressures. If your insurance policy covers out-patient testing in full, you can probably wait until after you are discharged to have further tests. These can be done by your primary care physician. Depending on the type of surgery, you may be able to arrange to have sutures taken out in the surgeon's office at the proper time.

If you are going to have surgery, the type of anesthesia used may affect your length of stay. Because general anesthesia tends to keep you in the hospital longer, you may wish to discuss the possibility of local anesthesia.

Some operations—those needing total muscle relaxation—must be done under general anesthesia, but many others commonly done under general can be done under local: most hernia repairs, for example. If you have a choice of anesthesia, you need to consider whether or not it will upset you to be awake and hear the surgeon discussing your operation with the assistants. Some people don't mind; others are made tense and fearful. (See Chapter Four for a discussion of anesthesia.)

Medical Admissions
A medical problem that is both a common cause of admission and a good candidate for early discharge is a heart attack (myocardial infarction). Until recently, it was common practice to keep people who had suffered heart attacks in the hospital for two weeks or more, but some interesting studies have made this lengthy a hospitalization questionable. For the patient who is in stable condition with no additional significant risk factors (arrhythmias, heart failure), recent studies indicate that there is little evidence that an extended stay is beneficial.

One study done at Duke University Medical Center[3] concluded that patients who were discharged after one week, with someone to take care of them at home, did as well as those hospitalized for nine to thirteen days. A study in England[4] showed that selected patients with heart attacks actually had a higher rate of survival if cared for at home from the beginning, instead of spending any time in the hospital.

We are certainly not suggesting you refuse admission for a heart attack. But if a lengthy hospital stay, once you are in stable condition, may not be as necessary or as helpful as was once assumed, it should not be surprising that many less serious illnesses may require no hospital admission.

STAYING OUT OF THE HOSPITAL

For many people, a brief stay is better than no stay at all. It may take a lot of energy to convince a traditional doctor that you'd be better off at home. And you must convince not only the doctor but also the insurance company. Most policies do not cover the costs of hiring visiting nurses, nor do they pay for other types of home help. The way our insurance policies are written not only limits our choices but also perpetuates the inefficient use of medical resources and increases the costs of care. If we had a well-planned and efficient system, we would reserve hospitals for what they do best: taking care of the seriously ill.

We expect that changes will occur because of the enormous and still-rising costs of hospital care. Nevertheless, if you want to avoid a hospital stay, you don't have to wait for a medical revolution. Here are some areas where you do have choices:

1. Surgery—Many procedures can now be performed in a doctor's office or in an ambulatory surgery center.
2. Tests—The reasons you're admitted for a work-up have to do with convenience and reimbursement. Tests can be done on an out-patient basis if you want.
3. Treatment—Many kinds of medical care can be given at home instead of in the hospital. (Of course, there has to be someone at home to help.)
4. Care of the dying—The hospice movement emphasizes home care (see Resource Directory).

Out-patient Surgery
(This topic is discussed at length in Chapter Four.)

Many types of surgical procedures can now be done outside of the hospital. In some instances, what was once a major operation has evolved into something much simpler. For example, patients with recurrent hemorrhoid problems used to spend up to a week in the hospital recuperating from a relatively major and very uncomfortable operation. Now, they can go to the surgeon's office for a "banding" procedure, and then walk home.

If the procedure you need cannot be performed in the surgeon's office, one alternative is a free-standing ambulatory surgery center, which means a facility that is not part of a hospital (free-standing) and which you will be able to walk out of (ambulatory) once the procedure is completed. Another is a hospital "day surgery" unit. Almost all cities will have one or both types of facilities.

Both types of units can provide well-equipped operating rooms, highly qualified support staff—such as nurse-anesthetists and anesthesiologists—and comfortable areas for post-op observation. A growing list of procedures can be done in an out-patient unit. The list includes gynecological procedures such as pregnancy terminations, D & Cs, tubal ligations; ENT procedures such as myringotomies or adenoidectomies; hernia repairs, at least in young children; varicose vein strippings; removal of pilonidal cysts; cosmetic surgery; operative arthroscopies; and bunion surgery.

Your best guide to the quality of one of these facilities is the reputation of the doctors who use it. If you are satisfied that the surgeon you have chosen is competent, you can assume that the facility is a good one.

Before deciding to go ahead with out-patient surgery, check your insurance policy to make sure you are covered. Insurance companies are beginning to realize that it is in their interest as well as yours to cover such out-patient surgery.

If you are in doubt after you read your policy, talk to the head of your benefits department at work. If you have an individual insurance policy, get in touch with your broker or call the company directly and ask for a benefits specialist. You or your physician may be able to convince the company to cover your procedure on an out-patient basis, since it will save them money.

If you prefer out-patient surgery, make sure that you choose a surgeon who can operate at an ambulatory surgical facility. You might ask your primary care physician to recommend such a surgeon. (Whether you need surgery at all is a different issue, which we discuss in Chapter Four.)

Out-Patient Tests and Treatment

Most health insurance policies will not pay for purely diagnostic procedures, in or out of the hospital. To help out patients, a doctor may shave the truth and admit them, listing the symptom for which the tests are being done as the reason for the admission. Actually, there is rarely any medical reason to hospitalize someone for tests—just about any test can be done on an ambulatory basis or, at worst, in a·special "short stay" unit of a hospital.

Keeping Children at Home

What is the best place for a child with a temperature of 104° F who needs medication every few hours, frequent temperature checks, and a humidified room? Many doctors favor the hospital, feeling it is a good safe place for people to be. Knowing that a sick patient is getting professional care sets the medical mind at ease, and since your doctor feels comfortable and safe in a hospital, he or she assumes you will too.

A doctor may, in an effort to make things easier for the parents, admit a child who could conceivably be cared for at home. If the thought of a hospital terrifies your child and if you are prepared to handle all the problems of home care, by all means ask if this is possible. Of course, many parents may not have the option of staying home to nurse a sick child.

Sometimes very creative solutions are available. One group of pediatricians became increasingly concerned by the large number of newborns being kept in the hospital for several days for treatment of jaundice. The one thing the hospital had that the home didn't was a piece of equipment called a bili-lite. The pediatricians devised a portable light system that parents could use at home and then convinced insurance companies to cover the cost.

Avoiding Admissions for Chronic Disease

Most of us can manage to survive a hospitalization in pretty good spirits, if the problem is cured. But if we have a chronic disease that requires a number of admissions, a return to the hospital may seem like a defeat. It is more important that people like this—children and teenagers in particular—stay out of the hospital if at all possible. Otherwise, their lives become centered on the hospital instead of on the home, or on work, or on school.

If home nursing care of some kind is needed but is not covered by your insurance, there may be a charitable agency that can provide it. For further help, there are support groups for people with serious chronic problems such as hemophilia, colostomies, or muscular dystrophy, and these groups may be helpful in pointing out the possibilities for home- and self-care.

Avoiding Admission for Someone Who Is Dying

Hospitals, which are dedicated to giving treatment and saving lives, are not places to die a peaceful death. If you or someone close to you is dying, you may want to explore the possibility of home-care, using private duty nurses when necessary. The hospice movement, which is just getting started in this country, is dedicated to helping people who are dying to be cared for at home or in a special facility designed to enhance the quality of life and prevent pain.

To find out if there is a hospice program or facility in your area, you can ask your doctor or a medical social worker at your hospital. Medicare now provides coverage for hospice care, as do many other health insurance policies.

IF YOU MUST ENTER A HOSPITAL
WHAT KIND DO YOU NEED?

The famous teaching hospital has a roster of brilliant researchers and is equipped with the latest technology, but how pleasant a place is it for its patients?

What about the brand new spiffy-looking hospital just opened by a group of doctors? It looks bright and modern and expensive. Is it adequately staffed?

If you live in a sparsely populated area or small town, there may be only one small local hospital. Is it good enough or will you be better off traveling to a larger, better-equipped, or more famous hospital even though you must leave family and friends behind?

Before you can decide whether a particular hospital is the right one for you, you must first know whether it is a teaching hospital, a community hospital, or a proprietary hospital, and what those terms mean.

A *teaching hospital* is involved with the training of doctors. If it is a *university hospital,* it will be a primary training site for a medical school and very closely identified with it. All the physicians on the staff of the hospital will also be on the faculty of the medical school. A university hospital is a good place for a patient with a problem that is very difficult to diagnose or treat. It will be staffed with superspecialists and have the latest diagnostic equipment.

A *university affiliate* is also a teaching hospital. Generally, physicians with privileges at a university affiliate will have faculty appointments at the medical school. Community, municipal, county, or veterans' hospitals may also be used to teach students from a given school, thus becoming teaching hospitals. Other hospitals may be sites for training specialists but not for teaching students; that is, they have interns and residents, but not medical students. In general, teaching hospitals are "tertiary care" institutions; that is, they are equipped to deal with the most complex kinds of diseases or surgery.

Community hospitals are designed to handle the usual problems that cause hospitalization. They do not ordinarily have advanced technology (burn units) and highly specialized physicians (pediatric neurologists). Sometimes referred to as "voluntary hospitals," these are not-for-profit institutions that are supported partly by contributions. Many community hospitals are also teaching hospitals, with interns and residents who receive part or all of their training there, usually in fields like family medicine, where the emphasis is primarily on diagnosis and management of the more common problems.

There may be some overlap among these types. In Manhattan, there are 700-bed community hospitals that in less populous places would be considered the main referral centers, attracting patients from hundreds of miles around. In a skiing area, a small hospital may have a fully-equipped orthopedics wing.

Proprietary hospitals are for-profit operations; they may be owned by an individual, by a group of doctors, or by a corporation. In some cities—New York is one example—public policy is such that no proprietary hospital can really compete with the university and voluntary hospitals and they have never taken hold. In other places, proprietary hospitals have flourished.

WHICH TYPE DO YOU CHOOSE?

You can get excellent care or terrible care at any kind of hospital, but there are a few useful generalizations that may help you identify the right place for the right problem.

The first thing to look for is the round-the-clock presence of doctors. One problem with a small community or proprietary hospital that has no teaching program is that there are no interns and residents to give continuous medical supervision. Some of these small hospitals do not even have a "house doctor" present at all times. Unless it has a reputation for unusually good critical nursing care, this kind of hospital should be avoided for any problem greater than elective surgery requiring only a brief stay.

If you have a "fascinoma" (a disease so unusual as to have physicians everywhere fascinated), you may well need the superspecialists of a major university hospital. If you have a more common problem, you may find the care is just as good and probably far more personalized in a reputable community institution. It won't be so large you get lost in the shuffle or so small that there is no review of your doctor's work. This advice runs counter to the impression you get from reading one of those lists of the best hospitals in the country, which are always composed of university hospitals.

Accreditation

Most hospitals are accredited on a regular basis by the Joint Commission on the Accreditation of Hospitals. Although the inspectors make real efforts to evaluate the quality of care provided by the hospital, they can only be sure of those facts that can be readily documented: e.g., whether the hospitals have written emergency procedures, corridors wide enough for stretchers, and x-ray machines that do not leak radiation. Thus accreditation inevitably becomes a minimum standard; there is no guarantee that you will get good care at an accredited hospital, but you must avoid a hospital that is not accredited.

CHOOSING THE HOSPITAL TO MATCH THE PROBLEM

TYPE OF PROBLEM	TYPE OF HOSPITAL	REASON FOR ADMISSION
Minor	Day Surgery Unit or any accredited hospital	Biopsies, cataract removal, D & C, minor hand or foot surgery, minor cosmetic surgery, pregnancy termination, tubal ligation
Routine	Well-regarded community or good proprietary hospital of any size	*Surgery for which the rate of post-op complications is low*: appendectomy, hernia repair, pacemaker insertion, thyroid surgery, vaginal hysterectomy, simple mastectomy
		Medical admission for control of diabetes, intravenous treatment of infection, uncomplicated heart attack, stroke
	Note: For both minor and routine surgical problems above, the skill of the surgeon is more important than the hospital	
Major surgery or serious medical problem	University-affiliated or well-equipped community teaching hospital with good reputation	*Surgical procedures with significant risk of post-op complications, or for which expert assistance is needed:* for example, all major abdominal operations (stomach, gall bladder, colon, abdominal hysterectomy), modified radical mastectomy, radical head and neck surgery, peripheral vascular surgery, lung surgery
		Serious medical problem such as complicated heart attack, diabetic coma, severe asthma, severe dehydration in infant, meningitis, initial course of chemotherapy
Very complex surgical or medical problem	University hospital or large community teaching hospital: consider traveling to find suitable hospital	*Extremely complex or unusual surgery, for which special equipment or surgical team is needed:* cardiovascular surgery, including coronary bypass surgery, brain surgery, spinal cord surgery, kidney transplants, severe burns
		Medical problems that are unusually difficult to diagnose or treat (usually multisystem diseases)

IF YOU HAVE A COMPLEX PROBLEM

The most critical decision would be which hospital to use if you have a very complex medical or surgical problem. (Examples are listed in the lower right hand corner of the chart on p. 95.) In this situation, your primary care physician may not always be your most reliable guide.

Although it is unlikely, we can't discount the possibility that your physician would feel compelled to recommend his/her own hospital, since the surgeons that work there are in the same referral network. One reason this is unlikely is that the direction of referrals is generally from primary care physicians to surgeons, rarely the other way.

What is more likely is that your physician is proud of the hospital and its many successes and feels that his or her familiarity with the staff will ensure you the best possible treatment. In truth, that inside knowledge is indeed important.

For serious problems the technological capability of the hospital and the credentials and experience of its staff are critically important. (See the Resource Directory for information on finding hospitals.)

Listen with an open mind if a doctor whom you respect feels you will get the best care in your own home town. One case we heard about not long ago concerned a child with a rare bone disease whose parents insisted on driving her to a medical center in Brooklyn, three hours from their home. When they got there, the famous specialist examined the little girl and then informed the parents that, in fact, the outstanding specialist in the country in that particular field was on the staff of one of their local hospitals.

If you have doubts, raise them. Your doctor should be able to give you specific reasons to support his or her recommendation. If you had been one of the parents we mentioned above, you might have been impressed had your doctor told you that the leading authority on your child's disease was on the staff of a local hospital, offered to show you journal articles, and cited that doctor's credentials.

In other situations, we have suggested you make allowances if your doctor seems defensive, but in this case you must absolutely insist that your questions be answered with facts and figures. You may want to know . . .

- the credentials of the specialist who will be handling your case (college, medical school, hospital training program and board status)
- the morbidity and mortality statistics for your problem when treated at the hospital your doctor is proposing
- what hospital has the best success rate for treating your problem, and how that rate compares to your local hospital (The best center may attract so many desperately ill patients that the success rate is lower than a lesser hospital. Centers that publish high mortality

rates are probably much better than hospitals that do not publicize their results at all.)

· whether there is a newer or better technique for treating your problem available in one of the top medical centers (places like the Cleveland Clinic, the Mayo Clinic, Massachusetts General Hospital, or Memorial Sloan-Kettering).

If your doctor does not know, he or she should be willing to find out for you. If your doctor does not seem forthright or helpful in response to these questions, you need to do further research. You can either find another doctor who will get you some answers or you can ask your present doctor to arrange for you to have a consultation at a nationally famous clinic or medical center.

An excellent discussion of how a physician made such a decision when he himself became a patient can be found in William Nolen's *Surgeon Under the Knife.*

HOW WILL THE EXPERIENCE AFFECT YOU?

Hospitalization is a traumatic experience for almost everyone. You enter a hospital, fearing or knowing that something is very wrong, and you must then hand over control of your body and destiny to others. In the impersonal and antiseptic environment of the hospital, where the staff tends to treat patients like children, it may be difficult to be one's normal adult self.

We know that people experience a kind of contraction of their world when they become sick. Attention and energy are focused on the body and its problems. Not only is it difficult to behave as a responsible mature adult, it may also be all but impossible to perceive the world in your usual adult way.

Eric Cassel, a physician interested in the ethical and philosophical problems of healing, recounts an experiment he made on a very sick patient who had been experiencing hallucinations after surgery.

> *I decided to duplicate a famous experiment conceived by the noted French psychologist Jean Piaget. I took two transparent specimen cups and a tall, thin test tube from the sink; filled the test tube with water; emptied it into one of the short, squat cups; and repeated the procedure with the other cup. Both cups now had the same amount of water, and the test tube was empty. I returned to the bedside and showed the cups to the patient. "Edgar," I said, "these two cups contain the same amount of water." When he acknowledged that, I told him to watch as I poured the contents of one of the cups into the test tube. Pointing to the filled test tube and the remaining cup of water, I asked, "Edgar, which one has more water?" To my astonishment, he*

pointed to the test tube. My middle-aged patient's response to this classic test of reasoning on the conservation of volume was the same as that of a child under six.[5]

Many of the problems you encounter will not be strictly medical. You may need either privacy or companionship, financial advice, emotional support, information. You may dislike the food or need a television set exchanged or adjusted. Following is a list of what you can do and the people who can help you cope with the extramedical side of your hospital stay.

1.   Think about whether you would prefer a private or a semiprivate room. Find out what the additional cost would be. Depending on the hospital and your coverage, the additional cost may be minimal.
2.   If you're not in intensive care, a private duty nurse can give you the kind of attention that may make you feel more comfortable and more secure. This service is expensive but in some cases may be well worth it, for example, for the first night or two after major surgery.
3.   Appoint a friend or relative to be your personal advocate. He or she can then go to bat for you if you are not getting what you need.
4.   If you are not happy with the food, ask to speak to the dietician. If you are not on a restricted diet, the hospital kitchen can probably give you substitutions for food items you don't like.
5.   Bring some small item from home—an old bathrobe you're fond of, a picture of someone you love—to provide a spot of familiarity in the impersonal hospital environment.
6.   Call the hospital Social Service Department for help with a number of problems. Hospital-based social workers are familiar with insurance reimbursements, follow-up or home-care, long-term rehabilitation, and nursing homes, as well as the kinds of family problems that can occur when people are sick.
7.   Pastoral counselors are another source of help. You need not be religious to use their services. They can be an alternative to the patient representative (discussed later on p. 113) and can also help you cope with problems you may be experiencing as a result of illness. Call the hospital chaplain's office or the Social Service Department to find one.

GETTING INTO A HOSPITAL

You've planned to have your hernia repaired at a hospital with a reputation for good nursing care. You choose the date of your admission carefully so that it won't conflict with birthdays, business trips, or your anniversary. You prepare yourself mentally for what lies ahead, and then the phone rings. It is the surgeon's office calling. "Sorry, we'll have to reschedule that surgery. The hospital doesn't have a bed."

Because the supply of hospital beds is limited and hospitals must reserve some for critical emergencies, you may find yourself either having to reschedule an admission or, if you or your problem cannot wait, going to a hospital that is not your first choice. If you must be sent to an institution where your doctor does not have admitting privileges, you will need a referral to another doctor for your hospital care.

Hospitals categorize admissions into three groups:

I. Emergency

Bleeding ulcers, heart attacks, diabetic coma, auto accidents—problems like these require immediate hospital care. Hospitals reserve a few beds especially for such cases.

If you come into an Emergency Room with a problem like this, you will be admitted or, if there are no beds, transferred to another hospital.

Note: If your doctor calls from the office to inform the hospital that you need to be admitted on an emergency basis, you may first have to go to the ER for an evaluation by the hospital staff.

II. Urgent

Problems like serious cardiac disease requiring catheterization or surgery, diabetes that is out of control, a chronic condition that has deteriorated.

You will be "on call" and must be prepared to present yourself for admission within a few hours of being notified that a bed is available.

Note: If you are awaiting hospitalization and realize that you are feeling very sick, let your doctor know. He or she may have you moved to the top of the list or arrange to have you admitted to another hospital that has a bed.

III. Elective

Most of the problems in this category are surgical procedures that can wait a week or more—hysterectomy, hernia repair, knee surgery, gall bladder removal.

You will be given an admission date a week or more ahead of time. Be prepared for a last-minute cancellation if the hospital has had to admit a number of more urgent cases.

USING YOUR PRIMARY CARE DOCTOR TO COORDINATE YOUR HOSPITAL CARE

You go to your family doctor, who refers you to a specialist; the specialist puts you in the hospital and takes over the case. What possible role is there for your regular doctor? We feel very strongly that the sicker or more helpless you are, the more you need a primary care practitioner involved in your care. The following case illustrates what can happen when the problems of a sick patient become subordinate to the demands of the hospital pecking order.

A five-year-old boy hospitalized with leukemia was being treated by an internist who specialized in hematology (diseases of the blood). His parents were quite understandably trying to save money, so they did not involve the child's pediatrician. All did not go well; the boy began to develop side effects from treatment and needed a generalist who could take care of sick children, not just sick blood cells.

The pediatric residents knew this and were doing their best, but they only had authority to care for patients admitted by a pediatrician; the private pediatrician was aware of the problem but felt correctly that she would seem unprofessional if she suggested to the hematologist or the parents that she be involved in the child's care. In the meantime, the child was deteriorating in the midst of all these rules and politics. Shocking, but it could easily happen anywhere.

Your primary care doctor understands how hospitals work and can prevent you from becoming a pawn in some sort of interdisciplinary power struggle. He or she can coordinate your care if you need consultations from more than one specialist and can make sure that you are seeing the right ones and getting the proper treatments on a schedule that suits your needs as well as those of the institution.

If you have the kind of problem that needs several elaborate tests, there may be a day or more between tests while you remain in the hospital, sitting idly in your pajamas, eating unpleasant meals at strange hours, and being exposed to undesirable bacteria. Since each test may have been ordered by a different specialist, no one doctor would be aware of this.

Your primary care doctor would, however, be alert to this confusion and either expedite the tests or discharge you and arrange to have some done as an "out-patient." (That is a doctor's word for you when you are not in a hospital; since lay people think of this as the normal state, you probably never considered having a special word for it.)

If hospital tests show any abnormality, most specialists would be loath to send you home. They will, though, if they know your primary care doctor will follow up on the abnormal test. You may also be spared unnecessary tests. The specialists may find something they believe must be explored, until your own doctor points out that you have already been checked out for that problem and been found normal.

Your primary care doctor can play a crucial role in helping you and family members understand your diagnosis and treatment, especially if you are very ill and have several specialists and/or subspecialists involved in your care.

After you are discharged, taking the prescribed medications, having the right follow-up tests, exercising, eating the proper diet, keeping the necessary appointments are all important to your cure; the more your doctor was involved while you were in the hospital, the better care he or she can give you now.

Finally, if you are dissatisfied with your postoperative care, you don't have a lot of leverage. After all, the surgery is over and done with and you are not apt to be a repeat customer. But if your primary care physician makes a request, you can be sure that the surgeon, who knows where referrals come from, will be responsive.

Children and Hospitals

Some hospitals have no separate children's floor—fine for the teen-ager who would rather be with adults than with young children and perhaps suitable for a school-age child requiring only a brief admission for elective surgery. But for preschool children, or any child needing an extended hospitalization, we recommend a hospital with a children's floor.

Try to find out which local hospital has a particularly cheerful pediatrics section, with a play room, recreational therapists, school teachers, and nurses with a special interest in children. Such an atmosphere tends to lessen anxiety and hasten recovery; a teacher prevents the school-age child from falling behind.

Hospital policies concerning parents "rooming-in" vary greatly. There is now a trend toward having a number of rooms designed to allow parents to stay overnight. Many hospitals without such special facilities are happy to let you stay, but you'll sleep on a cot or a lounging chair. Unfortunately, there are still a few institutions where you will be told it is against hospital policy to let parents stay; we know of one father, in such a situation, who plunked himself down next to his child's hospital bed and recommended that the nurse call the police to have him ousted. Of course he was allowed to stay.

If you would want to stay overnight in the event your child were hospitalized, check the policy of local hospitals now. That way, you will know which to choose in an emergency situation. Of course, if you find yourself in a hospital where you are asked to leave, you, too, can quietly but firmly make it clear you intend to spend the night; it is unlikely the police will be called.

One tip: even a hospital not set up for rooming-in will probably make an exception if you ask for a private room. Your health insurance will not cover the extra costs of such a room—as little as $10 a day or as much as $100—so be sure you can afford it.

WHO'S IN CHARGE HERE?

Remember the very sick patient in Chapter Two who kept asking who was in charge? As the number of specialists, subspecialists and Fellows involved in your care increases, so does the chance for confusion and even serious error.

A patient admitted as a "service case" is cared for by interns and residents who are responsible to the chief resident, who is in turn supervised by an attending physician serving as "attending of the month," and by the department chief. Private patients are the responsibility of the doctor who admits them to the hospital unless he or she turns the case over to someone else.

As we have noted, one of the tremendous advantages to you in having a good primary care physician is the support and information this person can provide if you must be hospitalized. He or she will visit you to see how you are progressing, will interpret tests and explain recommendations to you, and will coordinate the care provided by specialists.

What happens, though, if you do not have a primary care physician who stays actively involved? Suppose your personal physician, a general internist, admits you to the hospital and then calls in a surgeon. "This looks like a perforated ulcer to me," says the surgeon. "We've got to operate immediately." Your personal physician turns your case over to the surgeon for the operation. Here is where the trouble may begin. You develop a medical problem, and your surgeon calls in a subspecialist or two to have a look without letting your personal physician know. The consultants may also decide to call in their consultants.

> Mrs. D. went to see her primary care doctor with an unusually large skin growth. Her doctor felt it should be removed and, realizing it would require a skin graft, referred her to an excellent surgeon at a university hospital at which he himself did not have privileges.
>
> Mrs. D. expected a three- or four-day stay but instead spent ten days. Why? It seems that somewhere along the way the surgeon discovered an abnormality in her chest x-ray and called in some specialists. A series of tests were ordered. No one thought to mention these goings-on to the primary care doctor, who could have told them what they would discover after six hospital days and a number of tests. There was nothing wrong with the patient.

Who is in charge? Ultimately, you, the patient. No one can "order" a treatment or procedure without your permission. Do not hesitate to refuse that permission until you fully understand why a test or procedure is necessary.

HOW TO MAKE SURE
MISTAKES DON'T HAPPEN

Knowing that the possibility of confusion exists, you can make sure that you know who is in charge, understand what you are being treated for and why, and question anything that seems unclear or wrong.

1. Make a point of asking questions of everyone who is treating you—the doctor, the nurses, the anesthesiologist. You must know what to expect if you are going to recognize the unexpected.

2. Ask the nurses questions about medications—what each drug is and why it is being given. Ask whether you should alert them to change an I.V. bottle and how to know when.

3. The staff may miss or fail to follow an order. If you know that you should not eat for twelve hours before an operation, you won't assume that because you are being served breakfast you can eat it.

4. If you are too sick to cope with this approach, make sure you have a personal advocate. (Discussed below and on p. 113.)

5. Don't take any medication or allow any test or procedure that is unexpected. There is a possibility that this is intended for someone else.

6. Hospital staff may make you feel that they know what is best and that there is something wrong and "uncooperative" about you if you ask questions. Your health is more important to you than it is to the hospital, and you have every right to protect it.

CREATING A PERSONAL ADVOCATE

The man in the bed is thin and restless. He has difficulty focusing his thoughts, rendered hazy by the powerful pain killers he is taking. "They gave him the wrong flavor," says his wife, pointing to a full glass by his bedside. "He doesn't like the chocolate." She speaks to a nurse, who in turn finds out that the kitchen is out of the desired flavor but will order it.

A very small thing, but small things loom large for sick people. This same wife made sure that her husband was given the appropriate amount of pain medication. She asked the doctor how often her husband could have his pills, and in what dosage. "I carry some in my purse," she explained. "If for any reason the nurses don't come or won't give him enough, I will."

If you are sick enough to be in the hospital, you need to direct all your energies toward getting well. This is not the best time for you to have to manipulate, deal, negotiate, rationally discuss, or any of the other things you usually do to get what you need. You just want to be taken care of.

One way you can gain some control over the situation is to choose one person to represent you. This person will deal with the hospital staff, speak with your doctor, and relay information to friends and family members.

A little caution is in order here; sometimes the person who is the closest—parent or spouse—may not be the ideal choice for you. Choose someone who cares about you but is also able to be more objective, someone who will be able to empathize with your needs without mingling them with his or her own.

If you need more help from the nursing staff, fewer intrusions from medical students and well-meaning visitors, better explanations from doctors and technicians, your advocate can act as a go-between, explaining your problems calmly and pleasantly.

If you are seriously ill, you will get good nursing care, but you may have difficulty in finding out what is wrong and what is being done. Your personal advocate's role may be to get that information and make sure the hospital or doctor is helping you, not hurting you. (Vivid and painful examples of this problem can be found in *Heartsounds,* Martha Weinman Lear's devastating story of her physician-husband's battle with heart disease, and of his difficulties in finding compassionate and thoughtful medical care.)

Since you, the patient, may have quite enough on your hands coping with your anxiety and mustering all your energy to take walks, brush your teeth, and generally recuperate, you may find it very useful to have someone else track down your test results or ask why housekeeping is not responding to your request for a working TV.

We are being somewhat flippant here, but as we mentioned earlier in the chapter, people who are sick experience a narrowing of focus and may have a hard time behaving in their normal adult fashion.

THE IMPORTANCE OF NURSES

The difference between the skillful and attentive nursing provided in a hospital that values patient comfort and the routinized impersonal treatment that's dished out in some hospitals (both small and large) is enormous. Nurses know how to make sick people feel more comfortable. Whether it's physical care (a back rub or foot rub, soaks, a change of position) or their kindness and concern, good nurses make patients feel better and can even reduce the amount of pain medication needed.

"A close relative called me halfway across the continent," says a nurse who holds a high-level administrative job in a teaching hospital. "She was in a hospital where the care was pretty awful and she wanted some advice. After her surgery, she was in considerable pain from gas, something that happens quite commonly. There are ten things the nurses could have suggested that would have helped her. Instead she was told that nothing could be done. The problem wasn't that the nurses were too few or too busy. It was that they didn't care."

Some innovative hospitals have tried to improve patient care, and make nursing a better and more interesting job, by using a system called "primary nursing." Under this arrangement, each nurse, rather than doing one task for a large number of patients, is responsible for the total care of a few patients. If you are choosing a hospital, one with primary nursing would have a definite plus.

Whatever the system, do not assume that the nurses are too busy or too uncaring to help you. Good hospitals have enough nursing staff to take care of your needs. If you are uncomfortable, if you have questions, if you want a back rub or if you are feeling lonely or apprehensive, you can ask whether one of the nursing staff has some time to spare.

Night is the time when people are most apt to feel fearful, and although there are fewer nurses, they have less to do than the day shift and should be able to spend a few minutes with you.

Following Orders or Following Common Sense

Attendings (private doctors) have considerable authority; they write the orders and the nurses are legally bound to carry them out. How they are carried out and whether they are ever questioned—as they sometimes should be—depends on the nurses.

For example, the reason you may be awakened for a sleeping pill is that your doctor's order said "Dalmane® 15 mgs h.s." (hour of sleep), meaning "one 15 milligram Dalmane at bedtime." That legally requires the nurse to give you the pill; the doctor should have added "prn," which means "as needed." If the nurse notices the wording, she may question whether you should be awakened for the Dalmane, and the doctor can rewrite the order.

Nothing, however, requires nurses to discuss these orders; they have had far too many doctors react to their questions with irritation rather than responsive interest.

R.N.s, L.P.N.s, AIDES, ETC.

Not everyone in a white jacket is a doctor or nurse. Hospital staff members are supposed to wear tags with their name and function. If in doubt, ask.

Registered Nurses (R.N.s)	Training varies. 2–4 years of college plus 2–3 years of nursing courses.
Licensed Practical Nurses (L.P.N.s)	Work under direction of R.N.s. One-year vocational program in community college, more limited duties than R.N.s.
Nurses' Aides	Usually have had only short training course. (May be nursing students.) Give just physical care such as back rubs, baths, take temperatures and blood pressures.
Nursing Students	Should be identified by name tag. Have time to give a good deal of attention.
Clinical specialists. Nurse coordinators.	Highly trained nurses. Teach patients, help plan their care, prepare for discharge. For example, oncology nurse-coordinator gives chemotherapy drugs, does advanced nursing care.

In dealing with the nursing staff, it is important to have some sense of their hierarchy so that you will know whom to ask for help. Depending on how nursing care is organized in a particular hospital, the chain of command may vary somewhat. If you have requests or complaints, the person to start with would be the charge nurse, who is the head of a particular shift.

Supervising the charge nurse is the head nurse, responsible for all nursing care on all shifts in a particular unit. In most hospitals, the chain of command goes up from head nurse to nursing supervisor (there may be day and evening supervisors) to the director of nursing.

You are likely to get better results if you take your problems with nursing to a nurse who is in charge. If you try the nursing chain of command and are still unhappy, then make your complaints known to your doctor.

If you have identified someone to be your personal advocate, he or she will get the best responses by asking politely. Nurses are people— often undervalued and overworked ones—who very much resent the fact that they are ordered around by doctors. If the first approach is a demanding inquisitorial one, you are not likely to get very far. If you can avoid making requests during shift changes or at times when nurses are especially busy, you will get better results.

A hospital is good for patients largely to the extent that they receive good nursing care. To quote Lewis Thomas, notable physician-author of *The Youngest Science,* "My discovery, as a patient first on the medical service and later in surgery, is that the institution is held together, glued together, enabled to function as an organism, by the nurses and by nobody else."[6]

WHO ARE ALL THOSE VERY YOUNG PEOPLE IN WHITE COATS?

If you are a patient in a teaching hospital, you may begin to wonder just who is what? Are all those people who stop at your bedside to ask questions or examine you really doctors? They may or may not be: they may be medical students or nursing students or physician assistant students. They should identify themselves by name and function, but they may not. The bigger and more famous the hospital, the more of them there will be and the more casual they may be about introducing themselves to you. Yet there are advantages to some, if not all, of the extra attention.

Medical Students

One plus of having a medical student involved in your care is that they often have just one or two patients assigned to them: much of their time is spent in reading about whatever is wrong with you. They may discover something your doctor doesn't know or hasn't thought of. Furthermore, your doctor, who hopes that they do no such thing, will want to impress them and may do some extra reading in order to appear totally knowledgeable. If you are not extremely uncomfortable, you may not mind the careful attention the student pays to everything you have to say: no other medical person will be that intensely interested. You may also like the fact that you are helping in the education of a new young doctor.

If, however, you do not like being disturbed, discuss your concerns with your physician, who will try to minimize these disruptions.

Interns

Interns, now often called first-year residents, have graduated from medical school and are technically considered doctors, although most states will not give them a license to practice until they have completed a year of hospital training. Beware of being hospitalized in the month of July if you can possibly help it. On July 1, all the fourth-year medical students become interns, all the interns become residents, all the chief residents become attendings (fully trained doctors who have the right to admit "private patients"), and all the attendings shudder because they have a whole new crop of interns to get to know and teach.

The first week of internship, a young acquaintance of ours found himself working in the emergency room. A very sick patient was brought in, and the new intern started an intravenous and administered one or two basic drugs for the problem, but the patient did not improve. In desperation, our friend turned to the nursing staff. "This man is sick," he shouted. "He needs a doctor!" At least he had the good sense to realize that his new degree did not make him a "real doctor"; some interns just bluff their way through, sometimes to the detriment of the patient.

Despite their inexperience, there are advantages to having an intern involved in your care. He or she is in the hospital five or six days a week as well as two or three nights. Should you suddenly develop a complication, the intern knows how to begin emergency treatment while your doctor is being located. It is nice not to be bothered by extra questions and examinations, but if your condition worsens unexpectedly, that is a small price to pay.

Residents
These are young physicians receiving their specialty training. Depending on the specialty, the residency will last up to five or six years. Chief residents are in their final year of training and are apt to be very important in your care; they are usually up-to-date on all the latest trends in diagnosis and treatment and will be eager to impress your doctor with what they know.

The more involved the resident is, the better for you—so long as your doctor remains in control. Residents are knowledgeable but inexperienced. They will tend to overdiagnose or overtreat in their enthusiasm, a tendency that should be tempered by the attending (the private doctor).

In many teaching hospitals, however, the resident can seemingly exert more authority than the attending. Some institutions have a policy that your private doctor can only make suggestions, while the resident actually writes all the orders. In these situations, the resident is working under the supervision of an experienced doctor who has been designated "attending of the month" or some similar title. This attending will often be a well-known clinical specialist, a boon to you, especially if there is anything difficult or unusual about your case; but the attending of the month may be a well-known researcher, which from your point of view is practically useless. At all times you can certainly share your concerns with your doctor, who should be able to straighten out all of this.

Fellows
Then there are the Fellows. These are doctors who have completed a residency in a specialty (such as internal medicine) and are now taking additional training in a subspecialty (such as endocrinology).

When you are referred to a famous specialist in a world-renowned medical center, it is usually the Fellow being trained by that specialist who will really take care of you, although the specialist will send the bill. But the Fellow may know more than the specialist about taking care of your problem if the specialist is famous for research, not as a clinician.

Fellows, who are usually in their thirties, look and sound like "real" doctors. They are for the most part extremely knowledgeable and self-assured, sometimes too assured of their own expertise to realize how little experience they have. Therefore, they are not apt to call for help.

Ironically, it is when they do that problems may start. Fellows are subspecialists, studying the diseases of a particular organ system. If something goes wrong with a part of your body not included in your Fellow's specialty area, be it hematology, oncology, or cardiology, he or she will call on a fellow Fellow. The new "ologist," perhaps a gastroenterologist, nephrologist or a pulmonologist, may have a different view of what your problem is and what ought to be done about it. In these cases, the "ologists" may fall to squabbling, losing track of your needs and your confusion as they go racing off after the correct diagnosis.

Fellows can be extremely valuable when they are called on for help by your own primary care doctor, who can take their recommendations and modify your treatment accordingly. Because a generalist is more interested in helping you than in diagnosing a new syndrome, your care will be suited to your personal needs rather than to the advancement of science.

GETTING WHAT YOU NEED
IN THE HOSPITAL

The first step is to differentiate your needs from your wants. It would be wonderful to have a nurse available the instant you call, a careful explanation of exactly what is going on at every moment, excellent food served fashionably late, an undisturbed night's sleep, and a sophisticated, charming roommate who is unmarked by any sign of disease. Alas, none of this is likely in the forseeable future. Try to keep your requests realistic and limit them to things that really matter to you.

It helps to know what can be changed and what cannot. Meals are served at set times, but depending on your diet, the hospitals might allow you to eat food brought in from the outside. If you enjoy dinner at seven and a later dinner breaks up the time, making the evening shorter and less boring, you might have someone bring you a meal.

If you are a light sleeper or if you are irritated by the foibles of others, you may feel it is worthwhile to pay the extra money for a private room. If you must share a room and if your roommate is much sicker than you are or disruptive in any way, you can probably arrange to be moved, although perhaps not immediately. If you are a non-smoker, mention this before you are admitted. You do have a right to a smoke-free room, and the hospital should be able to arrange it.

Many top hospitals run at 100 percent of capacity, so when they tell you no other room is immediately available, they are probably telling the truth. Nevertheless, about 10 percent of patients are discharged every day, so the hospital should be able to transfer you the next day.

If you are concerned about getting uninterrupted sleep, ask your doctor to write orders for pain medication "prn" (as needed) and to specify that you should not be awakened for routine temperature taking, the 7 A.M. washcloth, or whatever else can wait.

If you want information, you might request help from the nursing staff. If the nurse who is caring for you does not adequately answer your questions, ask the charge nurse to find someone who will. Some nurses give very good physical care but explain things poorly. Or, the person you ask may be an aide or L.P.N. who does not have the information you need.

In general, you will get better results by explaining how something makes you feel than by criticizing the nurse's behavior or the hospital rules. For example, if you are being awakened at 4 A.M. to take an antibiotic, explain to the nurse that you feel much worse in the morning because you have trouble getting back to sleep. No doubt your doctor wrote that the drug was to be given "Q 6h," which means every six hours. Depending on when the drug was started and on hospital policy, that may mean 10 A.M., 4 P.M., 10 P.M. and 4 A.M.; and the nurse has to follow the doctor's orders.

If she or he knows this is affecting your recovery and wants to help you out because you are being so reasonable, at rounds in the morning, the nurse can ask your doctor to change the order to "QID," which means four times a day, allowing for much more flexibility. Even if it is medically necessary for you to receive the drug every six hours, a different schedule (perhaps 8 A.M., 2 P.M., 8 P.M. and 2 A.M.) might be more in tune with your particular sleep cycle. Even if nothing can be changed, you will probably feel better knowing that what is being done is an important part of your care rather than simply an annoyance.

PRIVATE ROOMS—PRIVATE DUTY NURSES

Unless medically necessary, neither will be covered by your health insurance, but if you have the financial means, there are times when you might want to use a private duty nurse or stay in a private room.

PRIVATE ROOM

Advantages
1. Quieter
   It is easier to sleep when you are feeling sick, easier to get work done when you are feeling better.
2. More flexibility for visitors
   Parents can usually stay overnight in a private room, even if "rooming-in" is not routine in the hospital. Usually there is no limit to the number of visitors, unless your physician specifies otherwise.
3. More peaceful
   No danger of being distracted by a thoughtless roommate or upset by sharing a room with someone who is seriously, perhaps fatally, ill.

Disadvantages
1. Cost
   The additional cost of a private room ranges from minimal ($10–$15 per day) to substantial ($50–$100 per day) depending on the hospital.
2. Loneliness
   Especially for patients facing a long hospital stay, or for people hospitalized out of town, or who for some other reason anticipate few visitors.
3. Safety
   Infirm, confused, or very ill patients may benefit from a concerned roommate who can call for a nurse or help answer a doctor's questions about the day's happenings.
4. Isolation
   Private rooms are frequently tucked away in corners far from the nurses' station. If there is any chance your condition could suddenly deteriorate, you may be better off where you'll be checked on more often.

PRIVATE DUTY NURSE

Advantages
1. Attention, comfort
   Someone whose only job is to care for you and make you feel better. The floor nurses may just not have the time for soothing back rubs, for example.
2. Reassurance
   Knowing that a trained person is always with you should anything go wrong.
3. Respite

For family members who are staying with a sick patient around the clock.
4. Prevention of catastrophe
If you are very sick, but not quite sick enough for the ICU, the continuous presence of an alert nurse could save your life. But be careful! Some private duty nurses are really not up-to-date on critical care.

If you want a nurse for this reason, discuss your request with the head nurse on the floor. It may be that one of the staff nurses would be happy to work an extra shift to make some extra money.
5. Advocacy
A health professional who is working for you can make sure the system responds to your needs.

Disadvantages
1. Cost
$80 to $120 per eight-hour shift. For very sick patients, the doctor may be able to justify "ordering" the nurse, which often means that insurance will cover the cost.
2. Unhealthy dependence
For chronic problems, the patient and family are going to have to learn how to manage for themselves, unless money is unlimited. And even then, the patient would probably do better to learn to manage as much as possible by him- or herself. In most cases, the sooner the patient and family begin this task, the better.

If you can afford it, a good compromise plan may be to have a private duty nurse to work the midnight-to-eight shift, giving the family a break and helping teach family and patient how to manage the problems for themselves.
3. Less attention from floor nurses
Inevitably, the floor nurses will pay less attention to the patient with a private duty nurse. This will pose no problem if all you need is comfort and attention—but if you are seriously ill, the floor nurse is more apt to be expert in caring for your problem, so less attention may mean poorer care.
4. Quality
As we noted above, the quality of private duty nurses is much more variable than that of hospital nurses. If you are seriously ill, be sure that any nurse you hire has been recommended by your physician or by someone else whose judgment you trust.
5. Lack of privacy
The constant care and concern over every minor problem that we so desire when we are either very sick or very young may become an annoyance when we are feeling better (or more mature). As the patient improves, he or she may find the constant presence of a nurse (or even a visitor) more annoying than helpful.

PATIENT REPRESENTATIVES:
WHEN YOU CAN'T GET WHAT YOU NEED

There is a new kind of professional who has been added to the staff of many large hospitals. Like the Swedish ombudsman designated to help citizens deal with the bureaucracy, the purpose of the patient representative or advocate is to represent the patient rather than the hospital and to find out what has gone wrong with the system. An effective patient representative will identify problems in the way the hospital works so that care can be improved for everyone.

If you have tried to work out your problems with the nursing staff or doctors and have been unsuccessful, you can hope your hospital has such a position. Call the switchboard to ask if a patient representative or advocate is listed. (He or she is sometimes a member of the Social Services Department.)

PATIENTS' RIGHTS

In this age of the informed consumer, hospitals have had to establish a patient's "bill of rights." Most hospitals will have a formal list of such rights, usually displayed prominently or otherwise available for the asking. Some of the items on the list are unenforceable, such as the right to be treated with dignity. Others are actual legal rights, such as the right to a written bill. Usually such a list will include the following points:

- the right to know who is treating you by name and function (for example, medical students should introduce themselves as such rather than let you think they are doctors)
- the right to give informed consent before any hazardous procedure is performed, which means that you should receive a detailed explanation of all risks and benefits (More on this subject in Chapter Eleven)
- the right to refuse a given treatment for yourself, despite the risks of such a refusal
- the right to be treated with dignity
- the right to confidentiality of your records
- the right to a detailed, written explanation of all fees and charges

If you feel you are being deprived of any of these rights, contact the patient representative or hospital administrator, or discuss the issue with your doctor. (Often people who feel they are being denied such rights are either those who don't have anyone they consider "their" doctor or those for whom the doctor is the problem.)

If neither the doctor nor the hospital administrator is helpful and you work for a large and/or influential company, you do have another source of help.

If there are serious deficiencies in your care, call your personnel office at work, report the problems you are having, and ask if anything can be done. If, for example, your company president were to call the president or chairman of the board of the hospital, this would undoubtedly lead to action. But don't "cry wolf"; your employer won't appreciate it, let alone the doctor or hospital. We are mentioning this avenue to make you realize that if you are sufficiently desperate, you can go outside the system completely to get results.

CHAPTER SIX

EMERGENCY!!!

If an emergency happened right now, would you know what to do and where to go? Would you recognize whether or not it *was* an emergency? By the time you finish reading this chapter, you will have some book learning on the subject, but we urge you to do more.

Investigate the emergency facilities in your community. Which hospital has the best emergency room? Is there anything that another hospital does better? Decide which means of transportation is safest . . . or quickest. To be truly prepared also means learning a few skills. At a minimum, you should know:

- how to do cardiopulmonary resuscitation (CPR) to aid victims of a heart attack, drowning, or electrocution
- how to do the Heimlich Maneuver (to save the lives of people who are choking on food or have an object lodged in the windpipe)
- how to stop bleeding

WHY YOU SHOULD KNOW THE DIFFERENCE BETWEEN URGENT AND EMERGENT

If you don't know the difference between a true emergency, which requires immediate action, and an urgent problem, which allows time for pondering alternatives, you will find yourself in a quandary whenever a serious medical problem arises. Is there time to call the doctor or should you rush to the hospital? Should this be treated at once no matter what the hour, the cost, and the inconvenience, or can you wait until morning to try to find a doctor?

If we can spare you an unnecessary and expensive trip to an emergency room or an hour's anxiety waiting for a doctor to call back, then we have achieved one of this chapter's goals. Knowing when something is *not* an emergency can save money and protect you against getting the wrong medical care.

WHAT DO *YOU* CONSIDER AN EMERGENCY?

1. You're sitting at the table, eating steak. A guest suddenly begins to choke.
2. You go in to quiet your fretful three-year-old son. His skin is burning to the touch; when you take his temperature, the thermometer registers 104° F.
3. You have been slightly queasy since eating a big picnic lunch a few hours ago. You vomit several times and can't seem to stop.
4. Your seven-year-old daughter falls and hits the back of her head on the coffee table. She begins to cry. Blood is suddenly all over the living room floor.
5. You wake up in the middle of the night with sharp pain and an urgent need to urinate. Your urine is blood red.

The only critical emergency on the list is the first example. There is no time to call a doctor or go to an emergency room. You must do something instantly; if you don't know the Heimlich Maneuver, you may have a dead guest. In all the other situations, there is time to think before acting, time to call your doctor and wait for a call back.

THE DOCTORS' LIST OF EMERGENCIES

1. Severe and uncontrollable bleeding
2. Serious difficulty in breathing
3. Choking
4. Poisoning
5. Severe chest pain
6. Convulsions
7. Heat stroke
8. Unconsciousness
9. Severe injuries; deep slashes that may have severed nerves or arteries
10. Any stabbing or bullet wound or other puncture that may have penetrated internal organs
11. Severe and extensive burns; chemical burns, especially of the eye
12. Sudden loss of vision
13. Diabetic acidosis or shock from hypoglycemia
14. Hypothermia (dangerously low body temperature)

If you have a problem that is not on this list, could it be a true emergency? The answer is similar to the one that real estate agents give when you ask why they advertise lavish homes without listing the price: "If you have to ask, you can't afford it." If you have time to wonder if something is an emergency, it is not.

At any rate, that is the way medical professionals think. To them an emergency is a situation in which seconds—possibly a minute or two—make the difference between life and death, or loss of limb or organ. So, for example, a very high fever does not by itself constitute an emergency. To the parent of a young child, that line creeping up the thermometer is terrifying. To the doctor, who knows that high fevers in young children are fairly common, it is the cause of that fever that may be a source of serious concern.

Young Infants Are Different

Infants, because they can get very sick very quickly, have to be handled differently from older children or adults. Always call your doctor if your new baby has a fever of 101° F or higher, or if an infant under one year has diarrhea that lasts more than one day. If a baby is vomiting (not just spitting up an ounce or so), losing weight, and/or is listless and sleeping all the time, there may be a serious problem.

WHAT TO DO ABOUT AN URGENT PROBLEM

If You Have a Primary Care Physician
Put in a call. If you feel your problem is urgent, say so. Either your own doctor or whoever is covering should get back to you within fifteen to thirty minutes. If you feel the problem is *very* urgent, make that clear to the person who answers the phone; he or she may advise you to go to an emergency room or may find a way to reach the doctor more quickly—by interrupting another call or by paging.

If You Do Not Have a Personal Physician
You have a more difficult decision. If the ER is convenient and the cost unimportant, the trip may be worth it. The only alternative, if you feel the problem needs immediate medical attention, is to find a doctor who will see you right away. This may be difficult, especially if you get sick late at night or on a holiday.

If you are not sure whether to wait until the next day to try to find a doctor who will see you or to pack yourself off to the ER, ask yourself what you want the trip to accomplish. Do you know what your problem is but want to start treatment immediately? Are you in pain? Or, are you terribly worried that you have something very serious?

If your problem is not on the emergency list, treatment can probably wait. Most pain is effectively treated with aspirin, or acetaminophen, or ice for a sprain. (See Chapter Ten for self-care measures.) As for anxiety, only you can decide whether having immediate medical attention is worth making the trip, waiting in the ER, and paying the good-sized bill you will receive.

You could try calling the ER to ask for advice, but the odds are very high that the person you talk to will merely tell you to come in. After all, they don't know you or your medical history and will want to protect you medically, and themselves legally.

WHEN TO CALL THE DOCTOR

The world seems divided between those who will suffer the torments of hell before "bothering" the doctor and those who through anxiety or thoughtlessness call in the dead of night with problems that could easily wait until morning. There is no simple and correct answer as to whether to pick up the telephone at two in the morning, but to get some sense of what your own instincts are, imagine you are one of the people we describe below:

1. You go in to check on your two-year-old daughter at two in the morning; she is restless and whimpering. She feels warm but you don't want to wake her, so you take her pulse and find it is 130. This doesn't seem right to you. Should you call the doctor?

2. You are a twenty-five-year-old man with a bad headache. It is now 5:00 A.M. Your head has been hurting since you went to bed, and the four aspirin you've taken in that period haven't helped. Should you call?

3. Your four-month-old baby has been awake and fussing all night. Now, at four in the morning, you notice that she has a badly swollen mosquito bite. Should you call?

4. Your fifty-five-year-old husband has been having sharp abdominal pains for several hours. He says he feels "very unwell." At midnight you call his doctor, who arranges to meet you at the nearby ER. You and your husband arrive but the doctor does not. Your husband appears to be getting sicker. It is a small community hospital with no ER doctor. The nurse says no treatment can be given until the doctor arrives. By now it is close to 1:30 A.M. Should you call the doctor again?

In the first three cases, the calls were made, quite unnecessarily, to the extreme annoyance of the doctors. (The physician who was awakened to hear about the mosquito bite tells the story often; he still can't get over it.)

In the fourth case, another phone call (which no one made) was imperative. The doctor was very explicit about meeting the patient at the hospital. In this situation, the nurse was professionally irresponsible.

She should have called the doctor, who—it turned out—had fallen back asleep after taking the call. The man's abdominal pains were caused by a perforated ulcer, and by the time treatment was started, it was too late. He died. Why didn't his wife call again? Was it mistaken politeness? Fear of the doctor?

MINOR EMERGENCY ROOMS

In our examples above, we assume that you have a doctor to call. What if you don't? Let's suppose you have moved to a new community and have not yet found yourself a personal physician. One evening your child has a rash and a high fever. You want medical advice but you hate to go to a hospital emergency room.

One good solution would be to find out whether or not there is a minor emergency room in town. There are presently some 400 or 500 of these facilities scattered around the United States, with many more on the drawing boards.

They are equipped to handle a wide range of problems; in fact, one specialist in emergency medicine who has worked both in hospital and minor emergency settings feels that eighty percent of the problems that the hospital deals with could be treated more efficiently, more comfortably, and for less money in a good minor emergency room.

If you are unsure as to whether your problem is minor or major, call the minor ER and ask. The doctor or nurse there will recommend you go to a hospital immediately if you have symptoms, such as severe chest pain, which suggest a critical emergency; or a serious problem, such as a broken hip, for which hospital facilities would clearly be necessary.

Qualifications
To date, there are no licensing requirements other than those that would apply to a physician in private practice. We suggest you ask the following questions:

Is there a registered nurse present whenever the facility is open?
Is there an M.D. on duty at all times?
Is this doctor board-certified in emergency medicine, family practice, or general internal medicine?
Are there skilled lab and x-ray technicians available?

WHICH HOSPITAL EMERGENCY ROOM?

Now is the time to find out which hospital emergency room is best. If you have a personal physician, you would go to the hospital where he or she could take charge of your care.

If you do not have such a physician, start by asking friends and neighbors which emergency room they would go to and why. You can call the hospital administrator for specifics on staffing and credentials.

Members of the fire department might know which ER is best. Private ambulance services are, of course, familiar with the facilities of all of the local emergency rooms. In some cities, a local newspaper or magazine may have rated emergency room services. (See the Resource Directory for a detailed discussion of ways to locate information on emergency care in your community.)

What follows is a list of factors to consider:

If you are considering a small hospital, does its ER have a doctor present all the time, or just a nurse, with a doctor who will be called if a patient is brought in?

If the small hospital has a full-time ER doctor, is he or she board-certified either in emergency medicine, family practice, or general internal medicine? If the doctor is a family practitioner or general internist, has he or she taken advanced training in emergency procedures?

If this is a medical center emergency room, staffed by interns and residents, with senior residents and Fellows in the hospital at all times and attendings on call, is it supervised by a physician experienced in emergency medicine? (This would be desirable.)

Does the hospital have an intensive, or critical care unit? Is it supervised by a qualified doctor at night as well as during the day?

Which hospital emergency room is best equipped to care for heart attacks? (One way to get this information would be to call your local medical society and find out at which hospital most of the cardiologists have staff privileges.)

Are the ER nurses certified in advanced cardiac life support?

Is there a coronary intensive care unit in the hospital?

If your child needs emergency care, is a pediatrician always available?

Does the hospital have a pediatric intensive care unit?

In the past few years, the specialty of emergency medicine has grown rapidly, and a topflight ER will generally have at least one doctor who is board-certified in that specialty.

The best emergency rooms are not invariably attached to the most prestigious institutions. A hospital with an excellent reputation for patient care may have an emergency room that is inferior to the high-powered operation run by a hospital located in an area where many serious emergencies occur.

We are thinking of a specific example here. If you were badly injured in an auto accident in New York City and were brought to Bellevue—a municipal hospital in the heart of Manhattan that seldom attracts "private patients"—you would get marvelous treatment in its emergency room, which is equipped to deal with all kinds of violent trauma.

BEFORE YOU LEAVE

If you live some distance from the hospital, call first; you may receive some useful advice for treatment you can give to prevent the problem from getting worse. And if the situation is anything short of critical, you will save time and confusion by making sure you take the information the ER will want when you arrive. Without insurance information, you may have to pay on the spot. If a patient cannot pay, hospitals will always evaluate and stabilize an obvious emergency, but in large cities, the case may then be transferred to a municipal or county hospital.

Things to take with you include:

· insurance identification card or policy
· such information as home and business phone, birth date, employer
· regular medications the patient takes
· if poison or pill overdose is the problem, take the container or bottle

WHO SHOULD GO?

The sicker the patient, the more necessary it becomes that he or she have someone to help negotiate the ER system. Young children and very sick adults are even better off with two people, one to stay with the patient and one to deal with the ER personnel. More than two helpers, however, would be unnecessary. Two people are especially recommended if you are driving to the hospital and must park the car.

HOW TO GET TO THE EMERGENCY ROOM

Ambulance vs. Taxi vs. Auto

You may be in a situation where you have no choice. If you lived alone, fell and broke your leg, then dragged yourself to a telephone— calling an ambulance would be the only reasonable thing to do. But many people assume an ambulance is best when that is not always so.

A New York doctor who lectured on drug abuse would often ask his teen-aged audience, "What would you do if, while walking down Broadway, you saw a man lying unconscious with a needle in his arm?" Almost everyone would reply, "Get to the nearest phone and call an ambulance." Yet in this situation, minutes may matter. Finding a telephone, calling, and waiting for an ambulance to arrive, and then transporting the victim to the hospital takes much more time than hailing a cab or, if necessary, stopping a passing car to get to the hospital.

Your decision may depend in part on the qualifications of the emergency network that serves your community. You need to find out whether ambulances carry advanced life support equipment and a crew of emergency medical technicians and paramedics, who are trained to treat cardiac arrest. (Anyone who watched the now defunct television show "Emergency" will have seen this type of setup.)

Call an ambulance if . . .

· the problem is a possible heart attack or potential respiratory emergency and the ambulance has special equipment
· you are unable to move the victim safely because of possible serious injury to the back or neck

If the ambulance does not have special equipment to deal with the emergency at hand, you would probably be better off with private transportation. It is faster and cheaper.

In New York City, regulations require the ambulance to take you to a specified hospital depending on where you are picked up. If it is a life or death situation, you will want to go to the nearest hospital, but short of that, you may have a strong preference.

If you live in a large city, even if you have your own car, a taxi may be your best choice, especially if parking near the hospital will be a problem.

WHEN YOU GET THERE

Upon arrival, it is usually simplest to have a patient who is in extreme pain or weak or dizzy remain in the car while the helper goes in and informs the receptionist of the situation. If necessary, the receptionist can then find the people and equipment—stretcher or wheelchair—to help move the patient and may also have him or her taken directly to an exam room. The patient who is well enough can walk in and take a seat, instead of standing outside the reception station, while all the arrangements are being made. Let the helper deal with the receptionist. There may be a wait or a number of routine questions to be answered.

If the patient has a doctor on the staff of the hospital, be sure to mention the fact. Many hospitals will go a bit out of their way for patients of a staff doctor and will try to involve that doctor in any decisions that are made about follow-up care or consultations.

When most adult patients are called in to see a doctor, no helper will be necessary. If the patient is a young child or is senile or confused, then someone will be needed to answer questions. If in doubt, ask the person whether he or she wants a companion during the exam. Your twelve-year-old child may possibly feel more confident and more in control seeing the doctor alone. Your spouse may have a concern he or she is uncomfortable discussing with you present.

If there are two helpers, plan your strategy. The person who is more assertive or knowledgeable should negotiate with the staff. The other person should perform other necessary tasks such as parking the car, making phone calls, and not least, comforting the sick person.

WHO ARE THE ER PERSONNEL?

The first person you encounter will usually be a clerk/receptionist. You can save time and frustration by giving a terse five-second description of the problem and then answering whatever questions are asked of you.

Next, you will probably talk to a nurse, whose job is to decide how quickly you should be seen and by which doctor. (Occasionally, you may talk to a nurse first, and in that case you will be asked medical as well as administrative questions.) Until you talk to a doctor, make your answers brief and to the point.

The Doctors
In most teaching hospitals, you are apt to see an intern or resident first; if your problem is minor, you may be treated by that person alone. If your problem is more complex, you will be checked by one or more additional doctors.

Be prepared to answer the same questions anew for each one. The fact that you are being asked questions you have already answered does not mean that the first doctor did not brief the second. Doctors prefer to take their own histories; they find the process of getting their own information helpful and are notorious for trusting no one but themselves.

If the sick person is very fatigued or uncomfortable, the helper should mention this to the doctor and offer to answer some of the questions.

IF YOUR CHILD NEEDS A PROCEDURE

A child brought in with a laceration will need suturing, and one with fever, stiff neck, and the sudden appearance of purple spots will need an emergency spinal tap. Commonly, the parent is asked to wait outside the procedure room. Quite understandably, many parents prefer to stay with their sick youngster. If you are the parent of a young child and feel strongly that he or she needs you there, say so. If the nurse turns you down, ask to speak to the doctor.

Some doctors, feeling that they work more efficiently without a parent present, will refuse your request. You will then have to decide whether you should continue to argue while necessary treatment is being delayed.

We would caution you that the doctor's discomfort at your presence might result in less skillful treatment. Also, older children sometimes feel more in control and are able to act more mature without a parent by their side. Before insisting on being present, ask older children whether they would like you to stay with them or wait outside.

WHEN TO ASK FOR A PRIVATE DOCTOR

The doctor who sees you should identify him- or herself by name and function: for example—Dr. William Smith, intern. If your problem is minor and Dr. Smith seems competent, fine. But if you are uneasy, doubt that the person giving care knows what he or she is doing, or have a serious problem that may involve an admission to the hospital, you will probably want to have a "private" doctor called in.

IF ADMISSION IS NECESSARY

If you already have a primary care doctor who is associated with the hospital, you simply ask to have that person called. He or she may handle the admission or may bring in the appropriate specialist to do it. If you do not have a physician on the hospital staff, life will not be so simple.

In many teaching hospitals, the house staff (interns, residents, and Fellows) are looking for patients, and so they will try to admit you as a "service case" (a patient with no private doctor). That way they will have primary responsibility for your care and the opportunity to learn more. They are not especially motivated to inform you that you can have a private doctor. You must ask.

Which Private Doctor?

Here's where things get tricky. Hospitals generally have physicians in each specialty on call to the emergency room in rotation. If you ask for a suggestion as to which doctor to choose, you will probably be given the name of the doctor who is on call that day. "Is that a good doctor?" you ask. The answer, of course, will be "Yes."

Alternatively, you may be given the name of the doctor who will let the house staff have the most involvement with your case, especially if you have an interesting problem. This may work out well; quite often the best doctors work most closely with house staff.

Sometimes, though, the house staff will recommend the least knowl-edgeable doctor, knowing that this is someone who must rely on them. Or they may recommend a young and inexperienced doctor they like because he or she "needs the business."

Here is a very good example of a situation you can avoid now by making sure that you have chosen a personal physician before you are faced with making the decision hastily and under pressure. Once in this situation, there is no good solution to the problem. You will probably have to go along with the hospital's recommendation.

DO YOU REALLY NEED TO BE ADMITTED?

Often people are admitted "just to be on the safe side" or for reasons that are nonmedical: to fill a bed or give some extra experience to a doctor in training. Ask the doctor who is suggesting you be admitted if he or she is a member of the house staff. If the answer is yes, you are dealing with someone who only sees people in hospitals and who is not in a position to offer the kind of office follow-up care that might allow you to go home to your own bed.

In such cases, you can ask to have a consultation with an "attending," a doctor in practice who is associated with the hospital. Ask whether you can be sent home on treatment and seen in the attending's office for follow-up care.

If you agree that a hospital admission is definitely necessary, you can ask to be admitted by a private doctor as a private patient unless you have little or no insurance.

Note: If money is a problem, you will be relieved to learn that if you are admitted to a major hospital as a "house staff" patient, there will always be one or more attending physicians assigned to monitor your care. In such situations, your case may become the province of some of the city's top doctors—at no charge to you.

WHY ARE YOU FORCED TO WAIT SO LONG?

Probably because you should not be in an emergency room in the first place. True emergencies will always be taken care of immediately. If it is a busy night, replete with auto accidents, shootings, suicide attempts, and heart attacks, you will wait there a long time with your earache. In fact, the less urgent your problem, the greater the chances the staff may forget about you almost entirely.

The doctors and nurses will take care of critical emergencies (heart attacks, uncontrollable bleeding) immediately and very urgent problems (possible appendicitis, head injuries) promptly. Most patient dissatisfaction occurs with problems that cause great discomfort or pain to the patient but are not considered emergencies by the staff: acute urinary tract infections, uncomplicated fractures of the wrist, lacerations that have stopped bleeding.

You should not have to wait to give a synopsis of your story, for without that, the ER staff has no way of judging how serious your problem is. Once you have answered a few questions, you may have to sit in the waiting room for a long time. Periodically, someone should tell you the reason for the delay, but if the doctors and nurses are busy saving lives, they may understandably be preoccupied.

Eventually, you will be ushered into an exam room. Again, you may wait quite a while—possibly because no one has told the doctor you are in there. After you are examined, you may have several more spells of waiting. The doctor may want to present your case to the senior doctor or have a consultant come in to see you.

ERs tend to do a lot of lab work, EKGs, and x-rays. If a test is ordered, you will first wait for the specimen to be collected, or for the film to be taken, and then you will wait for the results. And unless you have a critical emergency, waiting time can be substantial.

WAYS TO DEAL WITH LONG WAITS

Make Sure They Are Necessary
After you have waited fifteen minutes in the waiting room, you might ask the receptionist how long a wait to expect. You want this person— who may, in some instances, decide how soon you will be called—to be on your side, so a pleasant request for information is your best approach. Rather than saying, "Why hasn't my name been called yet?" you would do better to ask, "When do you think I will be seen?"

Remind the Staff that You Are There
A helper can be very useful in gathering information about delays and making sure you don't get lost in the shuffle. He or she can speak to the receptionist ("My friend is very anxious and in a lot of pain. Do you have any idea when he or she will be seen?") Similarly, if you have been waiting for some time in an exam room, you or your helper should check to make sure someone knows you are there.

Find Out Ahead of Time About Especially Long Waits

When blood is drawn, ask how long it will be before the results will be back. If the answer is thirty minutes, and you are not acutely ill, you might prefer to go to the hospital coffee shop and come back in thirty minutes.

Similarly, if you are told that a consultant is being called, find out how long it will take for him or her to arrive—it may be as long as an hour.

If you are going to be admitted, you may be waiting because a clerk has to come from another part of the hospital to get billing or other administrative information. Your helper may be able to go to the admitting office to fill out forms so that you can be taken to the floor more quickly.

HOW MUCH DO YOU WANT THE ER TO DO?

After you have been examined, what comes next and who should do it? Unless you have a true emergency, this is really your decision. We have already discussed the question of which doctor to use if you require further care or must be admitted to the hospital.

Remember that even if you have a problem that can be treated on an out-patient basis, the ER staff, which is geared to using the hospital's resources, will send you for further care to the hospital's lab and x-ray. Or the ER doctor may do a brief evaluation and then refer you to the clinic to be seen. Off you go to a new waiting area, where you may put in another hour or two. (You will not get credit for the time you have already waited in the ER.)

This may or may not suit you, so get the ER doctor to clarify how urgent your problem is. You may, for instance, be content with a less thorough evaluation than the staff wants to do. Let's say you rush to the emergency room because you are afraid your severe headache is the first sign of an aneurysm. Once you learn it is not, you may prefer to pursue the question of its cause with your own physician.

If you ask the ER doctor whether there is any reason why your own doctor cannot follow up on the problem the next day, he or she may agree this is perfectly reasonable. Whether the cause is a brain tumor or emotional stress, waiting one more day is not going to make a difference.

What if a problem needs immediate treatment? You still have some options. You do not necessarily have to get that treatment in the hospital. If, for example, you discover you have a fracture, you may save time by taking a taxi to the office of a nearby orthopedist rather than waiting at the hospital for the consultant on call to arrive.

Emergency Room Checklist

1. Call your own doctor if you can.
2. The more urgent the problem, the more quickly you need to get to the hospital. Go by the quickest form of transportation, not necessarily by ambulance.
3. Before you leave for the ER, gather as much information as possible and any necessary documents. An insurance I.D. card is extremely helpful.
4. Take a book or a few magazines with you. You may have time to kill.
5. Once there, if you are worried by delays or waits, ask the reason for the delay and how much longer you may have to wait.
6. One or two helpers for the sick person may make things easier.
7. Take a bottle of juice for a baby, a toy or puzzle for a child.

HOW TO HANDLE A CRISIS

An eleven-year-old girl out sledding runs into a tree and begins to bleed copiously from a long cut between her nose and lip. Fortunately her grandmother, having been a Girl Scout, knows what to do. She applies direct pressure to the cut with a clean handkerchief, then takes her granddaughter to the nearest emergency room and asks that the cut be repaired by a plastic surgeon. There is one on call; his clever stitches eventually become so faint as to be virtually invisible.

Here's an ordinary kind of accident. Knowing what to do can make a real difference in the outcome. Although this was not a life-threatening emergency, prompt action was necessary. Would you have known what to do in this situation or in a more serious one where your skill could save a life? Once again, we strongly advise you to take a course in first aid, including CPR and the Heimlich Maneuver. We will discuss some basic first aid information, but we caution you that manual techniques do not lend themselves to being taught by books alone.

WHAT TO KEEP ON HAND FOR EMERGENCIES, MAJOR AND MINOR

Do you have a box of Band-Aids in the house? Scissors? Some safety pins? Then you have the beginnings of a home emergency kit. Except for a few items, most people have what they need to deal with first aid problems. Soap and water will wash wounds. Cold water is good for burns. Bandages can be improvised from clean pillowcases, and splints from boards or even children's building blocks.

In the interests of preparedness, though, we suggest you have one place to keep essentials, a shelf or drawer that everyone in the family knows about. Here is where you should keep a book on first aid and a list of phone numbers—poison control, your doctor's office, the local emergency room, the fire department. We also suggest keeping these numbers near the telephone, perhaps written in the front of your telephone directory.

At Home

You can buy first aid kits at your pharmacy, or you can assemble your own supplies. There are two basic types of kit: a unit kit that contains enough of each item to treat a single injury, or a cabinet-type kit that contains more supplies. All sterile items in either kind of kit will be carefully wrapped. The manufacturers also supply wrapped refills for the kits they make.

Since the kits and refills are more expensive than assembling your own first aid supplies, we offer the following list:

- a roll of one-inch surgical tape
- gauze pads (4 x 4 and other sizes) to stop bleeding and make large dressings
- steri-strips or butterfly closures (used to hold the edges of a wound together) may prevent the need for sutures
- roll of gauze (to hold gauze pads over areas of bleeding or burns)
- a large triangular bandage or scarf (for a sling) and safety pins
- splints in several sizes—tongue blades for fingers, small light-weight boards to immobilize a broken arm or leg
- a bottle of syrup of ipecac when treatment of poisoning requires that vomiting be induced
- activated charcoal, for treatment of poisoning
- clean needles or tweezers to remove splinters
- cotton swabs (to remove a speck from the eye)
- elastic bandage to wrap a sprain (apply with light pressure only)
- scissors (round-tipped ones are safest) to cut bandage materials

(See pp. 218–219 under Home Pharmacy for non-emergency medications to keep on hand.)

Note: Those little bottles or ampoules of spirits of ammonia that used to be considered standard emergency equipment are unnecessary. They are intended to rouse someone who has fainted, but there is no reason to waft ammonia under the nose. Pinching is preferable in determining if an apparently unconscious person can be roused.

Traveling
Have a small first aid kit in your car. If you are a camper, you probably know how important it is to take one along into the wilds.

FOR SPECIAL PROBLEMS

In addition to the standard items everyone should have on hand, there may be some special ones you need, depending on your medical history or state of health. For example, if a member of your family is allergic to wasp or bee stings, you'll need a prescription for an Anakit®, which contains adrenaline to counteract the effects of the allergic reaction, plus a syringe and needle, swabs, a tourniquet, and antihistamine pills. If you live far from civilization, you will need more items on your shelf than if you live across the street from a hospital.

The following recommendations are intended to help you deal with some common emergency situations. Since every individual situation is unique, advice from a physician familiar with your particular circumstances should always take precedence over blanket recommendations of this or any other book.

BLEEDING

To Have on Hand:
sterile gauze pads and compresses
steri-strips or butterflies
adhesive tape

Most bleeding can be controlled. Do this first and then call the doctor for advice. Perhaps you can go to the office for further treatment, saving you the expense and long wait of an emergency room. If stitches are going to be required, you may want a particularly skillful surgeon to put them in, especially if there might be a scar on the face.

To control bleeding, clean the wound with soap and water and then apply direct pressure with a gauze pad, a piece of clean cloth folded up, or, if nothing else is available, a clean paper napkin or paper towel. Usually, only a freak accident would cause bleeding that is both severe and uncontrollable; for example, a shard of metal flying off a machine and severing the major artery that supplies blood to the brain or the upper part of your body.

A tourniquet, that old Scout standby, can be dangerous if you don't know what you are doing. The damage caused by stopping the blood supply to an arm or leg may make amputation necessary. Tourniquets are used to stop arterial bleeding—the blood spurts out rather than flows—and should only be considered if there is no other way to stop the bleeding. Once a tourniquet is applied, it must be left in place. Immediate care by a physician is imperative.

Scalp Wounds and Nosebleeds
These two kinds of bleeding alarm people out of proportion to the seriousness of the cause. Because the scalp is so well supplied with blood vessels, even a superficial cut may bleed very extensively. Quickly apply direct pressure. Allow up to five minutes, then release the pressure and see if the bleeding has stopped. Reapply pressure if necessary. If the cut is a half inch or longer, it may need stitches.

To apply pressure for a nosebleed, have the victim sit down and then pinch the nostrils together for five minutes. Almost all nosebleeds stop, unless the person has very high blood pressure.

Stitches
It will be obvious if stitches or sutures are needed to stop bleeding. But if the bleeding has already stopped, your main concern is what treatment will lead to the best cosmetic result. Small lacerations (one half inch or less) that do not gape open usually do well with butterflies or steri-strips. Longer or deeper cuts, and any facial cuts, may need suturing and should be evaluated by a physician.

Uncontrollable Bleeding: Is It an Emergency?
This type of bleeding is most apt to come from an internal source to which it is impossible to apply direct pressure. Finding blood in the urine, or stool, or coughing up blood may mean you have a serious problem. It will only be a true emergency if the bleeding is severe. Nevertheless, the appearance of any blood at all is liable to interfere with rational thought; in this situation, a powerful effort to remain calm will pay off.

If you have a doctor, put in a call. It will help your doctor evaluate the severity of the problem if you have some idea of the volume of blood that has been lost. Think of some unit, such as a measuring cup (8 ounces) and try to estimate how much blood you have lost compared with that measure.

> *To get some sense of what we're talking about, measure out a cup of tomato juice and begin to dribble it onto some cotton or gauze; a little juice will make a very large stain. Now dilute the tomato juice with an equal quantity of water and redo your experiment. The stain will look pretty similar for a given volume, even though the amount of juice is half as much. You would seldom be passing pure blood—it will usually be diluted with other bodily fluids or tissues. So if you estimate that you have passed a cup of bloody fluid—a huge amount—that probably means less than half a cup of blood, which would be two percent of your total blood, or one fourth of what you would give as a blood donor.*

If you determine that you have lost a small amount of blood, you do not have an emergency but rather an urgent problem. Seconds, minutes, even hours will not make the difference between life and death.

To sum up, if the bleeding is uncontrollable and severe—for example passing two cups of bloody fluid in a few minutes—you have a true emergency and should get to the nearest emergency facility in the quickest way possible. Anything less than that would be an urgent problem. You have time to call first for advice, unless you are far from help.

CHOKING AND SERIOUS DIFFICULTY IN BREATHING

To Have on Hand:
Vaporizer (For Croup)

Training:
Cardio-Pulmonary Resuscitation; Heimlich Maneuver
    A pediatrician nearly panics when he hears from his answering service that a mother has just called because her baby is having

difficulty breathing. Alarm bells ringing in his brain, he calls back instantly and learns that what the mother meant is that the child's stuffy nose is interfering with breathing. Colds, of course, do that.

There are various reasons why someone might be having serious difficulty breathing: a severe asthma attack, a heart attack, shock, brain damage, or drowning. The situation is an emergency and usually calls for a trip to the emergency room, or CPR, if the victim has completely stopped breathing.

Choking is the inability to breathe—not just coughing because of swallowing the wrong way. It is such an emergency that you would seldom have time to get a victim to the ER.

Learn to do the Heimlich Maneuver. It is easy to do and very effective. Developed by Dr. Henry J. Heimlich, it is a method that should be taught by a qualified first aid teacher.

But to give you some idea, here is a verbal description. The basic procedure involves standing behind the choking person and clasping your arms around his or her waist. One of your hands grasps the other, which is formed into a fist. You then apply sudden sharp pressure upwards. There are important variations for victims who are infants, pregnant, or unconscious.

At present, there is a good deal of controversy over the treatment of choking. Major organizations such as the Red Cross are still recommending back blows to dislodge the object in the windpipe. (Dr. Heimlich himself opposes back blows as dangerous, pointing out that they may force the object in even further.) The American Heart Association teaches a procedure called the chest thrust, adapted from the Heimlich Maneuver, with the idea of minimizing possible damage to the body caused by Heimlich's technique.

Death from choking occurs within three to four minutes. Because the Heimlich Maneuver is a proven and effective technique for a life and death problem, we think any possible risks are outweighed by its well-documented benefits.

Unconsciousness
If someone has sustained a head injury and has had even a brief spell of true unconsciousness, meaning that he or she could not be roused with a pinch or a shake, medical evaluation is necessary. But if the person is still unconscious, you must transport him or her as quickly as possible to a hospital emergency room. (You would use resuscitation techniques only if breathing stopped.)

If someone who has diabetes becomes unconscious, this must be considered a critical emergency. Get the patient to the hospital as soon as possible.

Fainting

Unlike an unconscious person, someone who has fainted can be roused. Fainting, light-headedness, or dizziness is best treated by having the person lie down in order to restore proper circulation to the brain. If you should feel faint, sitting down with your head between your legs accomplishes the same thing.

Although victims of fainting in books and films are always being plied with glasses of water and slugs of brandy, this is the worst possible thing to do. A person who has fainted cannot swallow properly and may aspirate the liquid, which could cause pneumonia or worse.

Stroke

Victims may suddenly lose the ability to move an arm or leg, or to speak. There is nothing you can do on the spot. Get the person to a hospital emergency room as fast as possible.

POISONING

To Have on Hand:
  syrup of ipecac
  activated charcoal

To Know: Emergency Room or Poison Control Telephone Number

Poisoning, including any kind of drug overdose, is an emergency. If a telephone is closer than the emergency room, call first, because there may be something you can do to begin treatment immediately. Never induce vomiting or give antidotes without medical advice.

Most emergency rooms have a telephone link with poison control centers and can give you the most up-to-date information. When you call, be sure to have on hand whatever container or vial the poisonous substance or drug came from. Take it with you when you go to the hospital.

CHEST PAIN

Significant chest pain is caused by a serious problem of either the heart or the lungs. Sharp pains associated with sudden difficulty in breathing may mean a pneumothorax (collapsed lung). A heart attack is generally not characterized by sudden sharp pain. The victim may break into a cold sweat and may complain of feelings of severe pressure or a crushing sensation. He or she may experience a sense of dread.

Whether or not chest pain is a critical emergency is perhaps the most difficult situation to judge. If the above very dramatic symptoms are present, it most definitely is. Sometimes, though, the victims of heart attacks will deny symptoms or attribute them to indigestion.

To some extent, you have to play the odds. Chest pain in anyone under thirty-five, or in a woman under fifty, is almost never a heart attack, unless there is something unusual about that person's genetics or health history.

Anxiety about chest pain can make the pain seem much worse. If you are in a low-risk age group, relax, take some deep breaths, and lie down for a couple of minutes. If the pain is unchanged, call your doctor. If you do not have or cannot reach a doctor, the safest thing would be to go to the ER.

Someone in a higher risk group, and certainly someone with a history of heart disease, who is experiencing severe chest pain should put in a quick call to the doctor, but head for the ER if there is no immediate call back.

If you must give emergency aid to someone who is having severe chest pain, one of the most important things you can do is to speak and act calmly and reassuringly. Panic affects the body; it can constrict blood vessels and raise the pulse rate.

CONVULSIONS

Most are of such short duration that they have ended by the time you get to an emergency facility. Unless the person is known to have a seizure disorder, he or she will need immediate medical attention.

If you are not sure where to go, you have time to make one or two calls. For example, should the convulsion occur in a child, you would be much better off going to a hospital where he or she can be seen by a physician (pediatrician, family practitioner or specialist in emergency medicine) who is familiar with this type of problem in children.

EYE INJURIES ARE URGENT

To Have: Cotton Swabs
Eye injuries should have medical attention fairly quickly. You can try to remove a "foreign body" in the eye—a piece of sand or grit. Lift the upper eyelid and roll it backward over a matchstick. You can then remove the speck very gently with a cotton swab or a corner of a tissue. If you are not successful, you must see a doctor or go to an emergency room for help within a few hours. Even a little piece of grit can scratch the delicate surface of the eye.

FEVER AND BROKEN BONES: YOU HAVE TIME

To Have on Hand:
Thermometer (Rectal for Infants,
Oral for Older Children and Adults)
Admittedly, young children are susceptible to febrile convulsions (seizures that may accompany high fever), but they will have the convul-

sion as the fever is rising, not after it reaches its peak. Therefore, a fever of 105° F in a three-year-old is not an emergency if the child is alert and responsive. If the child is inert and unresponsive, an emergency may well exist even if there is no fever.

A fracture may seem like a critical emergency, but it is not.

> A seven-year-old girl is attempting to do a cartwheel. Suddenly her parents hear a scream from her room. They rush in to find her lying on the floor writhing in pain, with her elbow at the opposite angle from normal. She is obviously seriously injured, but a few minutes will not make a difference. She is neither bleeding nor unconscious, so there is time to make a splint using her wooden blocks, to wrap the splint with a shawl, and then to bind her arm to her body by wrapping her tightly in a blanket. Immobilizing her arm does two things. It reduces pain, and it prevents further damage.
>
> Her parents call their doctor, who advises them to take the extra five minutes necessary to get to the hospital with the best orthopedic care.

HEATSTROKE

This is a medical emergency that occurs most often during heatwaves. Elderly people, or those suffering from heart disease or from alcoholism are especially vulnerable, as are people who do an unaccustomed amount of exercise in very hot weather. Infants who are left in a closed car in direct sunlight, or who are wrapped up too warmly when feverish are also at risk.

The victim should be taken to a hospital emergency room immediately if possible. Evaporative cooling rather than an ice bath is now the recommended treatment. If there is no ER nearby, you should put the victim in the shade, remove as much clothing as possible, and keep the skin wet and fanned. Ice packs are helpful; a handful of cubes wrapped in a cloth will do. Apply them at the neck, armpits, abdomen, and groins.

HYPOTHERMIA

A body temperature that is too low can be as dangerous as one that is too high, but this condition is not always easy to recognize. Victims may not shiver or even feel cold. In fact, some even feel sensations of warmth and will undress. Signs to look for are mental confusion, impaired gait, drowsiness, and combativeness.

According to *The Medical Letter*,[1] "Old age, lack of adequate housing, alcohol ingestion, and diseases such as convulsive disorders and diabetes are predisposing factors in urban hypothermia . . ." Prolonged exposure to cold air or water in the great outdoors can cause hypothermia in healthy people.

Get to an emergency treatment facility as quickly as possible. Gone are the days when you dumped someone in a hot bath or rolled them up in an electric blanket or sent a St. Bernard with a flask of brandy. Instead, victims should be handled cautiously and gently. Remove any wet clothing and wrap the patient in dry blankets.

Breathing and heart beat may be almost undetectable, but take great care and at least a full minute to establish whether CPR is necessary.

BURNS

First degree burns (redness only) and *second degree burns* (blisters) that affect only a limited area—the kind of burn you get from a hot stove or frying pan—can all be treated at home. Cover immediately with cold compresses or immerse in cold water. This will both relieve the pain and minimize the extent of the injury. All burns that are more severe will need immediate medical attention.

Chemical burns produced by corrosive substances must be treated *immediately* by continuously rinsing with water for at least fifteen minutes. Do this before you call the doctor or drive to the emergency room.

SOME COMMON NON-EMERGENCIES: STUBBED TOES, SPRAINS, APPENDICITIS

You have stubbed your fifth toe very badly; it is very painful, swollen, and possibly broken. An obvious case for immediate treatment, right? If you get expert help, your expert will take some tape and bind your broken toe to its neighbor. Why not do the taping yourself? You will reduce the pain by immobilizing the toe and save yourself time and money. If the pain persists for a day or two, and you want to know whether you did break the toe, you can arrange for a visit to a doctor's office. This advice does not apply to your big toe, for which you would need medical attention.

More serious is a badly injured ankle. But, whether you have sprained or broken it, the first treatment is the same: stay off your foot, elevate it on a footstool, and keep ice on it. Whether you rush to the ER or treat this problem at home will not affect the outcome, especially since it is better to avoid putting a cast on an extremity that is still swelling up from an injury. As long as you avoid putting weight on the injured leg, you are not hurting yourself if you do not get immediate attention.

Appendicitis is the first thing to enter the mind of someone who has an attack of severe pain in the abdomen. "I've learned," says one experienced physician, "that when my answering service tells me that someone has just called with possible appendicitis, that is the one thing it isn't. Appendicitis does not start out as a very sharp pain. Usually by the time I call them back the pain is gone." Sudden sharp abdominal pains are almost always caused by gas.

Appendicitis is an urgent problem, not an emergency problem unless you wait until the appendix is ready to rupture or perforate before calling for advice. Early symptoms include feeling increasingly unwell, losing all appetite, and increasing pain in the abdomen rather than a sudden sharp pain. Possibly there will be some vomiting, especially in children, and some fever. There is plenty of time to wait for a call back from your doctor. If you do not have a doctor and you have these symptoms, you will have to make a trip to the ER.

CPR

We recommend that everyone learn to do cardio-pulmonary resuscitation (CPR). Deaths from heart attacks have been cut by twenty-five percent in communities where a large number of citizens have been trained in this procedure. The sooner treatment begins, the better; but to be successful it must be started within four minutes or so after breathing stops.

CPR is also used on victims of severe electrical shock or drowning. If the drowning occurs in cold water, the victim may be revived even after thirty minutes or more of immersion.

If your spouse has had a heart attack, it is critical that you and any teen-aged children in your family learn this skill. CPR is taught by a number of agencies. Some do it free of charge; others impose a small fee. (See Resource Directory for information on how to find a CPR class.)

CHILD-PROOFING YOUR HOME: PREVENTIVE FIRST AID

Even better than knowing how to treat an emergency is knowing how to prevent one. Parents of infants and young children should go over their homes carefully, removing the kinds of hazards that can kill or injure. Although it has always been something of a mystery why the toddler who screams and cries when asked to eat string beans would drink bleach, it nevertheless happens with distressing frequency.

Put plastic socket covers in all unused electrical outlets.
Lock up cleaners, paints, and household chemicals, or place them out of reach on high shelves. There are special gadgets that can be installed on cabinets to make them childproof.
Make sure that knives and other sharp objects are kept well out of reach.

Small objects that can be swallowed, like pins and coins, can be dangerous. "Button" batteries are particularly hazardous.

Make sure that houseplants are out of reach. Some are poisonous when ingested.

Be careful of where you store medicines and vitamins. Some products, such as baby aspirin, have fruit flavors and may seem like candy. Keep them in a locked cabinet.

Are there heavy objects the child may pull over? (Tableclothes are especially tempting to little children.)

What about electrical appliances such as heaters?

Take doors off old refrigerators that are not in use.

Block off stairs with gates.

Keep lids down on toilet seats. Cases have been reported of toddlers who drowned face down in the toilet bowl.

Install window guards if you do not live on the ground floor.

Don't forget: use car seats for infants and young children at all times—seat belts for older children and adults.

SPECIAL WARNING: SUICIDE GESTURES AND THREATS ARE AN EMERGENCY

Any threat or attempt to commit suicide—especially by a child or teen-ager—is an emergency and must be taken seriously, no matter how manipulative it may seem. Some people seeing only a scratch on the wrist that is not even bleeding, or hearing that the person has taken six cold pills, try to make light of the situation.

The idea that someone you care about is desperately unhappy is painful and difficult to face. So difficult that yelling, preaching, scolding, joking, or ignoring are more common responses than an immediate attempt to get professional help.

If a person who is in therapy attempts suicide, you can start by calling his or her therapist—unless medical attention is necessary. The therapist will usually take over and tell you what to do next. If the person does not have a therapist, call an experienced mental health professional, if you know one, for advice on how to proceed.

Otherwise, your only option may be to bring the person to an emergency room. In this case, make sure beforehand that the hospital has a psychiatrist on call. An evaluation by a mental health professional is essential, and a 24-hour admission to the hospital for observation is often a good idea. Afterward, the patient will need some form of ongoing therapy to deal with the underlying problem and prevent a recurrence.

You can call your primary care doctor for advice, but you should realize that some physicians are not aware of the urgency of this kind of situation. Perhaps, like too many of us, they believe that "so-and-so is just trying to get attention" or "people who talk about it never do it."

(It is critically important to understand that talking about suicide is one of the signs of an impending attempt.)

A failed attempt, no matter how inept or obviously designed to be discovered, should be treated as an emergency. Many successful suicides were not actually intended to succeed. The person who is desperate for help or attention may miscalculate the amount of pills. The friend or lover who was supposed to appear at the door at a certain time is delayed.

Finally, if someone tells you in confidence that he or she is planning to commit suicide, you have the moral right—indeed, the moral obligation—to place that person's life ahead of your own discomfort at a breach of confidence, and to call for help. As a matter of fact, you can assume that the person confiding in you hopes you will do exactly that, no matter what protestations he or she may make to the contrary. Someone who is absolutely intent on self-destruction is not going to warn anyone about it ahead of time. If you have any doubts about the wisdom of this advice, read the affecting and sensitive book, *Vivienne, the Life and Suicide of an Adolescent Girl,* by Mack and Hickler (see Bibliography).

FIRST AND FINAL EMERGENCY ADVICE

In his book of medical black humor *The House of God,* Sam Shem gives a little professional advice that applies equally well in or out of the hospital. He suggests that the first step for doctors dealing with a cardiac arrest is to take their own pulse. In other words, before acting in an emergency, take a moment to make sure you yourself are in control—a few deep breaths, a momentary gathering of the inner forces. Ten seconds won't hurt the victim, but if it helps you to think more clearly, you will be far more effective, and *that* may make the difference between life and death.

CHAPTER SEVEN

DO YOU REALLY NEED A DRUG?

Each of us walks into the doctor's office with a set of private expectations. A woman tells her family she is going to see the doctor about a symptom that troubles her. She says she wants to know if there is something wrong or not. Privately, she wants no such objectivity. She is going because she hopes to hear the doctor say, "It's nothing. You're fine."

Her husband has a different agenda. He is sure he has a physical problem and he wants the doctor to give his symptoms a name, preferably a genuine hyphenated syndrome. If the doctor says, "I find nothing organically wrong; perhaps the stress you are experiencing in your family is contributing to your stomach problems," this man is going to be unhappy. That is not why he made the appointment.

One of the most common expectations when we are sick is that a visit to the doctor will result in a prescription. The doctor will examine us, name our pain, and give us a drug to make the whole thing go away. For many people, a visit that does not result in a prescription is somehow incomplete.

Beyond its medical efficacy, a pill or an injection or a lotion may represent the power of the doctor to cure, or may be a focus for the belief that we are really doing something to cure our illness.

This "placebo effect," the actual curative power of the patient's faith in the drug rather than the effectiveness of its chemical contents, has long been recognized. For most of the history of medicine, healers have prescribed such remedies as crocodile dung and worms and mistletoe and bezoar stones (crystallized tears from the eye of a deer bitten by a snake). Most of these substances have been placebos, although a few, such as digitalis (extracted from the foxglove plant), belladonna (from deadly nightshade), or morphine (from poppies) have become part of our modern pharmacopeia.

What's wrong with wanting a drug? Nothing at all. Some people feel that healing powers reside within their own bodies; others believe that if they ingest the right thing they will get better. If you belong to this second category and if you take a mild infusion of harmless herbs and flowers or a vitamin capsule (bearing in mind that not all herbs and flowers are harmless nor all vitamins safe in large doses), you can, at no risk to your health, enjoy the psychological benefits of feeling that you are doing something. For you, those benefits may be considerable. [We are discussing only the issue of placebo effect here, not the question of whether these treatments can cure.]

But if, in your need to take something, you manage to pressure your doctor into writing a prescription for a drug that isn't really necessary, you may have fulfilled an important emotional need at a price. The medicines that line the pharmacy shelves these days are powerful and carry a number of risks. They can cause everything from dizziness and drowsiness to deafness, kidney failure, and death. Generally, the more powerful the drug, the greater its potential to do harm.

At the other end of the spectrum are the people who hate swallowing pills, those who, having read one too many horror stories about the unknown and toxic effects of medication, regard any prescription with suspicion. This attitude can be protective unless it interferes with the proper treatment of those diseases that drugs treat effectively and safely.

In this chapter we will discuss what drugs actually do and why doctors prescribe them. Our goal is to help you avoid taking drugs you don't need, take correctly the ones you do, and steer clear of those that are dangerous or improperly prescribed.

WHAT YOU NEED TO KNOW
BEFORE YOU TAKE A DRUG

There you sit, examined, diagnosed, and waiting for the doctor's words of wisdom. He or she scribbles something on a prescription pad, hands it to you and says, "I want you to take two of these four times a day for the next seven days." You leave the office and go to the drugstore, hoping that you remembered correctly that it was two, four times a day for the next seven days rather than two every seven hours for the next four days. Fortunately, the pharmacist types out the doctor's instructions and also tells you to take the capsules at mealtimes. You pay and go home.

You wonder why you're taking these pills and why you have to take them with meals. Should you eat four meals a day in order for the medication to work properly? And suppose you feel better after four days; should you take the rest of the pills? Or, if you're not getting better, should you take four pills at a time instead of two? What if you forget one dose; should you double up or skip one? You can call the doctor's office and ask each question as you think of it—or save your effort and your doctor's time by asking careful questions about every prescription you are given.

HOW DO YOU ASK YOUR DOCTOR ABOUT A PRESCRIPTION?

The answer to this is similar to the answer to that well-known riddle of animal behavior: How do porcupines make love? The answer to both questions is "Very, very carefully."

For nonsurgeons especially, the choice of drug is a highly charged issue. Perhaps that is because for "medical" doctors—the internists, pediatricians, psychiatrists, family physicians, allergists, dermatologists, and various medical subspecialists—the prescribing of drugs tends to be the most powerful arrow in their quiver. Surgeons can cut you open, extract various parts, stitch other things together, insert new organs and "really do something." Nonsurgeons can stick needles and other instruments into various parts of your body, but in most cases, they do this to make a diagnosis, so it is not as satisfying.

Doctors are trained to *cure,* not care. Both their power to prescribe and their skill in choosing the right drug are critical to their sense of themselves as "real doctors" who have the power to make you well.

You ask, as you have every right to do, "Why have you prescribed this drug?" meaning, "What can I expect it to do for me?" But the doctor may hear, "Do you really know anything about drugs? How can I trust you to prescribe correctly?"

For some doctors, your simple request for information may be tantamount to questioning their whole being: all the years of sacrifice, the student loans, the 48-hour shifts, the life and death decisions, etc. Fortunately, once you have a comfortable relationship with your doctor, this need for caution will not apply.

To keep the doctor from becoming defensive, we suggest you start by making it clear that you want information by asking, "Could you tell me something about this drug?"—or "Could you explain exactly what this drug will do for me?"

QUESTIONS TO ASK

Once the topic is smoothly launched, the first thing you need to know is whether the drug is being prescribed to relieve your symptoms or to treat your illness. If the doctor tells you it is for symptoms, ask yourself if they are bothersome enough to treat. If so, then ask the following questions:

1. What kind of side effects and risks are there?
2. How effective is it?
3. How expensive is it?

SIDE EFFECTS AND RISKS

Drugs are poisons: helpful in the correct dose, ineffective in too small a dose, and dangerous in one that is too large. Through a long process of testing, researchers determine what they call a "normal therapeutic dosage range." Taken in amounts within this range, the helpful effects of a drug will be most significant and the harmful effects minimal. This is why you must take a drug exactly as prescribed.

Because they are poisons, you should avoid drugs unless they are clearly necessary. They all may cause side effects, things like drowsiness or nausea that will pass when you stop taking the drug. Side effects are not considered medically dangerous, yet they may endanger you. Antihistamines, for example, commonly cause drowsiness. If you became drowsy while driving, crashed into a tree, and died, your doctor would not consider your demise a drug-related death. In medical thinking, the drowsiness caused by the drug is not a risk.

Risks are the physiologically dangerous effects that a drug may have on your body. Some drugs have almost none; some will cause a reaction in a tiny handful of people; some are fairly dangerous for everyone—and are only to be used when all else fails. The antibiotic chloramphenicol is an example of a drug with serious risks. It should only be used for life-threatening infections. Why? Because one of the risks of this drug is that it may kill you by causing your bone marrow to stop making the white blood cells you need to fight infections.

TAKING DRUGS FOR SYMPTOMS

To treat passing symptoms, you would never take a drug that has risks; you might, however, decide to tolerate side effects, knowing that if they became sufficiently distressing you could always discontinue the drug.

In thinking about side effects you must take your way of life into account. For example, drowsiness is a much more serious problem to someone who makes a living driving a truck or a taxi than to a person who works at a desk.

Cost, too, may be a factor. Relieving a somewhat annoying but temporary symptom may not be worth the money to you.

If the expense or a particular side effect is a problem, mention these or other concerns to your doctor. He or she may come up with an alternative that would suit you.

TAKING DRUGS TO CURE A PROBLEM

If the doctor tells you that the drug is for treatment, then you must ask somewhat different questions:

1. If the drug has undesirable side effects, what can be done to minimize them?

2. What are the risks?
3. How is it administered?
4. How effective is it?
5. Is there an alternative with fewer risks or side effects?
6. Are there any special precautions to observe?
7. If the drug is expensive, is there a less costly alternative?
8. Will I have problems with any sort of interaction: with other drugs I am taking, with foods, alcohol, vitamins?

Many of these factors intertwine. For example, the cheapest drug may not be as convenient to take. Many drugs come in a sustained-release form; you have to take them only once or twice a day, rather than four times a day. Sustained-release drugs are usually much more expensive, perhaps costing $15 for a week of treatment instead of $5. If, however, you know you will never remember to take a drug four times a day, you may decide to use the most costly form.

Sometimes cost and effectiveness are intertwined. The doctor may prescribe an expensive drug that is only slightly more effective. For example, a drug may work eighty-eight percent of the time and be one-third the cost of a drug that works ninety-three percent of the time. If your problem isn't serious—a urinary tract infection, for example— you may prefer to try a cheaper drug first to see if it will work. If the expense is important to you, ask your doctor how much the drug costs and whether there is a satisfactory and less expensive alternative. (Of course, the few times the first treatment doesn't work and the second drug is necessary, this strategy will be more costly.)

You may be concerned about the method of administration, or how you take the drug. For certain problems, you have a choice between pills or a shot. Strep throat, for instance, can be treated with one injection of long-acting penicillin or with ten days of oral penicillin. Penicillin shots are painful, but if you know you are going to forget to take drugs on schedule, the shot might be worth considering. Gonorrhea, which until recently was always treated with an injection, may now be treated orally if you prefer.

When you need a drug for treatment, you may have to endure a side effect, but often there are ways to counteract any that prove troublesome. Find out what side effects may occur and be sure to tell your doctor if you experience one that bothers you. A different drug may then be tried in the hope that this particular formulation does not give you the side effect.

Special Precautions
Some drugs may cause abdominal pains if taken on an empty stomach; others won't work unless your stomach is empty. Some are lethal in combination with certain foods. The most noteworthy of these are the MAO inhibitors—used to treat certain types of depression—which

react dangerously with foods that contain tyramine (an odd shopping list that includes such items as aged cheese, ripe bananas, beer, and pickled herring). Others cause problems if you are exposed to sunlight (e.g., tetracycline, Butazolidin®, Retin-A®). Some drugs are to be taken until your symptoms go away; others must be taken for a full course of treatment or you risk a reinfection.

Pregnant women, in particular, must be especially careful in the use of any medication, prescription or nonprescription, especially in the first trimester. Nursing mothers, too, must take special precautions. Be sure to tell your physician and pharmacist if you are either pregnant or nursing.

Monitoring
If you learn that a drug may cause serious problems, ask your doctor whether there are some early signs to watch for. For example, if you are taking an anti-inflammatory drug that may cause a bleeding peptic ulcer, you should know beforehand to watch and report acid indigestion, stomach distress, and dark, tarry stools. These may be warning signs. For other kinds of drugs, regular blood tests will detect abnormalities at an early enough stage so that the drug may be discontinued before serious damage to vital organs occurs.

THE MOST IMPORTANT QUESTION

Of all the questions we have suggested you ask, the critical one is, *"What are the risks?"* Is there any danger to your life or health in taking this medication and if so, how statistically common are those risks?

Almost every drug can cause what doctors term an "idiosyncratic" reaction, one that happens only to a tiny percentage of people. Some drugs, however, have serious risks that are not all that uncommon. If there are no safe alternatives to a particular drug, then you need to ask two more questions.

What are the risks in not treating the disease?
How sure are you that I do have this disease?

RISK VERSUS BENEFIT

We discussed the question of risk versus benefit in Chapter Four in a surgical context, where we pointed out that if the risks of the surgery are great, then the condition it treats should be serious and the hope it offers substantial.

The same thing is true of drugs. The more risky they are, the more carefully they must be prescribed. Powerful drugs may have serious risks. They may cause damage to kidneys, heart, liver, and brain. They may kill you. For some antibiotics, for example, there is a very narrow margin between how much will kill only germs and how much will damage your kidneys. Drugs that help people with heart disease by thinning their blood may, if not administered carefully, cause internal bleeding.

Actually, we are involved on a daily basis with risk/benefit decisions without being aware that this is the case. Driving a car, taking an airplane, skiing, all carry certain risks—whether or not we think about them, weigh them in the balance, and decide that they are worth it.

For many people, taking a drug that kills one out of every million of those who ingest it seems more frightening than driving a car to the supermarket or skiing down a hill, two activities that may have less favorable odds. Perhaps it is because we fantasize that our own skill in driving or skiing will protect us but have no such confidence in our ability to swallow a pill in a special way that will prevent the danger.

DRUG INTERACTIONS

Any time you take a drug, you need to find out if it is going to be affected by other drugs you are taking or by what you eat or drink or smoke or otherwise ingest. Undesirable combinations may lessen the effectiveness of your prescription or cause serious damage to your body.

According to the March 6, 1981 issue of *The Medical Letter* (a newsletter we discuss later in the chapter), there are more than 400 known drug interactions. They involve such commonly prescribed medications as ampicillin (an antibiotic), which decreases the effectiveness of birth control pills, or antacids, which decrease the absorption of digoxin (a drug used to treat heart problems).

If you are aware that these interactions occur, you can avoid serious problems. Usually, your doctor will deal with the situation by adjusting the dosage of one of the drugs.

When your doctor whips out the prescription pad, ask what interactions you should be concerned about, if any. He or she is likely to have a tome called the *PDR (Physicians' Desk Reference)*, which lists side effects, risks, and interactions.

Make sure you mention everything you are taking—prescription or nonprescription drugs, vitamins, your daily three-martini lunch. (Alcohol is one of the worst substances to mix with medications.)

When you fill your prescription, go over possible interactions with the pharmacist.

Consult books like *The Essential Guide to Prescription Drugs* or *the People's Pharmacy,* which have lists of drugs and their interactions.

COMBINATION MEDICATIONS

If you need more than one drug to treat your problem, you may feel it would be simpler to take a single pill. Unfortunately, what you gain in simplicity, you lose in precision and safety. That single pill may contain ingredients you don't need and may be formulated in dosage levels that are wrong for your particular case. In addition, as you raise the number of ingredients, you also increase your chances of having an allergic reaction—or a long-range adverse effect if you must take drugs for a chronic problem.

There are some types of combination drugs that are useful; others that are not. To find out whether you really need the combination, ask your doctor or pharmacist the following two questions:

1. Do I need all the ingredients?
2. Are the dosage levels correct for my problem?

People who may have the most to gain from asking these two questions are those who must take drugs to control their high blood pressure and want to minimize side effects. Combination drugs may not allow enough flexibility in adjusting dosages.

There are exceptions to this rule, in particular Septra® or Bactrim®; in this case, each of the components (trimethoprim and sulfamethoxazole) alone is less effective in killing bacteria than the combination. Many birth control pills similarly are more effective if they combine more than one hormone. Most combination drugs, however, are designed merely to save you the effort of taking more than one pill. If your doctor is prescribing a combination medication, be sure it is more effective, not just more convenient.

WHAT IF YOU DON'T LIKE THE ANSWERS TO YOUR QUESTIONS?

If you have a doctor who is up-to-date on the subject of medication, reads *The Medical Letter,* or takes courses or attends lectures on pharmacology, you can safely use him or her as a source of information. If such a doctor doesn't already know the answers to your questions, he or she will either try to find the answers or refer you to a knowledgeable pharmacist.

If, no matter how tactfully you raise your questions, your doctor is unwilling to discuss the subject, you might very well consider changing doctors. You have a right—and really a responsibility to yourself—to find out everything you can before you take something with the potential for harm that many drugs have.

Some doctors are not especially thoughtful in the way they prescribe. They may rely for their information on the drug company sales reps. These are salespeople, not neutral and objective professionals. Doctors may prescribe drugs based on habit rather than well-researched information, or they may have a fondness for trying the newest product. Often, they are not as well-informed as a good clinical pharmacist, a professional whose role is discussed later in this chapter.

WHAT IS A THERAPEUTIC TRIAL?

Doctors may, at times, prescribe a drug when they suspect a certain problem but are not sure. In order to confirm the diagnosis, they have you take a "therapeutic trial" of the drug that would treat the disease they suspect you have. If you improve, then the diagnosis is confirmed.

Before you agree to take a drug for this reason, ask three questions:

1. Are the risks of the drug less than those of leaving the disease untreated?
2. Are there alternative methods for establishing the diagnosis?
3. Are the risks of the drug less than the risks of any of those methods?

WHAT DOCTORS MEAN BY "COMPLIANCE"

"Patient compliance" is doctors' lingo and embodies their view that desirable qualities in the people they treat are passivity and obedience. The nondoctor—as good a term for most people in the world as "outpatient" is for all the people who are not in the hospital—might call patient compliance, "doing what the doctor tells you to do." The assumption here is that the doctor speaks and the patient listens.

Despite the negative connotations of the term, the concept behind it does represent an advance in medical education; physicians in training are now learning about how important the patient's attitudes and knowledge are to successful treatment, especially when that treatment takes place outside the controlled world of the hospital.

When doctors talk about patient compliance, they generally mean the degree to which the patient will adhere to the regimen prescribed, usually a drug that must be taken in precise amounts at specific intervals for a given length of time. A lot of us don't take our medicine the way we should. Millions of dollars are spent on drugs each year by people who never use them at all!

Some people will faithfully follow their doctors' orders. Some won't. Many of us (including all doctors) want to know why a drug is necessary and what will happen if we don't take it. Teaching us these things is as much a doctor's responsibility as diagnosing and prescribing.

Whether or not your doctor is an effective teacher, your active participation is necessary to the success of your treatment. For your own sake . . .

Make sure you understand what the medication is, what it is supposed to do for you, and what possible side effects may accompany it.

If you experience unpleasant side effects, let the doctor know right away.

If you have not taken the medication, tell your doctor.

Try to figure out why you did not. Are the pills so large they are hard to swallow? Do you have difficulty remembering to take them more than once a day? (Many people do.) Is your drug-taking schedule confusing? If you must take one drug three times a day and another four times, you might have a hard time remembering all your doses. Do you dislike taking any medication? Do you hate taking the pills because they remind you that there is something wrong with your body? If you can verbalize the reason you did not take the medicine, your doctor may help you find a solution.

TEEN-AGERS AND THE DRUGS
THEY ARE SUPPOSED TO TAKE

Teen-agers, especially those with chronic diseases, often have a difficult time taking medications properly. While challenging adult authority is a normal adolescent response to life, it may interfere with health. If this is a problem in your household, you can do the following:

· Find a doctor who will deal directly with the adolescent.
· Find someone who enjoys the age group and is secure enough to handle challenges to his or her authority. The world's most brilliant physician won't do much good if the patient won't follow the treatment regimen.
· Let the doctor take the responsibility for what goes on. If parents are clever enough to remove themselves to the sidelines, they may also remove rebellion as a reason for failing to make medication.

DRUGS THAT ARE OVERPRESCRIBED

We are going to alert you to a number of drugs that tend to be overused. Some are drugs patients ask for; some are ones that doctors like to prescribe. Just as we warned you about the kinds of operations that are often performed unnecessarily, we suggest that you be especially careful about using the drugs we discuss in this next section. We will explain some of the wrong and some of the right reasons to use these drugs. Ultimately, your best protection is to ask questions and make sure you have been given a good explanation as to why you need a given prescription.

ANXIETY, SLEEPLESSNESS, PAIN:
WHEN SHOULD YOU TAKE MEDICINE?

Much of the energy of pharmaceutical science seems devoted to finding remedies for the stresses and strains of being alive and human. Sometimes a pill helps enormously; sometimes it interferes with solving a problem. If you are in pain from a disease or an injury, if you are going through a temporary life crisis and cannot sleep, if you are afflicted with anxiety and need medication in order to begin therapy, medication may be truly helpful.

Such limited and careful uses, however, cannot possibly account for the quantities of Darvon®, Valium®, Librium®, Dalmane, Seconal®, and Nembutal® that people consume. For years such drugs have been in the top ten of all drugs prescribed. (Until a few years ago, amphetamines given in order to suppress appetite or to "pep up" depressed "housewives" were also high on the list. Eventually, their dangers were recognized and strict controls placed on them.)

ANTI-ANXIETY DRUGS

Valium and Librium are much too frequently prescribed, a fact that received comic emphasis in the film *Starting Over*. When Burt Reynolds faints in a crowded New York department store (Bloomingdale's), his companion desperately asks the crowd that gathers, "Does anyone have a Valium?" Everyone does. (The movie is not far off the mark. If you doubt it, try asking as an experiment.) Jill Clayburgh, his co-star, then went on to dramatize the serious addictive possibilities of too much Valium in her portrayal of the heroine of the movie *I'm Dancing as Fast as I Can.*

Overprescription may occur when physicians misdiagnose emotional problems. For instance, Valium is often prescribed for people who have trouble sleeping on the assumption that anxiety is the cause of the problem. But if, as is common, depression is the cause of the sleeplessness, Valium, which acts as a depressant, will make things worse.

Another assumption that can lead to overprescription is the idea that just as a pain killer must be taken for physical pain, so must an emotional pain killer be taken to blot out feelings of anxiety or misery. All anxiety or misery is not necessarily bad. Immediately giving someone Valium because something sad or stressful has happened—death of a loved one, losing a job, starting college—may deaden feelings and prevent acceptance and adjustment.

If someone cannot manage during an intensely stressful time, a careful physician may prescribe an antianxiety drug for perhaps a week or so. After that, a consultation with a mental health professional will be much more helpful than refills of the prescription. (See Chapter Eight for more on Valium.)

THE PROBLEM WITH SLEEPING PILLS

· Sleeping pills become ineffective after a short period of time. Barbiturates may no longer help you sleep after a week; Dalmane will become ineffective after about a month.
· Because the body becomes tolerant of most sleeping medications, people tend to increase the dose, leading to addiction. Furthermore, some of these drugs have a narrow margin between the dose that may be needed by a chronic user and one that can kill. This problem may be compounded by the mental confusion the pills cause: the users forget that they took some only a short while ago. (This may have been the cause of Marilyn Monroe's death.)
· Chronic sleeplessness is a symptom of underlying anxiety, depression, or some other problem. Blotting out this important symptom prevents people from getting necessary care.

BEFORE YOU TAKE A PAIN KILLER . . .

Pain is actually one of your body's best natural defenses. It is a signal that something is wrong. Pain tells you to withdraw your hand from a hot stove or to keep your weight off an injured foot, and you respond correctly by snatching your hand away before the burn becomes too severe or limping so that the full weight of your body stays off the weakened foot.

Many of us, however, ignore equally important pain messages, such as recurrent heartburn or frequent tension headaches. Our body is signalling us to eat less or relax more, but instead we take medication to relieve the pain without doing anything to correct the underlying cause.

Since mind and body are not separate realms, chronic pain may also be a symptom of an emotional problem. Just because you cannot identify a medical reason for pain does not make it less real or any less necessary to attend to.

DARVON AND PAIN

Once touted as a non-narcotic pain medication, Darvon is now labeled "narcotic" in the *PDR*. This drug, which is chemically very similar to methadone, may lead to psychological or physical dependence. Its usefulness as a pain reliever, however, is not especially impressive. In fact, a number of studies have shown it to be not only less effective than aspirin, or acetaminophen, but also no more effective than a placebo![1] Many doctors, however, will tell you about patients for whom Darvon has seemed more effective than any over-the-counter pain relief.

What the properly designed studies take into consideration and what the doctors' reported experience does not, is the placebo effect. If you expect that your Darvon, which requires a prescription, is going to be more powerful than the aspirin or acetaminophen that anyone can buy in the supermarket, you may actually experience more pain relief. The experience is not imaginary, but the chemical effectiveness of the drug is.

Just because Darvon is ineffective does not mean it is a harmless sugar pill. An overdose can kill you, and habitual use in doses greater than prescribed can result in addiction. Why is this drug so commonly prescribed? Doctors will explain that patients demand it in the belief that this is the only thing that helps their pain.

Underlying the problem of Darvon is the question of what should be done about pain. If aspirin or acetaminophen will not do the trick, should you ask for a drug like this and should your doctor prescribe it?

Careful doctors want to know more about why you are having pain. If it does not seem to be caused by an identifiable organic disease, they may wonder if it might be caused by depression, which can be treated more effectively in other ways.

STEROIDS AND POWER

Many doctors feel that drugs are their "weapons" in what they perceive to be a "battle" against disease. In this martial metaphor, the newest and most potent weapon makes them feel the most powerful. What general would extol the virtues of bayonets if he (or she?) could get his hands on a heat-seeking missile, even though this latest invention may destroy the village in order to save it?

The use of a group of drugs known as *steroids* (compounds that are derived from or resemble hormones manufactured by the adrenal glands) is a good example of this "drug-as-power" attitude. One of the major discoveries in the history of medicine, this extremely powerful class of drugs has saved countless lives.

Steroids can, however, have extremely serious side effects. For example, prednisone, a commonly prescribed steroid, may raise blood pressure, reactivate latent tuberculosis, cause blood clots to form, inflame the pancreas, produce a peptic ulcer, or create a serious mental disturbance. Some of these adverse effects can lead to confusing situations:

> Karen, a young woman of twenty-four, developed a painful muscle spasm in her neck while on a trip. She saw a doctor who started her on a short course of prednisone. Several days later, she returned to New York. Her family and friends began to notice personality changes, culminating in her taking an overdose of Valium. She was admitted to a hospital where, at

first, her behavior was so bizarre that the doctors assumed she would have to be sent to a state mental hospital. But after observing her for a day and consulting with several internists and two psychiatrists, they wondered whether she had had a psychotic reaction to the prednisone. The drug was discontinued, and she returned to normal.

Why do doctors prescribe steroids if they can be so dangerous? Because they can be so effective for a number of conditions including:

- serious asthma attacks and other unusual allergic reactions, such as severe poison ivy
- arthritis caused by certain diseases, such as lupus
- certain heart problems, including postpericardiotomy syndrome (a complication of open-heart surgery)
- liver diseases, such as chronic aggressive hepatitis
- kidney diseases, such as nephrotic syndrome
- auto-immune reactions secondary to transplant surgery
- life-threatening illness for which nothing else works

In some medical centers, it is considered almost poor form for someone to die without being treated with "roids." This approach may be fine for the desperately ill; it is not so fine when it is applied to everyone else. Be suspicious of a doctor who jumps to steroids for problems such as asthma, heart disease, or joint pains without trying other forms of treatment first.

Furthermore, steroids must never be taken by anyone with an active peptic ulcer, an eye infection caused by herpes, or active tuberculosis.

THE OVERUSE OF ANTIBIOTICS: WHEN YOU NEED THEM AND WHEN YOU DON'T

Because antibiotics provide such clear examples of what drugs will and won't do for you, we have chosen to discuss them in some detail. Doctors overuse them and their patients overdemand them. The bacteria they are designed to destroy have not disappeared in the teeth of antibiotic warfare; in fact, some have developed more resistant forms.

Note: Technically, the term "antibiotic" refers only to some kinds of drugs that treat infections; the word "antimicrobial" is the broad term that should be used when such agents as Gantrisin® and Flagyl® are to be included. Since many physicians call all antimicrobial agents "antibiotics," we will use that term.

Many people don't know what an antibiotic really does. Ask yourself whether you would need one in each of the following situations:

· you have a painful sore throat
· you have an infected hangnail
· you have a high fever, you feel lousy, and you ache all over

In only one of these three cases would you necessarily need medication. If the area around the hangnail is red, swollen, and oozing a bit of pus, you have definite signs of a bacterial infection. It must be incised and drained, and probably treated with an antibiotic. The painful sore throat and the high fever, however, are likely to be caused by viruses, which will not respond to one of this family of drugs.

What does an antibiotic do? It kills bacteria; the colds and flus and sore throats and stomach aches that viruses cause cannot be cured by drugs. You may alleviate symptoms by taking something: for example, you can bring down a fever with aspirin or acetaminophen and soothe a sore throat with a lozenge or a hard candy. But you will never cure a cold with an antibiotic.

Antibiotics can save your life, but they can also kill you. When penicillin was first released, it represented one of the greatest clinical advances in medical history, saving thousands and thousands of lives; properly used it is still one of the most effective antibiotics. Penicillin, unfortunately, was widely overprescribed. Eventually, it replaced aspirin as the number one allergy-causing drug. In most cases the allergic reaction is a minor rash, but in a very small percentage of people, it is a quick death.

Chloramphenicol was another of the early antibiotics; it turned out to be not only extremely effective but also dangerous. Infants who received it often died. A very small percentage of adults who took it experienced a sudden and irreversible "shutdown" of their bone marrow and died. These days, "chloro" is reserved for life-threatening conditions in which the dangers of dying without the drug outweigh the dangers of dying from it.

Tetracycline was another of the early wonder drugs. It is a "broad spectrum" antibiotic, one that attacks a wide range of organisms. It too has its troublesome quirks. It can permanently stain the teeth of growing children; also, it should not be given to pregnant or nursing women. Outdated tetracycline that has been sitting around the medicine cabinet can cause a dangerous kidney disorder.

In a way, the most frightening result of overuse of antibiotics has been the development of flourishing strains of bacteria that are drug resistant. Now, for example, doctors have begun to find cases of syphilis that are extremely resistant to treatment. In hospitals, where powerful antibiotics are frequently used, there is a marked increase in infections caused by such resistant bacteria.

Sometimes the careless use of antibiotics can endanger health in more complicated ways.

Eight-year-old Jason is sick and feverish. His parents bring him to the doctor, who examines the child and prescribes tetracycline without identifying the cause of the fever. Jason goes home, takes his medicine, but doesn't seem to get any better. He complains of a stiff neck and is listless. His worried parents decide to drive to the nearest medical center.

The doctors there suspect meningitis but are confused when the results of a spinal tap are only slightly abnormal. They are dismayed to learn that Jason has been given an antibiotic.

Standing anxiously by their son's bed, the parents are told that although it is only a possibility that Jason has meningitis, there is no way the doctors can be sure. The tetracycline has interfered with their ability to make an accurate diagnosis. Therefore, to be on the safe side, they will have to assume that the boy has meningitis.

Finally, they explain that they will have to treat Jason with very powerful antibiotics, one of which will be chloramphenicol. Because they do not know which bacterium is responsible, they have to make sure that the drugs used will eliminate all the kinds of bacteria that could cause meningitis.

Doctors are rarely criticized by other physicians for *not* prescribing antibiotics—it is always for treating a cold or fever with tetracycline or for giving a penicillin shot without getting a culture first. Why do they do it, then? Some combination of sloppy medical thinking and a desire to please patients who want a prescription. Enough patient want this approach to create a thriving business in prescribing antibiotics.

COMMON PROBLEMS THAT MAY REQUIRE ANTIBIOTICS

Sore Throats

Except for those caused by gonococcus, the only bacterium that is a significant cause of a sore throat is the streptococcus (strep). And the only reason to treat a strep throat with antibiotics is to prevent the later development of dangerous reactions to the strep—in particular, rheumatic fever. The drug is not given to make you feel better. With or without it, your sore throat will go away.

Therefore, a careful physician will not treat your inflamed throat with an antibiotic without first doing a throat culture to document that the problem is indeed caused by streptococcus.

Some people are upset by all this caution and want to start taking medication right away in the belief that this will help the pain. It won't. If you insist on having a drug, your doctor may agree to write you a prescription for penicillin but will suggest you buy only two or three days' worth until you know you really need the whole course. (It takes ten days to eradicate strep.)

Some physicians prescribe an antibiotic after an examination in which they find you have fever, exudate (pus) on your tonsils, and enlarged, tender lymph nodes (swollen glands), in addition to an inflamed throat. They are, however, playing the odds without being aware of how unfavorable they are. Half the time these symptoms mean you have strep; half the time they don't.

If you still think a throat culture is unnecessary, consider the following scenario:

> Your daughter has had several bad sore throats, which Dr. S. diagnosed as strep without doing a throat culture. Now, you are told that you ought to consider a tonsillectomy. You take her to Dr. L., a well-regarded ENT (ear, nose, throat) specialist who learns of the history of three infections in the past year and recommends surgery. He performs a tonsillectomy, and unfortunately your child has a serious complication.
>
> Could the surgery have been avoided? Quite probably, yes. It is likely that one or more of those sore throats were viral, not strep—and tonsillectomy is not indicated for a history of viral tonsillitis. But without a culture, there was no way of knowing that strep was not the cause.
>
> (See Chapter Five for a discussion of tonsillectomy.)

Vaginitis

This problem may be caused by various types of organisms; some are bacteria, some yeasts, some protozoans. Before your doctor writes a prescription, he or she should examine a sample of the discharge under a microscope, and possibly send a specimen to be cultured. (Pap tests, which diagnose cervical cell changes that may lead to cancer, are often abnormal in the presence of an infection. You may need to have the test repeated when the infection is cleared up.)

Bladder Infections

Before prescribing an antibiotic, your physician should take a careful history, look at a urine specimen under the microscope, and possibly order a urine culture. If you have all the symptoms of a urinary tract infection and the results of the urinalysis are unequivocal, the doctor may save you money by prescribing an antibiotic without ordering a culture. The first time you have a bladder infection, this approach makes sense.

Anyone with recurrent urinary infections or confusing symptoms should not be treated without obtaining a culture. Sometimes, by the way, it is entirely reasonable for the doctor to take the culture and start the antibiotic before the results are back. As long as things are done in this order, no harm will be done. If the drug does not help, the culture will show what organisms are present and what drugs would be effective. You would then be switched to a different medication.

If you take a drug before you give a specimen to be cultured, treatment of your condition will be more difficult. The wrong antibiotic may be able to prevent growth of organisms in a culture medium without being effective enough to eliminate them from your body. Therefore, the lab report will be confusing. (This is the same problem as the "partially treated" meningitis we spoke of earlier.)

Ear Infections
These are exceptions to the rule of lab work first, then antibiotic. Since the infection is usually in the middle ear, the only way to collect a specimen would be to puncture the eardrum with a needle. Only a few research centers do this.

Eye Infections
These too are exceptions. Sometimes they are cultured, but because eye infections are commonly treated with a topical antibiotic, which is safer for your body, it is less critical to pin down the precise diagnosis.

Skin Infections
Problems such as impetigo that are treated with antibiotics should be confirmed by culture. A topical antibiotic alone is not sufficient for moderately severe impetigo; oral medication is needed.

Pneumonia and Bronchitis
A sputum culture is very helpful but is often difficult to obtain. Therefore, it is common practice to begin antibiotics based on a careful physical exam and possibly an x-ray.

Sexually-Transmitted Diseases (STDs)
Prior to treatment, a careful physical examination and lab tests should always be done. You may skip the lab tests and proceed directly to treatment if you learn that a sexual partner has been diagnosed as having a particular STD.

Diarrhea
This problem may be caused either by a virus or by a bacterial infection. Unless there is a positive culture for the latter, you should not take an antibiotic.

Abscesses
These are usually incised and drained, then treated with antibiotics, sometimes given by injection. Unless the infection is exuding pus, there may be nothing to culture.

Sinus Infections

Serious infections with pain, swelling, redness, and sometimes fever (not just stuffy feelings in the sinus areas) are generally treated with an antibiotic after the diagnosis has been confirmed with an x-ray.

FILLING YOUR PRESCRIPTION

Your Drug Profile

Just as a careful physician takes a complete medical history before making a diagnosis, a good pharmacist should take a complete pharmacy history, or drug profile, before filling a prescription. The pharmacist should ask if you have ever taken this drug, or a similar one, before, and if so, whether you had an adverse reaction; what other medications—prescription, nonprescription, vitamins—you are presently taking; what allergies you have to drugs or other substances; whether you have a history of a significant medical problem, such as a bleeding ulcer; and whether you have a chronic disease, such as hypertension or diabetes. Only then can he or she fill your prescription properly.

If you are being cared for by more than one physician, the pharmacist may be the only professional who has your complete drug history, a record that serves as a safeguard for your health. By knowing about past reactions to drugs and checking for possible adverse interactions, the pharmacist can make sure that the drugs you take are as safe for you as possible. An allergic reaction to medication means, at a minimum, that you have wasted money on the prescription; it may also lead to additional physician visits, and in some cases, even hospitalization.

What Will It Cost

To determine which pharmacy to use, call the pharmacies that would be convenient for you and ask what each charges for the three or four medications your family is most apt to need. We did this as an exercise, and the chart below gives the details of what we learned.

We chose Septra, an antibiotic commonly prescribed for urinary tract infections; Ortho-Novum® (birth control pills) because of the chance to save a considerable amount of money on this monthly item; Monistat®, a vaginal cream used to treat monilia; and Diprosone®, an expensive but very convenient and effective steroid cream for atopic dermatitis (an itchy and uncomfortable skin disease).

We called three discount stores and three community pharmacies for prices and also asked if the pharmacists kept drug profiles. Stores A, B, and C on the chart belong to discount chains. Stores D, E, and F are community pharmacies. We found that the most expensive pharmacy charged thirty percent more than the least expensive!

To test prices in your area, you can use our shopping list or draw up

	Store A	Store B	Store C	Store D	Store E	Store F
Septra (Double-strength) 20 tablets	$11.71	$13.59	$11.79	$14.00	$14.95	$12.10
Ortho-Novum 1/35 (21 tablets)	8.49	8.75	8.19	12.35	12.40	9.20
Monistat	10.78	12.23	11.29	12.65	12.60	12.25
Diprosone Cream (45 grams)	15.17	18.90	15.69	18.85	20.15	19.16
Totals	$46.15	$53.37	$46.96	$57.85	$60.10	$52.71

your own. Try to include one prescription that must be refilled. The potential for savings on a continuing prescription in a year is considerable.

It would be nice to find that the pharmacy with the lowest prices also keeps and uses a drug profile, but this is an unlikely combination. The big chains have the biggest discounts and their pharmacists have the least time for service.

Although our shopping list could be filled more cheaply at either of two discount stores (A and C), we would pay a few dollars extra to shop at store F, where the pharmacist kept drug profiles and counseled customers on interactions and the proper use of the drugs they purchased.

If the only pharmacies that take profiles are at the high end of the price spectrum, you may be better off keeping your own drug profile and shopping at the least expensive store. In addition, you can protect yourself by buying a good book on drugs and consulting it before buying any medication, either prescription or nonprescription. (See Resource Directory for sample drug profile and Bibliography for book recommendations.)

Take your profile with you and insist that the pharmacist review it before filling your prescription. Wherever you shop, you should ask the following questions:

1. How should I take this drug?
2. How should I store it?
3. What are the side effects and risks?
4. Under what circumstances should I discontinue the drug or call my doctor?
5. What possible interactions should I be alert for?

THE NEW BREED OF PHARMACISTS

There is a new field called clinical pharmacy, designed for students who are primarily interested in the health care aspects of their profession. Clinical pharmacy programs stress the needs and problems of patients, and their graduates are particularly concerned with the effective, appropriate, and safe use of drugs.

Most clinical pharmacists work in hospitals, prepaid health plans, community health centers, or student health services. They keep careful records of patient drug use, check for possible interactions, counsel patients, keep the medical staff up-to-date on issues of drug safety and efficacy, and make sure that drugs are not being improperly prescribed.

A good clinical pharmacist will make sure you are taking the right drug and dose for your problem and will call a doctor who has prescribed incorrectly to see that your prescription is changed. If you receive care at a health care center that employs a clinical pharmacist, you are in luck, especially if you must use several drugs.

SHOULD YOU TAKE GENERIC DRUGS?

A single drug may be manufactured under many names. It will always have a generic, or chemical name, and some number of trade names, depending on how new it is. For seventeen years after a drug is introduced, it is protected by patent. It then enters the public domain. Penicillin V, for example, is the generic name of a drug that was first marketed in 1953. It is now supplied to the public under its generic name as well as a long string of trade names such as Betapen VK®, Ledercillin VK®, Pen-Vee K®, Robicillin-VK®, Veetids®, etc. Generic drugs are usually, but not always, less expensive than the brand names.

States differ in their laws affecting the dispensing of generic drugs, and you should find out your own state law. In some, for example, pharmacists must fill the prescription with the least expensive effective form of the drug they stock, unless the doctor indicates otherwise. In other states, there is no law governing generics.

Be aware that there is considerable disagreement in the medical community on the issue of generic drugs. Some physicians feel strongly that certain brands of drugs are more effective than others. Pharmacists may object to making routine generic substitutions on the grounds that some generic drugs are poorly manufactured.

The big questions in this debate are "bio-availability" and "quality control." Bio-availability refers to the amount of drug that actually reaches the part of your body that needs it. A capsule contains a given amount of an active ingredient, but this does not guarantee that the stuff will actually arrive at its intended destination. Depending on how it is manufactured, your digestive system may trap it and get rid of it before it has done you any good.

Quality control has to do with the care with which a medication is manufactured, stored, and dispensed. A well-informed and conscientious pharmacist is apt to know more about these factors than most doctors. He or she will know the reputation of the company that manufactures the generic, the comparative bio-availability of chemically comparable drugs, and the price.

In making decisions about drugs, you will encounter yet another confusing aspect of our medical care system. The community pharmacist with all the helpful knowledge is a businessperson, not a consumer advocate. By recommending the cheapest effective generic, he or she may stand to lose money. And, too, just because a drug is a generic does not mean that it will cost less. There are some that even cost more.

Without going to pharmacy school, how are you ever going to decide whether you are saving money at the expense of your health? Our suggestion would be to listen carefully to the style of argument. A pharmacist who maintains that all brand names are better than all generic drugs might well have a financial incentive to sell you the brand names. A doctor who says, "I always prescribe this drug and it works very well," or, "You don't want to take a chance on a drug without a big company in back of it," has not given you an adequate answer.

If, however, you ask your doctor for a generic and are told, "For this particular drug I believe that the most effective form is the one I am prescribing because . . . ," followed by precise reasons, you might well follow this advice.

DON'T UNDERESTIMATE THE OTCs

Over-the-counter, or nonprescription, drugs may do the job as well as a much more expensive prescription medication. Drugs are sold through a doctor's prescription not necessarily because they are stronger or more effective but because they are more dangerous, especially if misused. In fact, many of last year's prescription medications are now being sold over the counter. Because OTCs are relatively safe does not mean they are completely harmless and risk-free. People with significant medical problems such as high blood pressure must be especially careful about taking *any* medications and should check with their physician before treating themselves with OTC drugs.

OTCs treat the kinds of problems that you can diagnose and take care of yourself such as:

· athlete's foot
· poison ivy
· pollen allergies
· infected pierced ear lobes
· mild to moderate acne
· colds

· dandruff
· skin problems such as mild eczema (atopic dermatitis)

The real problem with OTCs is their vast and duplicative array. How do you choose among the endless variations and combinations on the themes of pain, itching, pimples, and congestion? Your best source of information would be either your physician or a good clinical pharmacist if you can find one. Doctors who recommend OTC drugs are helping their patients by saving them money and by teaching them how they can treat a minor problem themselves. (See Bibliography for more sources of drug information.)

SHOULD YOU EVER TAKE A NEW DRUG?

If you have an unusual problem, if the tried-and-true remedies have failed, you may be a candidate for a new drug. Otherwise, there would be little reason to use one.

While the FDA approval process for new drugs sets a certain standard of safety, there is really no substitute for long-term experience with large numbers of people. The longer a drug has been around and the more people who have taken it, the more chance there is to see if it has unsuspected or long-range ill effects. *The Lancet,* a highly respected British medical journal, carried an article with a useful list of questions to ask about any new drug.[2]

Is it more active, microbiologically, than existing compounds?
Is it less toxic than related compounds?
Is it pharmacologically superior to similar agents? (For example, is it better absorbed from the gut; does it penetrate better into infected tissues?)
Is it cheaper than existing agents of similar efficacy?
Do comparative trials indicate superiority over existing agents?

That last question may save you money. Many new drugs simply duplicate those already on the market and are usually more expensive.

THE MEDICAL LETTER:
THE INSIDERS' GUIDE TO DRUGS

For many years, physicians looking for reliable information on drugs have turned to a biweekly newsletter called *The Medical Letter.*[3] It accepts no advertising. This publication has a remarkable track record in sifting through the evidence and coming up with valid conclusions about what drugs are effective and safe. Most of the time, *The Medical Letter* finds that the new, highly touted drugs offer no advantage over well-established ones. When it says that a new drug is worth using, the recommendation is usually for limited situations only.

If you are concerned about a particular medication, this is a first-class source of information, the *Guide Michelin* of drugs. To those who are serious about the restaurants of France, we need say no more. To those who are serious about what kinds of chemicals they put into their bodies, we suggest checking to see what *The Medical Letter* has to say. (See p. 242 for suggestions on how to find medical information.) If your doctor subscribes to it, you have a good indication that he or she is both careful and up-to-date.

CHAPTER EIGHT

MENTAL HEALTH: WHO CAN HELP YOU FIND IT

Psychotherapy—do you want it, want more of it, or want nothing to do with it? For some people the word itself has a mysterious ring. Those who have had some, and have benefited from it, think everyone else ought to try it. Those who need it, and run from it, think anyone who suggests it is trying to label them "crazy." The puritans in our midst fear that getting professional help would somehow be a sign of moral weakness. More liberal thinkers feel that a good dose of insight might improve us all. There tends to be a wider range of reactions to the idea of psychotherapy—some enthusiastic, some doubtful—than to treatments for other health problems.

It is easier for some of us to see a physician for a lingering physical ache or pain that interferes with our lives than it is to consult a mental health professional to treat an emotional problem that interferes just as seriously but in different ways.

Although we think skillful help is valuable and good and *helpful,* we are not suggesting that every emotional difficulty requires a trained professional and a three-year course of therapy. In this chapter, we will try to help you assess just what kinds of problems would lend themselves to treatment. We will also sort out the basic categories of care and care givers, with some guidelines as to cost and credentials. Much of the chapter focuses on psychotherapy, but we will also discuss hospitalization and the use of psychotropic drugs.

WHEN DO YOU NEED THERAPY?

You call a physician when a pain or symptom persists or when you have a sudden severe problem such as a broken leg or internal bleeding. The same holds true of emotional difficulties. We all experience

common reactions to problems and obstacles: anger, frustration, anxiety, guilt, helplessness. These are part of the typical expectable range of human experience. If these reactions are recurrent, persistent, and/or disruptive, preventing us from working and loving and enjoying life, then we might consider getting professional help.

For example, if you are depressed and unhappy because someone you care about is sick or has died, you expect that these feelings will lift in time. Talking to people who are close to you can help you deal with such feelings. If, however, you cannot begin to mourn or cannot stop, you might benefit from counseling.

What do you do if someone tells you that you need therapy? Much depends on who does the telling and why, and whether or not you agree. If, for example, a co-worker tells you that your anger annoys everyone around you and you really should get help, you might want to find out if there is any truth in this. Are you aware of being angry? Do other people experience you as being angry a good deal of the time? Have you ever had a supervisor mention this to you or perhaps even lost a job because of your temper?

In the end, you alone must make the decision to change or seek help. Going to a therapist because someone, be it spouse or boss or lover or parent, thinks you ought to is almost sure to lead to a disappointing experience. Therapy is a kind of working partnership that won't work if you don't do it for your own reasons.

TWO COMMON REASONS TO SEEK HELP

Depression
The least severe form of depression is the mood we call "the blues," a sad, let-down feeling that lasts for a while, then lifts and disappears. It may be provoked by situations you would least expect to cause sadness, such as holidays. Usually, people deal with this kind of mild depression on their own.

A more serious depression is harder to manage without help. Approximately ten to twenty percent of women and five to ten percent of men will have, at least once in their lives, depression serious enough to benefit from treatment.[1]

> Vera B. isn't sure why she is so jumpy and tearful. To help make ends meet, she has returned to work, but her husband and two young children still need an awful lot of attention. She snaps at her kids and has severe arguments with her husband. She isn't hungry and has great difficulty sleeping. Whenever she talks to her friends, they make the same suggestion: quit the job. She can't, though. Her family needs the money. Matters have come to a head because a mild criticism by her boss caused her to burst into tears and run out of the room. Over-

whelmed, she discusses her situation with her doctor, who suggests a consultation with a therapist and provides her with the name of one.

What do you do if you can't seem to shake that "down" feeling; if you find yourself waking up each day feeling irritable, tired, hopeless; if you find that you just aren't interested in anything? These feelings, if persistent, are symptoms of something more serious than a transient mood and should lead you to consider having at least a consultation with a mental health professional.

Often these feelings prevent people who are experiencing them from acting. Be prepared to insist that a close friend or family member who is exhibiting symptoms of depression seek professional help.

The most severe type of depression takes the form of intense sadness and a more pronounced withdrawal from the outside world. The afflicted person may want to stay in bed all day and refuse to talk with other people. He or she may have suicidal thoughts. This kind of depression is extremely debilitating and requires professional intervention. In some instances, medication may be required.

Checklist of Symptoms
If you or someone close to you exhibits one or more of these symptoms, and the feelings persist, you are probably dealing with depression.

sad mood
crying spells
feelings of hopelessness and helplessness
recurring feelings of guilt
not finding pleasure in anything
inability to concentrate, problems with memory
disturbances in sleep patterns (inability to fall asleep, to stay asleep, or to stay awake)
changes in appetite (usually a loss of appetite but sometimes overeating)
loss of sexual interest
suicidal thoughts or behavior
increased physical complaints (with no medical basis) such as lack of energy, backaches, stomach upsets
increased irritability
loss of interest in activities that were once pleasurable

Anxiety
Everyone experiences anxiety from time to time, and in fact, the desire to decrease the amount we feel may motivate us to make positive changes in our lives. But if you find that symptoms provoked by this

state begin to appear too frequently or become unusually intense, you should seek professional help. Symptoms of anxiety are the same as those we associate with the physical reactions to fear:

perspiration
racing heart beat
tense muscles
upset stomach
dry mouth
jitteriness

Unlike fear, the cause is not easy to explain. If you ask an anxious person, "What's bothering you?" the answer is likely to be, "I really don't know."

Anxiety may play a part in almost every kind of psychological problem, including depression. It may be present all the time, intermittently, or may appear out of nowhere and seem almost to take over. In severe cases, it leaves its victims so agitated that they are unable to concentrate or get through their daily routines.

Depression and anxiety are two common afflictions, heading the list of reasons why people seek therapy. There are, however, as many reasons as there are people for wanting professional help. The emotional obstacles to a full and satisfying life are as real and as painful as physical problems and should not be ignored. If you are at all hesitant about going to a therapist, or wonder how to find one, you can begin by discussing your concerns with your primary care physician. If you are religious, you might talk to your priest, rabbi, or minister, many of whom have had training in counseling.

If the person you first talk to in any way belittles your fears or tells you that you just have to be strong, this is most likely someone with very negative ideas about the concept of professional mental health care, or ignorant of how to deal with emotional problems. Beware of any doctor whose idea of treatment is merely to dispense sleeping pills or tranquilizers on a regular basis.

OTHER REASONS TO SEEK COUNSELING

self-destructive behavior such as abuse of drugs or alcohol, compulsive gambling, obesity
repeated sexual problems
chronic, repetitive, disruptive problems in dealing with other people
serious problems in dealing with your children
persistent irrational or peculiar thoughts (other people are out to get you, strange things are happening to your body)
repetitive and uncontrollable behavior such as continual handwashing

    hearing or seeing things that are not there
    prolonged marital and/or family problems
    difficulty adjusting to physical disability or pain
    stress-related physical symptoms or illness
    continued feelings of low self-worth or of failure to live up to one's
      potential

WHO CAN HELP YOU

You will have a choice, sometimes a confusing one, among a variety of mental health workers, some of whom are trained, some merely self-proclaimed. We'll start and stop with those who have recognized credentials. Although their certificates will not guarantee that you have found the "right" person, you will have at least some basis for selection and real protection against the dubious and possibly dangerous quacks who dwell on the fringes of the mental health field.

"Psychotherapist" is the general term that covers several different mental health professionals. There are four predominant groups who are specifically trained to deal with emotional problems: psychiatrists, psychologists, social workers, and psychiatric nurses.

Psychiatric Nurses
Most work in community mental health programs or in in-patient psychiatric units in hospitals. They are generally trained to do crisis intervention and counseling rather than long-term therapy. There are only a handful in private practice.

Social Workers
Those who have been trained in clinical practice (as opposed to administrative, organizational, or medical social workers) probably provide more psychotherapeutic service at lower cost than any other professional group, especially in clinics or other institutions. In addition to working in such facilities, many social workers have private practices.

Psychologists
There are many different types of psychologists—school, industrial, experimental—but only two specific groups are trained to offer psychotherapy to adults: clinical psychologists and counseling psychologists. (School and educational psychologists are often trained to do counseling with children.) Their fees may be higher than those of social workers but are generally lower than those set by psychiatrists. Psychologists are trained to do psychological testing in addition to counseling.

Psychiatrists
Because of their medical school training, psychiatrists are the only mental health professionals who can prescribe medication and do

medical procedures such as electroshock therapy. They are also trained to evaluate and treat emotional problems that arise as the result of organic disease. While psychiatrists are not necessarily better suited to doing office-based psychotherapy, they are especially well equipped to deal with the kinds of problems that require hospitalization and drug treatment.

FINDING THE RIGHT THERAPIST FOR YOU

Credentials are a good place to begin. What you are looking for is a well-trained professional who has the correct background and licensing. Should a therapist be reluctant to discuss credentials or make you feel uncomfortable for asking, you would do well to seek someone else.

Once you have found someone with appropriate credentials you have established a kind of bottom line, but you still do not have any guarantee that you have discovered a person you can work with. The first consideration has to do with *you*. Do you really want to change and do you feel that therapy can help you? The next consideration has to do with your feelings about the therapist you choose.

Most studies of the effectiveness of psychotherapy have concluded that except for some specific problems best treated by behavior therapies (phobias, obesity, smoking), there is no substantial difference in the success rates of different schools of psychotherapy. (We will discuss those schools later in this chapter.) Although still in an early stage, current research indicates that a successful outcome depends most on the following factors:

- the therapist's experience, flexibility, and sense of professional responsibility
- his or her personal qualities, such as empathy, acceptance, warmth, and respect for people
- the client's desire to be helped and his or her trust in the therapist
- the "correctness" of the match between client and therapist

Earlier in the book we discussed the human and personal, as opposed to the purely professional, qualities of your physician. Therapists too are human. They are subject to the same biases and stereotypes we all are. Through training and through their own therapy, they attempt to examine their own responses and prevent biased reactions from interfering with their treatment of patients. Like most of us, though, they get along best with those who are most like them (in social or economic background, education, etc.).

If you wonder whether a therapist's background or possible prejudices would affect you, raise your concerns. Many therapists will not answer intimate questions about their personal lives, but they should be willing to discuss how you would work together.

For example, if you are a woman and sexism is a concern, you could

TRAINING AND CREDENTIALS TO LOOK FOR IN THERAPISTS

PROFESSION	DEGREE	TRAINING	LICENSE CERTIFICATION
Psychiatrist	M.D.	college (4 yrs) medical school (4 yrs) internship (1 yr) psychiatric residency (3 yrs)	state medical license board certification by American Board of Psychiatry & Neurology
Psychologist	Ph.D. or Psy.D.	college (4 yrs) graduate school (3 yrs) clinical internship (1 yr)	for clinical/counseling psychologist: state license (in most states, only Ph.D.s can be licensed, in others M.A. is sufficient) ABEPP: diplomate status (similar to board certification for M.D.)
Social Worker	M.S.W or D.S.W	college (4 yrs) social work school (2 yrs, includes supervised field experience) advanced doctorate (2 additional yrs)	CSW: awarded by Academy of Certified Social Workers
Psychiatric Nurse	R.N. and M.S.	college (4 yrs) graduate work (1–2 yrs)	none

ask for the therapist's views on the subject. By the way, don't assume that only men have stereotyped or out-of-date ideas about the role of women: one psychiatrist who has carved out a niche for herself commenting on women's issues actually holds the most traditional ideas imaginable on the possibilities for middle-aged women of satisfaction in love and work. Any client of hers over forty exposed to this underlying and pervasive pessimism would require a large amount of fortitude to do more than resign herself to her inevitable decline.

If you are homosexual, you might quite reasonably want to know how your proposed therapist feels about that. Although homosexuality is no longer classified as a disease, some mental health professionals still seem to consider it one.

If you are of a different race, nationality, or cultural background from your therapist, you might wonder how well this person could understand how your background affected your responses.

Some therapists will answer questions about such concerns directly; others may want to know why you are asking. But no matter how they begin to discuss your questions, they should in the end give you a good idea of where they stand. If, after several sessions, you do not feel satisfied with the answers, you have not found the right therapist.

COLLECTING NAMES

1. Friends
Some people ask friends who are in therapy for the name of their therapist. A word of caution here: the perfect therapist for your friend may not be ideal or even right for you. If the person has good credentials, start with a consultation visit to see for yourself.

2. Your Primary Care Doctor
You can ask your primary care physician for a recommendation, bearing in mind that he or she may tend to recommend a fellow M.D.: a psychiatrist. That's fine if you have a problem requiring medications or hospitalization. If you don't, you may find a psychiatrist's fees too high. Since they are no more skillful as psychotherapists than other mental health workers, you might want to ask your doctor to suggest a qualified social worker or psychologist too.

3. Organizations
If you are unable to gather names from people you know, you can contact one of several organizations to obtain lists of qualified professionals from which you can make a selection.

Call or write to the county mental health society or county mental health groups maintained by the various professions, such as psychology, psychiatry, and social work societies. Departments of Psychiatry,

Psychology, or Social Work at large universities or hospitals are another source of names (see Resource Directory).

ARRANGING FOR A CONSULTATION

Before you decide on a therapist and undertake a course of treatment, you need a consultation: one or more visits in which you and the therapist discuss your problems and what types of treatment, if any, you should have. If the person you consult recommends therapy, generally he or she will offer either to be your therapist or to provide you with names of others.

When you call for a consultation, mention the person who referred you and ask specifically for a consultation visit. You may also ask what the fee will be. Many therapists will give you the figure for a consultation but will want to discuss their regular fees in person. This is because they have a sliding scale that depends on the ability of the client to pay. When you first call, you could ask whether the regular fees are fixed or are flexible.

Schedule consultations with one or possibly two therapists. If you line up consultations with a list of names, you will waste money and risk confusion.

The Consultation Visit

This may extend for two or three sessions and is a process of discovery. The therapist will be trying to assess the severity of your problems and how best to work with them. This time can also be used to discuss some of the specific and practical issues on your mind: credentials, fees, confidentiality, how the sessions will be conducted, whether the therapist has any particular slant or bias. You will also be gathering emotional information: do I like and trust this person and can we work together.

Fees and Schedule

You will want to know not only how much per session but also when the therapist wants to be paid. Ask how missed sessions are handled. Some therapists will bill you regardless of the reason you missed a visit; others will not charge if you call within a specified time period to cancel. A few therapists (usually psychoanalysts) expect their patients to vacation when they do. Whatever the arrangements are, they should seem fair to you.

If you have any concern about whether your insurance will cover your therapy, now is the time to determine whether the therapist meets the policy requirements. While some policies cover licensed social workers, many specify that you use either a psychiatrist or a licensed psychologist. (See Chapter Twelve for more information about insurance.)

In addition, responsible therapists will provide their patients with a way to get in touch with them in a crisis, will give advance notice of vacations, and will supply the name of another therapist who can be called if the patient needs to talk to someone while the therapist is away.

Confidentiality
This is the basis of a trusting, safe relationship and most professionals are extremely scrupulous about it. If the therapist takes notes, or makes video or audio tapes of your sessions, you have the right to know why. Such recordings can only be made openly and with your knowledge and consent. In addition, no information about you can be given out until you have signed a "release of information" consent form. (Any unethical behavior in this area can be reported to the state licensing board and to the therapist's professional association.)

Clues to a Successful Partnership
Yes, first impressions are not always correct, but they are powerful and they generally guide our behavior for quite a while. There are dozens of messages you will be receiving; their sum will make you decide either that you may have found the right therapist or that you had better keep looking.

Notice the office arrangement. Does it seem sloppy or professional, warm or cold? How does the therapist greet you? Is he or she on time for the appointment? As you talk, do you feel respected and attended to or are you being interrupted before you finish what you want to say?

Therapy is a verbal give and take. Can you tell this person what's on your mind? Do you understand what he or she says to you? As you discuss the reasons that have led you to consider therapy, do you feel this is someone who agrees with what you feel your problems are, or do you feel you are on separate tracks?

You do not have to like every single thing about your therapist or agree with every assessment—after all, you are there to get a different perspective—but you do need some gut sense of mutual respect; you need to feel this is someone whom you trust and can talk to about personal and painful matters.

IF YOU NEED HELP AND ARE LOW ON CASH

So far we have been discussing private practice, which is the most expensive way to get treatment. The advantages are that you can select your own therapist and will most likely be able to continue treatment with that person as long as you wish.

There are alternatives. Many hospitals, universities, and psychotherapy training centers have mental health clinics with sliding fee scales (the bottom end may be very low, the top almost as high as private practice). Because their primary goal is training, there are some drawbacks from the patient's point of view. There are also some advantages.

Drawbacks:
· You will be assigned a therapist
· Therapist may leave during the course of your treatment
· There may be a waiting list and therefore a delay in beginning treatment

Advantages:
· Costs will be considerably lower
· Therapist will be closely supervised by an experienced professional

It is possible to get very good, affordable treatment in such a setting. Should you find you do not work well with the assigned therapist, you can certainly request that you be transferred to another.

THE DIFFERENT SCHOOLS OF THOUGHT

So far we have discussed psychotherapy in general without any attempt to distinguish one type from another. In fact, there are hundreds of different approaches, some far more established than others. Most therapists today, however, utilize all or part of the few generally accepted types of treatment we are going to discuss.

The particular approach used will affect how the sessions are conducted, how your problems are interpreted, the frequency of your visits, and the length of your treatment.

This section of the chapter is for your general interest; trying to choose a therapist on the basis of theoretical orientation may prove somewhat difficult since so many practitioners are eclectic; that is, they combine different approaches based on what they think a particular patient needs.

Psychoanalysis
This is the method most closely derived from the work of Sigmund Freud. Analysts believe that by uncovering the repressed and painful conflicts of childhood that continue to influence adult life, people will be able to minimize their effects.

Jim has been passed over for promotion at work several times. The older men who were his superiors told him his quick temper and angry fights had cost him the position he desired. In analysis, Jim explored his anger at his father when he was a child, anger he had "forgotten" that he had ever experienced. His analyst helped Jim make a connection between those childhood feelings and his present difficulties with older, gray-haired men whom he identified with his father.

Since the goal is to evoke memories buried in the unconscious mind, psychoanalysis uses special techniques to improve access. People in analysis lie on a couch and say whatever comes floating into their minds (free association), whether it makes sense to them or not. Although these thoughts may seem to be random, they are often connected. The psychoanalyst helps the patient to examine those connections, and also to interpret dreams and to examine the feelings the patient has toward the analyst. During treatment, the role of this type of therapist is to remain essentially neutral, expressing few opinions, revealing little that is personal.

Psychoanalysts (who are not necessarily psychiatrists) are therapists who have received advanced training in analysis from a special psychoanalytic institute or center.

Psychoanalysis is a lengthy and expensive process that works best for bright and verbal people who are deeply committed to it. Patients are seen three to five times a week over a period of three to seven years. Fees range from $45 to $125 a session. Because of the cost and demands of this type of treatment, it is not widely used.

Psychoanalytic Psychotherapy
The goal of this approach, too, is insight, but the methods are different. The therapist takes a more active role and is more concerned with the patient's ability to cope with present problems and difficulties with other people. Unlike psychoanalysis, the couch and free association are generally not employed. Patients are seen from one to three times a week, and treatment lasts anywhere from a few months to several years. Many of today's therapists use some aspects of psychoanalytic psychotherapy in their work.

Behavioral Psychotherapy
Behavior therapists believe that people have problems not so much because of early traumatic experiences but because of faulty learning. What has been improperly learned can be relearned; that which has never been learned can be taught.

People who enter behavioral therapy set goals with their therapist as to what behavior is to be changed. They then make a contract specifying what the patient and therapist roles are to be, the fee, and how much time will be involved. The behavior therapist develops specific exercises for the client to learn in therapy and practice in everyday life. This approach is most useful for treating such concrete problems as smoking, obesity, and phobias (fear of flying, of elevators, of heights, etc.).

Cognitive Therapy

This variant of behavioral therapy is based on the idea that emotional difficulties are a consequence of habitual illogical thinking and perceptions. The therapist helps the client to perceive and think more realistically.

The Humanistic Approaches
(Human Potential, Existential)

The emphasis is on building self-esteem through personal growth and development. Humanistic psychologists believe that we fail to reach our full human potential because we block off those parts of ourselves we feel are somehow unacceptable to others. The goal of this type of therapy is to help patients remove these blocks in the safe and approving atmosphere of the therapist's office.

There are many theories grouped under the heading "Human Potential," with names like Gestalt therapy, Rogerian therapy, and Existential therapy. They all tend to focus on present behavior, with the goal of helping people become more aware of their full selves, more responsible for the choices they make in life, and for undertaking change if they are dissatisfied. In many of these types of therapy, it is common for therapists to play a very active role, making suggestions and expressing personal beliefs and opinions. These therapies may be very brief or may continue for several years. Sessions are usually once or twice a week.

NEW OR "RADICAL" THERAPIES

Of course, all of the approaches we have just discussed, from Freud down to the present, were challenged and questioned when they were new. The problem for someone who is seeking help now is how to choose a care provider with some degree of safety and confidence. Probably the best guideline is to look for basic credentials and stay away from the miracle cure, the weekend that will change your life (it probably won't), or the latest psychological fad.

We believe that because human problems are complex, the person who promises you a quick and total "fix" will turn out to be a quack. Brief therapy or counseling can be extremely useful, but responsible practitioners will not promise that they can change long-held attitudes and heal deep emotional wounds with a flick of some psychological or quasi-religious wand.

ALONE OR WITH OTHERS

Up to this point we have discussed only individual therapy. Depending on your particular needs, your therapist might suggest a different modality for you, either in addition to individual therapy or instead of it.

If cost is an issue, check your insurance. Some policies only cover individual therapy.

Couples/Family Therapy

This approach is based on the idea that one person is never totally responsible for all the problems in a given human interaction: it is the couple or the family as a unit that has the problem, and all those involved must be treated. People who feel they are having problems with their marriage may find couple counseling to be quite helpful.

Often family therapy will be recommended when parents ask for help and advice about a child who is causing trouble of some sort. The therapist may feel that the child is really a barometer of difficulties that the family as a whole is experiencing. A family therapist may meet with family members separately as well as together and will often ask to include members of the extended family, such as the grandparents.

This approach focuses on specific problems and is generally short-term, lasting from several sessions to several months. It may be more expensive per session than individual therapy, with fees ranging from $40 to $100, but that fee includes all the family members.

Group Psychotherapy

How can other people with problems help me? Many people wonder about this when presented with the idea of entering group psychotherapy. Therapists who lead groups feel that this may be the best setting for someone who has problems in dealing with others.

Here, in a situation that is a kind of safe version of the real world, an individual can explore, test, and experience responses from other people under the guidance of a trained therapist. A good group therapist will help the individual group members focus on their own individual concerns as well as on the interpersonal problems that arise.

Groups, usually composed of five to ten members, are led by one or sometimes two therapists. Some groups are composed of people with similar problems (drugs, obesity, work); others have members who may share similar characteristics (all adolescents, all women).

Probably the most common type of group contains a variety of people with different kinds of problems. In addition, groups may be open (a new member is added when an old one leaves) or closed. Group therapy may be less costly than individual therapy, with fees ranging from $10 to $50 per one- to two-hour session.

PROBLEMS OF CHILDREN AND TEEN-AGERS

With rare exceptions (e.g., childhood autism or schizophrenia), the emotional problems of children and teen-agers are related to some aspect of family life. Whatever the problem, whether it's school phobia, anorexia nervosa or "attention-deficit disorder" (the new term for hyperactivity), the involvement of other members of the family in evaluation and treatment is usually very important.

Where do you turn if your child is exhibiting disruptive or upsetting behavior? If you have a family physician or pediatrician who has shown an interest in behavior, you might make an appointment to discuss your child's emotional problem. He or she may be helpful or may refer you to an appropriate therapist. If you go to a therapist, we believe you will have the most success with someone who has training in family therapy.

If you are a teen-ager who is having trouble with family, school, or life in general, we suggest you talk to an adult you can trust: this person could be a school counselor, your doctor, or a priest, minister, or rabbi. Your friends may be sympathetic, but they do not have the training or experience to give you the help you need.

SEX THERAPY

Almost all people experience some kind of sexual difficulty at one time or another, a fact that is not especially surprising when one considers the complexity of the human sexual response. An occasional sexual difficulty doesn't mean very much. Sexuality may be affected by many factors: emotional state, physical condition, medication, illness.

Typical problems include inhibited sexual desire, inhibited sexual excitement, inhibited orgasm, premature ejaculation for men, pain on intercourse or vaginal spasms for women. These are things that can be dealt with very effectively by a well-trained sex therapist.

If one or more of these problems become habitual, then you might want to consider sex therapy in order to restore enjoyment to an important area of life. The therapist you choose should have specific training and certification in treating sexual disorders (see Resource Directory).

Any good sex therapist will start by taking a detailed history of your problem and will ask if you have had a medical examination in order to rule out any underlying physical causes. If there is any question of a physical basis for your problem, the therapist will insist you have a medical examination by a qualified physician. Even if your therapist is a psychiatrist and therefore an M.D., he or she will most likely suggest that you go to another doctor for your physical.

Many sex therapists see sexual problems as something shared by both partners in a relationship; some will not treat you without your partner, others will want to talk to the two of you at some sessions. Together with the therapist, you and your partner will examine the emotional aspects of the problem and consider its effect on your life. Most sex therapists suggest a series of exercises that you practice privately with your partner.

Beware the therapist who suggests having sex with you or your partner, watching you have sex, or performing a physical examination if he or she is not a physician. There are *no* justifiable reasons for doing these things, and such behavior on a therapist's part would be highly unethical.

EVALUATING YOUR THERAPY

When you feel that your therapy is going well, when you gain and use new insights to improve the kinds of choices you make in dealing with others, in coping with work, in finding and developing new interests, there is just no question but that the process is worth it.

What should you do if you feel that nothing is happening? "Is this really helping?" you wonder. "Am I getting anywhere or am I just spinning my wheels—or am I getting worse?" These are the typical questions people ask when they feel a lack of progress. They may question whether therapy itself is useful or they may be dissatisfied and angry with a given therapist and wish to change.

We will try to show you a way to find answers to these questions, hoping that you will bear in mind how tricky it is to generalize in this area. The problems that people bring into therapy are of varying difficulty; some can be helped greatly, even dramatically, in a fairly short period of time, and others only imperceptibly over several years.

The kind of problem you bring to therapy, and the type of therapy you are in, will determine how easy it will be for you to weigh the success of your treatment. If, for example, you are seeing a behavioral therapist for a particular fear, you will have worked out as part of your treatment a clearly defined goal, the specific steps you will take to achieve it, and how much time the process will take. To evaluate the treatment, you need only ask yourself: Is that fear lessening?

If you have entered therapy because of a crisis in your life such as the death of someone very important to you or the loss of a job, you can ask yourself if the therapy is helping you to deal with your situation more effectively. If you are in family or couple therapy, you know whether the treatment is helping you make changes in your relationships.

Long-Term Therapy
Suppose, though, that you enter therapy with long-standing problems that are not so specifically defined as the loss of a job or a fear of heights. Suppose you want help because you are constantly anxious or have difficulty forming satisfying love relationships.

In long-term therapy, you may find that it takes some time to define your goals. You may also find that those goals change as your therapy progresses. The question to ask in this situation is, "How am I doing so far?" If you find that you are feeling better about yourself, getting more positive responses from other people, coping better with routine problems, then you have a fairly straightforward answer.

Progress in therapy is sometimes very difficult to assess. Human beings are complex and so are their problems, which do not disappear systematically. In hindsight, you may see that your therapy was a kind of spiral, moving upward even though it took occasional small dips downward.

The way you work with your therapist is the first thing to think about if you feel you are having problems with the therapy itself:

> When you began therapy, did this person take time to collect a lot of information about you and what is important to you?
>
> Are you in agreement about the nature of your problems?
>
> Is this someone who truly listens to what you say?
>
> Does he or she use the information you offer to help you understand your problems more clearly?

If your sessions leave you feeling that you and the therapist are not on the same wavelength, and if, whenever you point this out, the therapist insists that yours is the wrong one, the chances of progress are not very good, regardless of who is wrong and who is right.

How do you feel about your therapist? The strong feelings and reactions you have are an important part of therapy. Therapists expect them and use them as a tool to help you understand relationships outside of therapy. There are times when you are likely to be annoyed, dissatisfied, even angry with your therapist.

What is important is what underlies these shifts in feeling. Do you have a sense of trust and a belief that you and your therapist can discuss negative feelings and then continue to work together?

When Is It Time to Change Therapists?

We have already discussed some basic considerations such as how you are treated as a person, whether you feel your confidences are secure, whether you are seen on time. What is of absolute importance is that you deal with a true professional, with a professional code of ethics. This code requires that the interests of the patient be paramount.

Therapists who discuss their own interests rather than your problems are demonstrating a lack of concern. A therapist who suggests having sex with a patient is a prime example of unethical behavior, and this is one situation where it is absolutely necessary to change therapists without further ado.

If your therapist seems habitually bored or tired (some have been known to fall asleep during sessions), you may need to look for another therapist. At the other end of the spectrum is the therapist who seems to have outbursts of anger or other very strong reactions out of proportion to what you say or do. It is important that you tell the therapist that these reactions upset you.

Your therapist's response can help you decide whether you have found the right person to help you. If he or she listens to what you have to say and discusses the matter willingly and openly so that you both come to a better understanding, then you are probably on the right track. If, however, you have a therapist who either openly or covertly refuses to discuss the things that are bothering you or habitually makes you feel that whatever your concern, it is "your" problem, then you need to consider finding someone else.

When Have You Had Enough Treatment?
We can't really tell you to wait until all your problems are solved, because therapy will not solve all of your problems.

When to stop is entirely your decision, albeit a difficult one. Therapists sometimes suggest that it may be time to stop; more often, though, they will wait for a cue from the patient. Most therapists recommend that you focus on the way you are solving or enduring your problems when you think about ending therapy. Are you finding more effective and less self-destructive methods for dealing with difficulties? Do you feel better, happier, more self-confident?

The time to stop may come when you realize that the specific situation that brought you into therapy is much improved. If, for example, you and your spouse fought constantly and were unable to discuss any of the things that caused the fights, you might stop therapy when you realize that now you only fight occasionally and are talking more calmly and openly about your problems.

We recommend that you discuss your decision with your therapist, who may feel that this is a reasonable point at which to stop therapy or who may convince you that you need more work. Common reasons to end prematurely are a reluctance to talk about uncomfortable feelings, or anger at the therapist.

ALTERNATIVES TO PSYCHOTHERAPY

Should everyone who has a problem go into therapy? While research has shown that many people can be helped more quickly if they are getting professional care, this is not the only way to get help or even the one that is most desirable for everyone. Therapy is expensive, for one thing. Well-trained therapists are in overabundant supply in the major cities, but they may be few and far between in rural areas.

Some people have found that reading and thinking about a problem can give them insight. Bookstores have shelves lined with self-help books on almost every imaginable subject, from parenting to depression to choosing a new vocation. Suggestions you find in these books may help you make changes in your life.

Many people have found enormous relief from having to do battle alone against a difficult problem by joining a peer self-help group. Alcoholics Anonymous, for example, is composed of people with the same problem who offer support and encouragement to one another, and it has been very successful.

There are groups for people with serious medical problems, weight problems, drug problems. There are senior citizens groups and organizations for divorced people such as Parents Without Partners—the list goes on and on.

To find out what kinds of self-help groups exist in your community, check your newspaper (many will carry notices of meetings in the community calendar section), the yellow pages of your phone book, or a community service agency such as the YM/YWCA. Your primary care physician may also be helpful in finding out what is available (see Resource Directory).

If you suddenly need someone to talk to, there are any number of crisis intervention services nowadays. Many communities have suicide prevention services, rape crisis centers, shelters for abused women. Most of these services are staffed by trained volunteers under the supervision of professionals. Many are telephone services that are operated around the clock.

Note: There are some emotional problems that require a different kind of intervention from "the talking cure." In this next section, we are going to discuss psychiatric drugs and hospitalization. If it is difficult to make rational and informed decisions with a disease that seems purely physical, imagine how difficult it is to do so when you are emotionally disturbed.

PSYCHIATRIC DRUGS

Drug therapy is an attempt to change behavior by altering body chemistry. Certain drugs have proven to be very effective in giving relief from the symptoms associated with severe disorders such as schizophrenia. As with any medication, there are always risks to be considered along with the benefits.

With growing public concern over the widespread use of some of these drugs, particularly Valium, it seems important to make a distinction between the legitimate help a psychiatric drug offers and the unthinking abuse that can lead both to dangerous dependence and undesirable side effects.

In addition, these drugs may produce jerking movements, tremor, jitters, or stiffness and rigidity—a group of side effects that resemble symptoms of neurological disease but are really a result of the drug. These reactions may appear within days or weeks after the medication is begun. Such symptoms should be reported to the physician so that other drugs may be prescribed to counteract these side effects.

Antipsychotic Drugs
(major tranquilizers)

Uses	Common side effects
hallucinations	listlessness
panic	drowsiness
disturbed thinking	dry mouth
delusions	blurred vision
unreasonable suspiciousness	constipation
excessive excitement	urine retention
	low blood pressure

A more serious side effect of the drugs and one difficult to treat is tardive dyskinesia, a condition that manifests itself in a series of grimacing, sucking, and smacking movements of the mouth, as well as body jerking. Only a small percentage of those who take these drugs develop this condition, which may persist for a long time or vanish after a few weeks or months. Onset generally occurs either during or after prolonged use of antipsychotic medication.

These drugs should be prescribed only by a physician highly experienced in using them. Dosages must be carefully adjusted for safety and optimum effectiveness. While some professionals are strong advocates of these drugs and others deplore them, we urge an attitude of enlightened caution. If you don't really need them, obviously you are better off without them; this is true of any drug from aspirin to ampicillin. If the medication is used to enable someone walled off from the world by terror or hallucination to interact with people and to work toward a more normal existence, the risks are clearly worth taking.

Antidepressants
(for serious depression)
These drugs will not make someone euphoric, or high, but they will alleviate abnormal depression in many cases. As one woman remarked, "Although I still felt sad, sometimes miserable, I could function. I could get up in the morning, go to work, and manage to get through the day. Without the drugs, I simply lay in bed."

There are several types of antidepressant medication. Some have been used for a number of years; others have only recently become available. Which drug the psychiatrist prescribes depends on the kind of depression being treated and on the age and physical condition of the patient.

MAO (monoamine oxidase) inhibitors can cause a sharp rise in blood pressure, which may in turn lead to a stroke; consequently, they are given only to people for whom no other drug would be effective. *Tricyclic compounds* are less risky. Side effects include dry mouth, dizziness, blurred vision, constipation, or urinary retention. Some of the newer drugs are either more effective for certain problems or have fewer risks and side effects.

Whatever the medication, it must be carefully prescribed and the dosage should be adjusted to suit individual needs. The tricyclics do not work immediately; they may take anywhere from three days to three weeks to begin to help alleviate depression.

Anti-anxiety Drugs
These medications act rapidly to calm anxiety and are intended for short-term relief of minor problems. They should be used sparingly under the supervision of a physician who understands what they will and will not do.

Valium (diazepam) is the most popular drug in this category and the most widely abused. Even though much attention has been focused on the problems of this type of medication in books such as Barbara Gordon's *I'm Dancing As Fast As I Can,* there are still physicians and their patients who feel that a pill is the answer to every sort of stress and nervous tension. Valium and similar medications interfere with normal responses. There are side effects such as drowsiness, fatigue, nausea—sometimes blurred vision, rashes, and headaches. When mixed with alcohol, the anti-anxiety drugs produce a state of confusion that makes it impossible to drive safely or do other tasks that require alertness.

There is also a serious long-term problem: these drugs may become a habit. The user abandons any attempt to solve the root cause of the anxiety and begins taking more and more of the "magic" pills.

Why would a doctor prescribe them? Patients want them. The doctor wants to do something to make the patient feel better, and the pills work.

To be safe, no one should take an anti-anxiety drug unless it has been prescribed by a physician experienced in its use (usually a psychiatrist), who will continue it for only a short period of time. Prescribed in conjunction with psychotherapy, the antianxiety drugs can help people who are suffering stay calm enough to begin a process of working on their problems.

Some dentists suggest that very apprehensive patients take a small dose of Valium before certain procedures in order to raise their threshhold of pain. This may work well for some people and does not pose a problem if only a small number of pills are prescribed.

Lithium
(for chronic manic-depressive problems)
So far the experts don't know precisely how lithium works, but they have demonstrated that it can be very helpful in preventing extreme mood swings. It must be used with extreme care, taken exactly as prescribed, and carefully monitored through regular blood tests. Any

vomiting or diarrhea should be reported immediately, since dehydration can be dangerous to patients on lithium.

IF YOU ARE WORRIED ABOUT PSYCHIATRIC DRUGS

Throughout the book we urge those of you who are concerned about any aspect of medical care to discuss the situation with your physician. We would give the same advice if you are unhappy with the use and effects of these drugs, but because of the nature of psychiatric problems, the person who is the patient may not be able to do this.

If you are a concerned relative, you may be able to arrange to meet with the doctor and talk over the situation. If you are not satisfied with the reasons a doctor gives for administering a particular drug, you can always ask for a second opinion from a consulting psychiatrist.

OTHER SOMATIC TREATMENTS

Two treatments that are more extreme than the use of drugs are psychosurgery and electroconvulsive or electroshock (ECT) therapy, popularly known as shock treatment.

Psychosurgery

The aim is to prevent violent and aggressive behavior by cutting the connection between the frontal lobes and the rest of the brain. Far more common in the 1950s, the procedure, known as a prefrontal lobotomy, is now rarely recommended. It can cause death and may leave those who have received it so dull, slow, and tranquilized that they seem like zombies.

Electroshock (ECT)

In the past, this treatment has been used too freely on far too many people and has acquired a bad reputation. Those who have read Ken Kesey's book *One Flew Over the Cuckoo's Nest* or have seen the movie version will undoubtedly have strong negative feelings on the subject. Nevertheless, for people with severe and life-threatening depression, whose illness cannot be helped by psychotherapy and/or antidepressant drugs, ECT may offer the hope of alleviating the condition with fewer risks than alternative treatments.

Nowadays, the way electroshock is administered has changed. Patients are given a muscle relaxant to prevent injury from convulsions, general anesthesia so that they have no memory of the experience, and much lower doses of electricity so that memory is not as severely affected.

People who have had the treatment suffer from recent memory loss—they cannot remember what happened immediately prior to, during, and after treatment. Usually, memory returns, although for some people it does not. ECT can, on rare occasions, cause cardiac arrhythmias. In addition, the risks associated with the use of general anesthesia must be weighed against the risks of allowing a debilitating depression to continue. If you are involved with the care of a family member or close friend for whom ECT is recommended, you should ask to have a second opinion from a board-certified psychiatrist who is affiliated with a major medical center.

PSYCHIATRIC HOSPITALIZATION

Psychiatric hospitalization most frequently occurs because an individual needs intensive, comprehensive help quickly. The goal is to provide a total therapeutic environment free from the usual day-to-day stresses.

During a hospital stay the patient may receive various treatments:

- individual psychotherapy
- group therapy
- drugs or ECT
- recreational and occupational therapy

Most psychiatric hospitalizations are voluntary, but there are occasions when a person who is a danger to self or society is placed in a psychiatric institution, usually under the certification of one or two physicians. The rules for involuntary hospitalization vary from state to state. To protect the individual, the federal government has published a "Patient Bill of Rights," which hospitals receiving federal funds must honor (see Resource Directory).

Just as there are different kinds of medical hospitals, there are also a variety of psychiatric facilities—private psychiatric hospitals, V.A. hospitals, state and county mental hospitals, and general hospitals with psychiatric divisions. Health insurance, if it covers psychiatric hospitalization at all, commonly covers treatment in a general hospital only.

To find out about a psychiatric hospital, ask your primary care physician or a mental health professional the following:

Is it accredited by the Joint Commission on Accreditation of Hospitals?
Is there a mandatory length of stay?
What are patients' rights and privileges?
What are the rules for visiting?
What is the discharge procedure?
Is the hospital approved for Medicare, Medicaid, and other third party payments?
How is payment to be made?
What kinds of therapeutic services are offered?

What are the credentials of the staff?
Will the admitting psychiatrist be allowed to work with the patient?

Psychiatric units are usually set up so that one mental health professional has direct responsibility for the treatment of the patient. Since a psychiatric hospital is a medical facility, there will always be a physician with direct medical responsibility.

Frequently the psychiatrist who arranges to admit the patient has privileges at the hospital, but this is not always the case. Some facilities do not allow psychiatrists to work with their own hospitalized patients. If continuity is important, you should ask before an admission whether your own or the staff psychiatrist will be in charge of treatment.

CHAPTER NINE

CHILDBIRTH: THE BEST WAY FOR YOU

Tacked to the bulletin board at the nursing station is a peach-colored piece of paper headed "Routine Labor Care." On it are listed the rules that the nurses must follow for all women who come into the hospital to have their babies. Under the heading "anesthesia and analgesia," rule number two states, "Check with the doctor's routine orders for sedation." The nurses do just that. If Dr. Y. has left instructions that all of his patients are to get a shot of Demerol®, the nurses are bound to carry out his wishes. If you are Dr. Y.'s patient, the nurse may insist that you have medication "because that is what your doctor ordered." Technically, she is right, but of course Dr. Y. didn't order it specifically for you.

Do you want to choose the way you give birth? The message of the peach-colored paper is clear: the time to talk about issues like pain medication and prepared childbirth, episiotomies, and rooming-in is at the very beginning of pregnancy.

This is an interesting, albeit unsettling, time to explore the question of the best way and the best place to have your baby. By "best way" do you mean the safest, the least painful, or the most family-centered and personal?

Maternity care has gone through enormous changes, and undoubtedly there are more to come. Right now, a passionate and political debate is raging over the "right" way to do things. The "medical/technological" school of thought focuses largely on the health and safety of the infant. Professionals favoring this approach—mostly obstetricians—recount truly terrible stories of newborns whose brain damage or death could have been prevented had the mother chosen a proper hospital setting.

The "family-centered non-interventionist" school (advocates are generally found among doctors, nurses, and lay people who favor what is often termed "natural childbirth") are concerned about possible risks associated with technology. When interventions are practiced routinely, not reserved only for those situations where they are indicated, will they do more overall harm than good?

Perhaps in five or ten years, there will be an unequivocal body of facts. Right now, you will have to make a decision without having data that compare the risks for low-risk patients in the following categories:

· hospital births using fetal monitoring
· hospital births without fetal monitoring
· maternity center births
· home births

We do have certain opinions on the subject and we will list them here.

Preparation for childbirth is essential.
The father ought to be as much involved as possible.
Medication should be used only because the mother herself wants it.
The absolute priority is the health of mother and child.

Alternative birth centers (either in or out of hospitals) offer a welcome compromise between the generally safe but frightening traditional hospital and the freedom from intervention and family setting of a home birth.

THE WORLD OF THE OBSTETRICIANS

Not so many years ago, a young intern who announced that a mother had just delivered her baby was sternly reprimanded by the OBGYN resident who was supervising his work on the obstetrics floor. "Mothers do not deliver babies; obstetricians do." There is more than one generation of obstetricians out there who believe precisely that. And there are women who want to be their patients, who want someone to make all the decisions, and who feel reassured by a take-charge approach.

Yet physicians are relative newcomers to a field that historically has been the realm of midwives. Throughout much of the history of medicine, a woman in childbirth was much safer with a midwife in attendance than she was with a physician. In the middle of the nineteenth century, Ivan Semmelweis, an Hungarian physician, noted that women who were directed to the clinic that trained physicians instead of the one where midwives worked, "prayed to be allowed to die at home, and gave themselves up for lost" (quoted by author Diana Scully in her book *Men Who Control Women's Health*).[1]

Semmelweis was distressed by the awful toll of childbed fever. In his famous experiment, conducted between 1844 and 1846, he instructed his medical students to scrub their hands before examining each patient; they did, and the death rate dropped dramatically.

But when he presented these findings to his colleagues, he was ridiculed, attacked, and ignored. Doctors then and now do not like to think that they have been killing their patients; some of the resistance of established medicine to change can be traced to the physicians' understandable wish to believe themselves faithful to the Hippocratic principle, "First, do no harm."

Despite these beginnings, modern obstetrics can justly claim vast improvements in safety for both infant and mother. That obstetricians see the hospital as an ideal setting for childbirth should come as no surprise when you understand how they are trained and with what emphasis. Their special area of expertise is in treating the complications of childbirth. They have seen all sorts of emergencies, and they know just how far things can go wrong, and how serious the consequences can be.

What the profession as a whole has been slow to acknowledge is that the atmosphere in which physicians work and the interventions they practice may actually interfere with their dual goals: a healthy mother and a normal baby (unless you define a healthy mother as a woman who is enjoying an uneventful recovery from a cesarean section that may have been unnecessary).

Thoughtful obstetricians have begun to reexamine both their role as the "deliverers" and the kinds of standard practices that interfere with what nature has designed the body to do. They have also begun to devote more attention to the quality of the experience from the point of view of mother, father, and family. A handful have been pioneers in working for change in the hospitals where they practice.

Unfortunately, they have been opposed by present-day traditionalists: the doctors who routinely order the same medication for all obstetric patients; who always follow set procedures such as shaving patients and performing episiotomies; and who insist that women give birth lying flat on their backs with their feet in stirrups (the lithotomy position). The types who in the era of Semmelweis didn't want to wash their hands are as reluctant as ever to question old habits.

WHY YOU NEED TO DO YOUR HOMEWORK

"I had a cesarean section," says a young doctor, "and I couldn't get out of bed. But the nurses were very uncooperative about bringing the baby in for breast-feeding. The hospital paid lip service to good maternity care, but even though they had a rooming-in program, my baby was with me only half of the day. When he had to have treatment for jaundice, they took him over to another building, to the neonatal intensive care unit. In order to see him and nurse him, I had to get myself and my IV pole over there. There was no one to help me."

This is an interesting example for those people who entertain fantasies that doctors command the best possible care. The doctor in this case was a patient at one of those hospitals that pops up on lists of the ten best. Her husband, even though he was a physician, was not allowed to be present for his wife's cesarean. Hospital rules.

How had this couple been caught in this situation? A combination of unpredictable events and some bad luck. She had embarked on labor attended by a midwife at a free-standing birth center, but was transferred to a hospital when it became clear she needed a cesarean section. Because the obstetrician "backing up" her midwife was doing a procedure at a nearby medical center, he could not deliver her at the community hospital she preferred.

What is to be learned from this? Do your homework ahead of time and be as prepared as possible for the unexpected. These young physicians were so sure that childbirth would take place in the encouraging atmosphere of the birth center that they never thought about where their obstetrician might be if they needed him.

HOW DO YOU WANT TO HAVE YOUR CHILD?

Healthy, of course. How do you feel about childbirth? Mothers-to-be, do you want the most possible control over what happens to you, or would you feel more secure following traditional, set procedures? Do you insist on having your baby without a hint of any sort of pain killer, or are you terribly afraid of pain and hope to be made insensitive to the slightest twinge? Fathers-to-be, do you want to coach your partner when she enters labor? Do you want to be present when your child is born? Or does the whole thing make you feel slightly queasy? How you answer these questions and a number of others will determine what kind of setting you choose and what kind of obstetrical care you seek.

Some choices, though, are safer than others, and all things are not possible for everyone. There may be no midwife or maternity center in your community. You may have health risks or psychological needs that make a hospital the best and safest choice for you from the outset. If problems develop during labor, you may require medical intervention you had hoped to do without. Says an experienced obstetrician who is highly innovative and who serves on the board of his community's free-standing birth center, "I make sure all my patients know that if a serious problem develops, they may very well have their baby in a hospital."

PREPARED CHILDBIRTH IS FOR EVERYONE

Whatever way you choose to have your baby—and whether you think you need it or not—we strongly recommend that all prospective parents take a prepared childbirth class. Recalls one mother, "I took a Lamaze class because I decided I would try to have my baby without drugs, thinking I could always ask for something. My baby was premature, and the doctor didn't want to give me anything. Thank God I took that course."

Any good class that prepares parents-to-be will offer a thorough explanation of the exact physical changes of pregnancy and the process of childbirth. Ignorance in this case is definitely not bliss; in fact, fear of the unknown will increase pain and may, according to some experts, actually slow labor. Women who know what to expect and who view birth as a normal process rather than a mysterious medical problem are apt to need much less medication.

The three methods that are generally taught are those developed by three obstetricians: Grantley Dick-Read, Robert Bradley, and Fernand Lamaze. Read, an English doctor, was the first to develop a formal system of childbirth education, based on his perception that the less fearful the mother, the easier her labor and delivery. Bradley, an American, was influenced by the work of Read and added to it his own emphasis on the use of the father as coach during childbirth. All three methods emphasize the use of relaxation techniques.

Best known and most widely taught in the United States is the Lamaze method. Dr. Fernand Lamaze, in addition to teaching women about childbirth and giving them exercises to help them learn how to relax during childbirth, also developed specific methods of breathing coupled with a light self-massage technique. Part of the aim of the breathing techniques is to overload the memory banks of the cerebral cortex (the message center of the brain) so that it will fail to register pain messages. [If you are a singer, or trained in abdominal breathing techniques, you may have a difficult time with the chest-breathing taught by this method.]

Your obstetrician, family physician, or nurse-midwife will be able to recommend instructors; almost every community will have one or more prepared childbirth programs. If you should encounter an obstetrician who tells you that this is not worthwhile or necessary, change doctors. It is hard to imagine a family physician and impossible to conjure up a nurse-midwife who would not highly recommend prepared childbirth.

In selecting a program, remember that it will reflect the philosophy of its designer. For example, if you take a childbirth course at a hospital where patients routinely get pain medication, your instructor won't spend a lot of time teaching you how to have a nonmedicated birth. Almost all classes include information on what to expect if you should need a cesarean section.

HOW MUCH INTERVENTION DO YOU WANT?

Women can give birth unassisted in a field. If there are no problems, if the baby is strong and healthy, and if the mother knows how to tie and cut the cord, no technology is strictly necessary. There are some risks: for example, if the baby were born with the cord wound tightly around its neck, resuscitation would be necessary to save its life.

Of course, it would be extremely unwise to give birth this way. At a minimum, whenever a woman gives birth she should make sure that she has the services of a trained and licensed birth attendant, and that suction equipment to clear out the newborn's nasopharynx, and clean instruments to cut the cord, are available.

From the array of additional techniques and equipment that now exist, you may wish to choose those you feel will help you and reject others you feel interfere. The problem is not the existence of new childbirth technology but the way it is used. For women who have uncomplicated pregnancies and routine deliveries, very little in the way of mechanical assistance or drugs may be needed; others with known risks in their medical history, or problems during pregnancy, may want and need technology to provide an extra margin of safety.

ELECTRONIC FETAL MONITORING (EFM)

In many hospitals, women in labor are routinely hooked up to a machine that continuously records the fetal heart rate. The purpose of the machine is to provide a warning at the earliest signs of fetal distress so that steps can be taken before any damage is done to the fetus.

There are two kinds of monitors. The external fetal monitor consists of two belts strapped over the abdomen. One records the fetal heart rate; the other indicates the occurrence of a contraction. This information is passed to a printout device or a screen. The internal monitor is both more accurate and more invasive: in order to insert it, the membranes must first be ruptured. Two slender catheters are then threaded through the vagina and cervix. One is clipped to the fetal scalp (or other presenting part) to record the heart rate, and the other is inserted farther into the uterus to record the force of the contractions.

Proponents of the monitor claim that it decreases neonatal mortality and reduces the risk of brain damage by giving an early warning of fetal distress. The widespread use of this technology is based on these supposed benefits; however, careful studies were not done prior to introduction, and evidence now appearing suggests that actual experience does not bear out these claims.

For example, a researcher who examined data from hospitals in Vermont found that at a university hospital using EFM, there had been a thirty percent drop in the newborn death rate between 1969 and 1974. He then looked at a group of hospitals that did not use EFM in that time period and found a similar decrease.[2]

In Denver, two studies looked at differences in outcome between mothers who had EFM and those who were examined every fifteen minutes by nurses using stethoscopes.[3] There appeared to be no difference in outcome (the health of the baby) between the two groups.

What is most disturbing is the potential for harm that routine use of this technology holds. What are the disadvantages of monitoring?

It is subject to mechanical error, giving false indications of fetal distress twenty to forty percent of the time.

It may be used by physicians who are not properly trained to interpret the data it yields.

Because of the above factors the widespread use of EFM has contributed greatly to a soaring C-section rate.

It immobilizes a woman in labor.

It may lead to a reduction in the amount of direct nursing care that women in labor receive.

Internal monitoring is invasive. There is a slight risk of fetal or maternal infection.

Internal monitoring requires that the amniotic sac be ruptured. This may cause abnormally strong contractions, detrimental to the fetus.

Whether or not to use a fetal monitor is a subject you should discuss with your physician ahead of time. If you plan to deliver in a hospital that monitors routinely, you will need the support of your doctor if you would prefer not to be monitored.

Once you enter the hospital, should you refuse fetal monitoring you will probably have to sign a form releasing the hospital from legal responsibility. Having to sign such a form may cause anxiety if you do not have a well-thought-out position.

Chain of Events Distorting Childbirth

Events	Routine administration of intravenous fluids	Confinement to bed	Stimulation with oxytocin or aminiotomy
Origination	Because of use of general anesthesia in delivery	For women with cardiac and respiratory problems only	Only when medically indicated (e.g. atonic uterus)
Consequences /Hazards	Adds to pathologic environment Eliminates need for liquid food by mouth Precipitates metabolic acidosis	Slows down engagement of fetal presenting part Decreases maternal circulation Leads to postural hypotension Promotes waiting for each contraction (no distractions) Reduces effectiveness of contractions	Elicits stronger, longer contractions with shorter relaxation periods between, making it difficult for mother to cope Presents risk of possible cerebral ischemia and birth trauma for fetus

WHY LYING IN BED
IS NOT THE BEST WAY TO LABOR

Since hospitals have customarily confined women in labor to bed, the introduction of the monitor may not have seemed like much of a change on this score. The women were lying there anyway.

An interesting study[4] by Roberto Caldeyro-Barcia, an obstetrician with an international reputation, examined the effects of maternal position on the progress of labor. He found that labor was thirty-six percent shorter for women having their first baby (and twenty-five percent shorter for other women) who were allowed to stand, walk, sit, or lie down as they chose. For delivery, the women used a table with an adjustable back and hand grips to help in pushing.

Of those who were given a free choice of position, ". . . only 5% preferred to lie down; 95% preferred to stand, walk or sit." An upright position did not lead to an increase in the incidence of fetal head compression, late deceleration of heart patterns, or caput succedaneum (swelling in or under the scalp in newborns).

"ACTIVE MANAGEMENT"

This is an obstetrical phrase that includes a whole group of interventions. If an obstetrician actively manages your labor, you don't just sit, walk, stand, breathe, and push. Instead you may have the amniotic sac ruptured and oxytocin administered (both done to speed up labor), pain medication, an electronic fetal monitor, an episiotomy, and forceps. You will lie down during labor and assume the lithotomy position for the actual delivery.

Sandra F. Johnson, R.N. writing in *The American Journal of Mater-*

Chain of Events Distorting Childbirth

Events	Use of analgesics/anesthesia	Use of forceps
Origination	Subsituted for emotional support from family. Used when medically indicated (e.g. prolonged labor)	For complicated or arrested second stage of labor
Consequences /Hazards	Produces lethargic mother who is unable to respond actively to the labor process and narcotized infant with possible respiratory and neurological complications	Necessitates lithotomy position and episiotomy May lead to possible damage of infant's facial nerve or brachial plexus or to intracranial hemorrhage

continues on next page

nal Child Nursing[5] demonstrates how one intervention can produce the negative effect that makes another intervention necessary; "The many distortions of the childbearing process described here are directly or indirectly related to one another."

THE LITHOTOMY POSITION

Here is an impossibly strange and difficult thing to do, even more bravura a feat than singing a major aria while lying on a couch. Yet many hospitals still require women to give birth while lying flat on their backs with their knees held up in stirrups.

Early surgeons used this position to extract kidney stones (*lithos* is the Greek word for stone); it was an eighteenth-century French obstetrician, Francois Mauriceau, who popularized its use for childbirth as a way to make things easier for the birth attendant, not the mother.

The lithotomy position is not only uncomfortable; it may also be hazardous to the fetus. Dr. Caldeyro-Barcia points out that it causes the weight of the uterus to press on the blood vessels that supply the placenta, "resulting in a fall in maternal arterial blood pressure, which can lead to fetal asphyxia."[6]

Hospitals with up-to-date maternity departments will offer an alternative to this form of delivery such as an adjustable delivery table or a special birthing bed.

Furthermore, many forward-looking physicians feel that enemas do not have to be given routinely and that there is no reason whatsoever for shaving the pubic area since the birth passage itself is not sterile.

Chain of Events Distorting Childbirth

Events	Supine-lithotomy position	Episiotomy
Origination	Convenience for active management of birth by obstetrician	Result of developing a table with stirrups and using forceps for delivery Lack of patience in waiting out the course of labor and training in basic measures to comfort woman and facilitate second stage of labor
Consequences /Hazards	Requires mother to move at difficult time from labor room to delivery room table Inhibits mother's voluntary efforts to expel infant Increases tension of perineal tissues May lead to supine hypotension with resulting decrease of oxygen to fetus	Requires strapping mother to table and shaving perineum to maintain sterile field Necessitates at least local anesthesia Initiates painful postpartum recuperation, thus leading to more pain medication

FORCEPS

Forceps, if they are properly used, are generally safe, although they can cause problems, such as a temporary facial paralysis in the newborn. Often, the reason they are necessary is because the pain-relief method chosen for childbirth has relaxed the muscles that normally work to expel the fetus.

An interesting study published in *The Lancet*[7] showed that a number of women who were interviewed a year after a forceps delivery felt dissatisfied with their experience of childbirth. Said one, "I felt no sense of achievement."

PAIN RELIEF

Childbirth in many ways resembles an athletic feat requiring strength and endurance. How difficult it is for you will depend to a large extent on how well prepared you are, what physical shape you are in, how relaxed you are, and whether you have a supportive companion throughout labor.

No two labors are identical even for the same woman. One may require no medication, while another is so long and difficult that pain relief is clearly necessary. If you want to minimize the chances you will need drugs—and there are good reasons to avoid them if possible—you can do many things ahead of time and during childbirth to make the experience as comfortable as possible.

If this is your first child, learn everything you can about childbirth, in precise detail. Take a prepared childbirth course. Tour the hospital. Look at pictures of childbirth. Fear of the unknown can make you far more susceptible to pain.

The breathing and relaxation techniques taught in these classes are effective in reducing discomfort.

Even if this is not your first child, you will probably benefit by taking a prepared childbirth class. You don't need to learn how babies are born, but the relaxation exercises and breathing training are important.

Make sure that you have someone who is trained in prepared childbirth to stay with you throughout labor and delivery. This may be the father, a friend, a nurse-midwife, or an obstetrical nurse. Women who have good coaching need less medication than those who labor alone.

Even someone untrained but supportive is better than no one. A study of the benefits of companionship was reported on in *The New England Journal of Medicine*[8]. Labors were shorter, averaging 8.8 hours for women with companions as opposed 19.3 hours for those without. Furthermore, those who had no companion had more perinatal problems (meconium staining, fetal distress, C-sections) and their babies were more apt to be hospitalized during infancy with pneumonia or diarrhea.

The more you can move around, the shorter and more comfortable your labor will tend to be. If you are using a hospital, find one that will not confine you to bed. (At birth centers and in some innovative hospital programs, patients can explore different positions to find the most comfortable.)

TAKING MEDICATION IS A PERSONAL DECISION

Medication is an important topic to discuss with your physician or midwife at the outset of your relationship. Your choice of health care provider may depend on the response you get when you raise the subject. Some doctors have set routines; others are far more flexible.

If you decide to use a midwife, find out what types of pain relief she is trained and licensed to supply. If, on the other hand, you want to be able to have epidural anesthesia, neither a midwife nor an obstetrician nor a family practitioner can administer it. You will need the services of an anesthesiologist.

HOW SAFE ARE DRUGS?

Physicians used to believe that many drugs could safely be used for childbirth because they would not cross what is termed the placental barrier. Alas, this proved to be an illusion. Drugs cross the barrier with ease and can have such undesirable effects as slowing the fetal heart rate or causing difficulties with breathing at birth. Drugs may also lower maternal blood pressure, thereby affecting the amount of oxygen the mother is supplying to the fetus.

New knowledge has led to a lowering of the recommended dosages of some drugs and to the abandonment of others that are not considered either safe or effective. Scopolamine (which produced "twilight sleep") is no longer used by responsible practitioners, and general anesthesia is given only for emergencies.

Most women find it reassuring to know that if they need medication to help them through a difficult labor, it is available and, if used carefully, can be considered safe.

TYPES OF MEDICATION

General Anesthesia

Nowadays, general anesthesia is used mainly for emergency cesarean sections, which must be performed within minutes. If more time is available, most obstetricians arrange for the woman to receive medication that is safer and that allows her to be awake to see her new baby.

Inhalation Anesthesia
· Low concentration of a gas such as nitrous oxide
· Self-administered
· Does not appear to have significant effects on either mother or fetus
· Used during delivery

The advantage here is that a woman can use pain relief as she needs it by holding a mask over her nose and breathing. If she becomes drowsy, her hand relaxes and the mask drops away.

Local Anesthesia
· Given by injection
· Blocks pain in specific area
· May be very short-acting
· Rapidly enters fetal blood supply
· Affects fetal heart rate

A *paracervical block* is given before the cervix is completely dilated, lasts up to an hour, and is used to reduce pelvic pain. The injection may be repeated.

Pudendal blocks are injections given during delivery to numb the perineal area. They are also used to relax the vagina and perineum if the obstetrician decides to use forceps for delivery.

Spinal Anesthesia
· Injection of local anesthetic into spinal canal
· Fast acting
· Interferes with pushing
· May make it necessary to use forceps for delivery
· May be used if forceps delivery is considered desirable
· May lower mother's blood pressure
· Does not enter fetal blood supply
· Considered very effective as pain relief
· May cause postpartum headache

A woman who has a spinal should not labor on her back. The weight of the uterus pressing on the blood vessels that supply the placenta may interfere with the amount of oxygen that reaches the fetus.

Epidural
· Injection of local anesthetic into space surrounding spinal cord
· Requires anesthesiologist with special training
· Can be used for cesarean section
· Takes up to fifteen minutes to provide pain relief

· May cause drop in maternal blood pressure; therefore woman should not labor on her back
· Increases probability forceps will be needed

Only an anesthesiologist who has been specially trained to do this procedure should be used, so you would need to make sure that the hospital you will be using has one who will be available. A "lumbar epidural" (referring to the lumbar region of the spine) is now preferred to the "caudal" because it requires less medication and affects a more limited area.

A possible consequence of spinal, and improperly administered epidural, anesthesia is a severe and persistent headache. If this should happen, report it to your doctor promptly; there is now a fairly simple treatment called a "blood patch." Some of the patient's blood is injected into the site of the puncture, where it clots and forms a seal. This should be done before discharge from the hospital.

ANALGESIA

Some of the drugs used to relieve pain work not by blocking it but by making the woman in labor feel calmer or drowsier. Demerol (meperidine) is a synthetic narcotic that is often given in combination with a tranquilizer. Nowadays, only small doses are given.

Since the drug enters the fetal bloodstream, the baby may be drowsy and narcotized if the drug is given too close to birth. Another drug can be administered to the newborn to reverse those effects.

Discuss the risks and benefits of pain medication with your physician or midwife long before your baby is due. There is no way to know ahead of time what a given childbirth will require. Women who have described themselves as being cowards and fearful of pain have given birth without needing medication. Other women who have assumed they would need only breathing exercises and a strong will have experienced extremely long and difficult labors: as the hours went by, they finally decided they needed a little pharmaceutical help.

If you are fortunate enough to have a supportive physician or nurse-midwife who sees his or her role as helping nature rather than running the show, and if you have chosen a place to give birth that emphasizes family-centered care, the chances are that you will not be encouraged to take unnecessary medication.

WHERE DO YOU WANT TO GIVE BIRTH?

In choosing where to have your baby, you may have to make some compromises. The usual trade-off involves sacrificing some degree of comfort and familiarity for the advantage of increased safety.

Are you looking for a homelike and relaxed place to give birth? The traditional hospital, with its inflexible routines, fragmented care, separation of mother and infant, and exclusion of family, is probably the worst place. But the hospital also has what you need if complications develop.

Do you want a home birth? If you stay home, you will have no problems with rules about the presence of fathers and siblings, and the setting will certainly be familiar. It may or may not be safe or feel safe, depending on your pregnancy and labor.

You may decide that the best compromise would be a free-standing maternity center, where you could have your baby with minimum medical intervention yet still be near a hospital. Is there one in your community and does your particular set of risk factors fit its requirements?

HOW YOUR RISKS AFFECT YOUR CHOICES

Before embarking on a detailed exploration of childbirth alternatives, you might take a minute to think about the question of risk. Your age, habits, state of health, socioeconomic status, and previous experience with childbearing all affect your statistical chances for having a normal pregnancy and a routine delivery.

If you are assigned to a low-risk category, however, you do not have a guarantee that nothing will go wrong, and if you are at high risk for complications, you may still enjoy a perfectly normal childbirth.

There is no uniform nationwide system for assigning risks, but the following are examples of single factors that carry a high risk.

· Rubella in the first three months of pregnancy
· Bleeding during pregnancy
· Rh sensitization
· Diabetes

There may be a combination of factors that place a woman at risk for complications. For example, if you are over thirty-five or under seventeen, smoke a pack of cigarettes a day, and have been taking tetracycline while pregnant, you are at high risk.

A middle-income woman between the ages of seventeen and thirty-five, with no medical problems, no past pregnancy problems, who does not smoke or drink, is not overweight, and has taken no medications during pregnancy would be considered a low-risk patient.

These are all physical risks. Recently, there has been more attention paid to the emotional factors that can affect pregnancy and childbirth. The Center for Research on Birth and Human Development in Berkeley, California has worked out a risk assessment format that takes into account feelings and beliefs, relationships and personality.

For example, an independent woman who enjoys sex, wants a baby, and is happily married is less likely to have problems than an unhappily married woman who is dependent and mistrustful.

If you know ahead of time that you have physical or emotional problems that may affect your pregnancy, we suggest you choose the setting and a caregiver that offer the greatest safety should complications develop.

HOW WILL THE SETTING AFFECT YOU?

The physical setting in which you have your baby may affect how long your labor lasts, how difficult your delivery is, and how you feel about the entire experience. Anxiety and tension can interfere with contractions, thereby prolonging labor. If you fear hospitals, these feelings might contribute to a more difficult childbirth. If, on the other hand, a hospital makes you feel safe, do not choose a home delivery because intellectually you think it's the thing to do.

If the setting is the most important factor for you, start by investigating *where* before you think about *who*. For example, if you want to deliver in a hospital, that decision may preclude the use of an independent nurse-midwife; at present, relatively few hospitals allow nurse-midwives to practice obstetrics. If you want to have your baby at home, you will have a difficult time finding an obstetrician to support that choice. You may, however, find a nurse-midwife or possibly a family physician to assist you.

Medical professionals agree that for "high-risk" patients, those whose problems greatly increase their chances of having childbirth complications, the hospital is the safe and reasonable choice. If you are in this category or if you would simply not feel secure giving birth anywhere else, you have narrowed your range to the question of which hospital to use.

CHOOSING A HOSPITAL

Until recently, hospitals have treated labor and delivery in much the same way that they deal with surgical procedures. Patients undergoing surgery are wheeled from their own rooms into the operating room, then to the recovery room, and then back to their rooms on the surgical floor. Visitors wait in a waiting room.

Soft lights and soothing music and homelike decor are not part of the atmosphere of an operating suite. Loved ones do not provide the support of their presence during an appendectomy, and no joyous family members are waiting to capture on film the removal of a diseased gallbladder or the repair of a hernia.

In hospitals, anesthesia and pain medications are the rule: they make surgery possible. Surgical pain has never been popularly viewed as something that can be overcome by the powers of the mind (although some interesting experiments with hypnosis and acupuncture suggest that this is indeed possible). There is no consumer demand for "natural open-heart surgery."

But recognizing that childbirth is a natural event, some of the more forward-looking hospitals have begun to reorganize the way it is conducted. In one city, all three hospitals that have obstetrical services now offer birthing rooms. They have been led in this direction by people who want to have their babies in a caring, supportive atmosphere.

Because you need or want a hospital setting does not mean you must abandon the idea of doing things your way. Hospitals differ greatly in the kinds of maternity care they offer, the rules they impose, their physical layout, the way that obstetrical nurses are trained, and who is allowed privileges—to list a few of the variables. You might want to choose the hospital that seems most desirable to you and then look for a good obstetrician, family physician, or nurse-midwife who practices there.

Choosing the hospital first makes a lot of sense if you are going to use the services of an obstetrician or family physician. In most cases, these doctors do deliveries in rotation with a group of perhaps two to four associates; the chances are at best fifty-fifty that the doctor who gives you your prenatal care will be there when you give birth. (In New York and a few other large cities where competition for patients is intense, some obstetricians try much harder to guarantee that they will deliver their own patients and will also arrive early in the course of labor.)

Here are some questions to ask about a hospital you are considering:

1. How far away is it? Will there be a lot of traffic on the way?
2. How hard is it to find parking?
3. What is the physical setting for childbirth? Is there a homelike birthing room available if you want one?
4. What is hospital policy on the presence of fathers throughout childbirth?
5. If you would like a friend or family member other than your husband to serve as your labor coach, is that allowed?
6. What is the reputation of the nursing care on the maternity floor?
7. Will you have a private or semiprivate room?
8. Does the hospital have a no-smoking policy? Can you request a nonsmoking room or roommate?
9. Can mothers keep their babies in the room if they wish?
10. After childbirth, does the hospital allow children to visit?
11. What does the hospital do to help nursing mothers?
12. Is there encouragement for a brief length of stay (twelve to twenty-four hours) if that is what you wish?
13. Will you receive hands-on instruction in how to care for your newborn at home?

Before making your choice, glance through our chapter on choosing a hospital, but bear in mind that an excellent overall reputation will not guarantee the quality of a given department. You will still have to ask specific questions about maternity care.

A tour is a good way to get a sense of what a hospital is like. Most hospitals will arrange for tours by expectant parents. (Call the community relations department for information.) On the way there, make note of how long the trip is taking and whether there is a traffic problem en route, or difficulty parking. The problems of getting to a particular hospital may rule it out as a choice; a liberal policy encouraging fathers to participate may do you very little good if the baby arrives while its father is still struggling to find a parking space.

When you visit, try to get a feeling for the place—how relaxed is the atmosphere, how friendly, how humanly, as opposed to technologically, up-to-date. Notice whether staff members are gathered around the nurses' station chatting with each other or are dispersed among the rooms on the floor, attending to patients. Can women in labor walk around or are they confined to their beds?

Notice the way things look. Are the rooms antiseptic hospital-white and bare or are they homelike? Is there a comfortable chair for the person who will be your labor coach?

Will you be able to keep your baby with you if you wish? Hospitals have come up with various types of rooming-in plans. The most flexible allows the mother to have her baby with her whenever she wants and to turn it over to a nurse when she wants to sleep or have visitors.

If babies are kept in a newborn nursery, find out if they are brought to mothers on the hospital's set schedule or whether some other arrangement is possible. If you are planning to nurse, the question of where your baby is kept becomes especially important.

Hospital-Based Birthing Rooms

Consumer preference has led the way in making hospitals more flexible and more human in their maternity practices. One of the results of the demand for more family-centered childbirth is the creation within the hospital of a birthing room or suite to be used by people who want to avoid many of the traditional hospital rules and interventions.

The term "birthing room" means different things in different institutions. In some, it is an austere hospital room with a birthing bed and nothing more. In others, it may be a comfortable suite, with a lounge that can be used by the family during labor.

The advantage of a hospital birthing room as opposed to a free-standing maternity center or home birth is the availability of the hospital's personnel and highly specialized equipment for emergency care should a problem arise.

MORE QUESTIONS TO ASK AT THE HOSPITAL

1. Can I labor and deliver in the same room, possibly in the same bed?
2. Are labor rooms private or will I be put in with someone else?
3. How is the bed or delivery table designed? Can I be propped up or will I be forced to deliver in the lithotomy position (flat on the back, with legs up in stirrups)?
4. What is the hospital's policy on fetal monitoring? Is it used routinely or only in selected high-risk situations?
5. Are all the maternity facilities (including the operating room for cesarean sections) on the same floor and in the same wing?
6. What is the cesarean section rate?
7. If I have a cesarean will I be able to see my baby as much as I want?
8. Can my husband or labor coach be present for a C-section?
9. Can I hold and nurse my baby right away? If not, how long must the baby be in the nursery before it is brought to me?
10. Can the father hold the infant right after it is born?

Evaluating the answers to many of these questions will be easy. You don't need special expertise to decide that you prefer a smoke-free atmosphere or easy parking. You don't need a course in obstetrics to know that you would like someone close to you to be with you during childbirth, or that you want to be able to hold and nurse your baby without having to wait for some set hour.

Hospital Cluster System

The Cybele Society (see Resource Directory), an organization devoted to educating physicians in the importance of family-centered obstetrics, has promoted an innovative way to design hospital maternity care so that *all* women, not just those who have been labeled low risk, can enjoy a more nurturing yet medically safe environment.

The Cybele Cluster System is a self-contained unit. One room is used for labor, delivery (even a difficult one), and postpartum care for mother and newborn. A group of these rooms are clustered around a central core that contains a nurses' station, a family lounge, storage space, etc. Operating rooms for cesarean sections are part of the unit.

At present, the system has been adopted by only a handful of institutions, but because it offers advantages of economy and convenience, the number may increase significantly.

If you have a choice of hospitals, you may have to juggle sets of factors. Hospital A may have acres of parking and a liberal policy on rooming-in, but the fetal monitor may reign supreme. Hospital B may have a birthing room that seems ideal, except there is a monumental waiting list to use it. Be prepared to decide which factors on your wish list are the most important to you.

HOW DOES THE HOSPITAL C-SECTION
RATE AFFECT YOU?

The cesarean section rate is very high in some hospitals. A figure of twenty percent or more indicates that far too many procedures are being performed; it also indicates that this hospital has yet to grapple with the problem of preventing unnecessary C-sections.

Some hospitals may have higher rates than others because they admit more high-risk patients: women with diabetes and heart disease, young teen-agers, older women, drug addicts, heavy smokers and drinkers. The patient population will obviously affect the rate, but it still should not be over twenty percent. (There are medical centers with a large high-risk population and a much lower rate than this.)

Your individual situation and the way in which your own physician makes decisions is obviously paramount; nevertheless, if you enter a hospital that has a high C-section rate, you increase your statistical chances of having this procedure. Physicians—especially obstetricians with their large malpractice premiums—are very influenced by the behavior and attitudes of their colleagues. If everyone else at a hospital does a cesarean section in certain circumstances, it is unlikely that your physician will buck the trend.

HOW ARE THE NURSES TRAINED?

The attitude and skills of the nursing staff are of supreme importance in determining how well things go for you in the hospital. Your doctor will probably be there for only a small percentage of the time it takes you to have your baby. For most of labor you will rely on the hospital nurses to help you, coach you, and make sure that you get the kind of treatment you want.

Are there nurses on all shifts trained in Lamaze or other prepared childbirth methods? The nurse who is untrained in, and unsympathetic to, prepared childbirth will inevitably undermine a woman who is attempting to have her baby without medication. What about the nurses who care for mother and child after delivery? Are they knowledgeable about breast-feeding? If there is a central nursery, will the nurses bring your baby to you on your schedule or theirs?

The attitudes of the nursing staff will also greatly affect the way the father is treated. Nurses who have been trained to work with prepared couples will encourage him to be present for labor and delivery and will make sure that he is involved in coaching.

HOW LONG MUST YOU STAY?

Some hospitals, in an effort to fill empty beds on the maternity floor, have tried to counter the trend toward shorter stays by such dubious gimmicks as a candlelight dinner scheduled for the evening of day three. There is no medical reason for a mother and infant who are in good shape to stay for more than a few hours after birth. A stay of one day or less will save a good deal of money, reduce the exposure of mother and child to hospital bacteria, and return them to a more comfortable and familiar environment. If continuing care is necessary, it can be provided at home by a visiting nurse.

A woman with two or three young children at home may view a hospital stay as a welcome vacation. If insurance covers everything and if she is not concerned about such problems as set routines, limited visiting hours, and risk of exposure to infection, there would be no reason to press for an early departure. She might find, though, that having some help at home—either a supportive family member or friend, or a housekeeper—to free her simply to rest and take care of her new infant would be a better and more pleasant solution.

HOME BIRTHS

There is an enormous amount of controversy on this subject. Advocates, mostly lay people, declare that home is the best, safest, kindest, and healthiest place to give birth. In support of their arguments they point to countries such as the Netherlands, where home births are commonplace and safe. Their opponents, mostly physicians, fear unnecessary infant deaths and maternal damage, and point out that the speed with which things can go wrong in labor, and the instant need for skilled care for an infant who is born with abnormalities, demand a hospital setting.

If safety is the first priority, the opponents may be right. Obstetricians and pediatricians can cite case after case in which only speedy intervention saved the life of the newborn.

Until all hospitals can provide the kind of care that people want, though, there will be couples who choose their own bedroom over the impersonal coldness of the traditional hospital labor room.

The key to making a home birth as safe as possible is the presence of a well-trained birth attendant, and no one should attempt a home birth without one. A study published in *The Journal of the American Medical Association* showed there were 3 newborn deaths per 1,000 home births attended by a licensed lay midwife as opposed to 30 deaths per 1,000 unattended home births.[9]

FREE-STANDING BIRTH CENTERS

There are now about 100 of these facilities throughout the United States, and many more are being planned. They have been established in response to consumer demand for a place with some of the safety features of the hospital (life-saving equipment, trained personnel) without the rigidity of hospital rules or the emphasis on technology.

A good birth center has a homelike and relaxing atmosphere and a supportive staff. The birthing rooms look like bedrooms, and there is a lounge or living room and a kitchen that family members can use. You will be able to bring children with you if you wish. The staff should include certified nurse-midwives and nurses trained in obstetrics, with pediatricians and family physicians or obstetricians to back them up.

Birth centers offer prenatal care, postpartum and newborn care, and classes in prepared childbirth. They accept only those women who are at low risk for complications of childbirth.

Some physicians have become enthusiastic supporters and enjoy assisting at births in this kind of setting. Others, who are opposed to the concept, will cite horror stories; and it is certainly possible that a given birth center has a poor record. What the opponents will not do is give you comparable incidents that they know have occurred in their own hospitals.

Does a birth center seem ideal to you? Find out if there is one in your community. (See Resource Directory.) Is it properly staffed? Can patients be transferred swiftly and smoothly to a nearby hospital—one with a neonatal intensive care unit—if problems develop? If the answers to these questions are yes, and if you are healthy and anticipate a normal birth, this would be a perfectly sound choice.

CHOOSING A CARE GIVER

Once you decide on how and where you want to have your baby, your next step is to find the physician or midwife who will give you the care you need. Since regular prenatal care is extremely important to the health of both you and your baby, you should choose this person very early in your pregnancy.

You may have the world of childbirth choices at your command or you may have some limits, imposed by the fact that you live thirty miles from the nearest doctor or that you are forty-five, have high blood pressure and diabetes, and are pregnant with triplets. If you live in a rural area, there may be only one or two doctors to choose from and no nurse-midwife.

There are really two parts to maternity care: the prenatal checkups and advice that help keep you in good health during your pregnancy, and the actual childbirth. Women who receive good prenatal care have far fewer problems during pregnancy, fewer complications of childbirth, and healthier babies.

As you begin the process of choosing the person who will give you care, remember that there are certain qualities that will be particularly important to you. If you have lots of questions and want detailed answers, you must find someone who has enough time to sit down and talk to you. The famous obstetrician with the crowded waiting room may never have more than two or three minutes to spend in discussing your concerns.

If you want to be able to make decisions about the use of medication during labor and delivery, you need someone who thinks it appropriate for you to have opinions. If you want to have your baby at a maternity center, make sure this is something the care giver you are talking to is willing and able to do.

Obstetricians
(Sometimes referred to by the initials OBGYN, which stand for obstetrician/gynecologist.) Their training prepares them to deal with serious complications of pregnancy and childbirth, and to perform cesarean sections. As a group they tend toward intervention and the use of technology in childbirth and, with some exceptions, are not enthusiastic about such innovations as the use of a birthing bed, family participation, hypnosis for pain control, or soft lights in the delivery room. (In fairness, bright lights do make it easier for the physician, if not for you or your newborn.)

These generalizations apply to OBGYNs only as a group. Some of the leaders in humanizing birth and ridding it of unnecessary interventions are obstetricians.

If because of medical risk factors or preference you decide you need an obstetrician, you may find one or more in your community with a flexible approach and an open mind. If there are only one or two, you would probably want first to select the person to give you care and then plan to use the hospital where that doctor delivers.

Repeat Cesarean Section

Once you have had a C-section, must you forevermore give birth this way? Not necessarily. Much depends on the reason for the C-section and the way in which the surgery was performed. If you would prefer to deliver your next baby vaginally, raise the issue at your first meeting with the doctor. Some obstetricians are absolutely opposed to the idea; others will be perfectly happy to consider it and have helped many women who have had a C-section to have normal vaginal deliveries.

Specialists in Family Medicine
These practitioners are trained to provide prenatal care and to do normal deliveries; some have additional training in performing cesarean

sections. They are more apt to be flexible in responding to their patients' requests. Family practitioners can take care of a normal newborn as well as the mother, and are by training interested in the family aspects of childbirth such as parent-infant bonding, the relationship of the parents to one another, and the effect of the newborn on the family group. In choosing a family physician, you have the potential to use him or her as the primary care doctor for the entire family. Should you develop serious problems either during pregnancy or childbirth, your doctor would call in an obstetrician.

Certified Nurse-Midwives

These R.N.s have taken a special program that trains them to do routine deliveries and give comprehensive care to low-risk women and to normal newborns. Their training focuses on childbirth as a normal event, and they see themselves as helpers rather than orchestrators of the process. Nurse-midwives tend to spend more time with their patients during prenatal visits than do physicians, and are present for a longer time during labor and delivery. They will transfer women who develop problems to the care of a physician.

Regulations governing how they practice vary. Most states allow nurse-midwives to practice independently, but many hospitals do not grant them privileges. Therefore, if you want to use a midwife and also want a hospital delivery, you may have to shop around. (See Combinations section below.)

Lay Midwives

There is no uniform standard of training and certification of lay midwives at present. Some are highly experienced; others have been present at only a handful of births. Because the meaning of the term "lay midwife" is so variable, we would urge you to proceed with caution if you are interested in using one. Has she completed a formal training program or is she self-taught? How many births has she attended? How many deliveries has she actually performed. If your state licenses lay midwives, is she licensed?

In some states—Arizona, for example—efforts are being made to upgrade and standardize the training of lay midwives and require certain levels of training for licensure.

Combinations

Some innovative doctors now work with nurse-midwives as part of their practice. Patients can choose either the midwife or the physician for prenatal care and delivery. One obstetrician who is exploring new ways to organize his practice in order to give patients maximum care and attention works with a nurse-midwife and has added a nurse trained in counseling, who can spend time with patients who are having nonmedical problems that may affect their pregnancy.

Note: If you have strong feelings about the way you have your baby and have succeeded in finding a provider who shares your views, you are still not home free. Remember that most doctors do deliveries in rotation. Often doctors who work together have similar approaches, but this is not something to take for granted. Ask!

DETECTING FETAL ABNORMALITIES DURING PREGNANCY

New technology is now available to detect genetic abnormalities in the fetus and problems in its development, size, and position. Whether or not you need this technology will depend on your age, health, family history, and the progress of your pregnancy.

Ultrasound

Using a machine that employs ultrahigh frequency sound waves rather than x-rays to make a picture, the radiologist or obstetrician can create either still photos or a "real-time picture" of the fetus, shown on what looks like a TV screen. At present, the procedure is considered to be entirely safe.

Why use it? The scan will yield some important information including:

- the size of the fetus (helpful in determining the expected date of delivery and how well the fetus is developing)
- its position
- the cause of bleeding
- certain abnormalities such as hydrocephalus or a missing limb
- whether what seems like a very large fetus is actually two or three

Amniocentesis

This procedure, performed when a woman is 16 to 18 weeks pregnant, is used to determine whether or not a fetus has certain types of congenital abnormalities such as Downs syndrome, meningomyelocele (an open spine) and Tay-Sachs disease. Using ultrasound equipment to visualize the fetus, the physician passes a thin needle through the wall of the uterus and extracts some amniotic fluid, which is then analyzed in a laboratory. This procedure also reveals the sex of the fetus. If a couple finds out that the fetus is afflicted with the kind of genetic defect that will cause early death, severe mental retardation, or other serious abnormalities, they may then choose to terminate the pregnancy.

It is recommended that all women over thirty-five and those couples either of whom has a family history of such genetic defects as hemophilia, Tay-Sachs disease, or certain forms of muscular dystrophy have this test. If you fit the above criteria but would never consent to an abortion under any circumstances, there is no reason to have an am-niocentesis.

PROVIDER SUMMARY

PROVIDER	SETTING USUALLY USED	CONSIDERATIONS
OBGYN	hospital	• necessary for very high-risk patients • can do C-section if needed • rarely agrees to do out-of-hospital delivery • usually works in rotation • highest fees
Specialist in Family Medicine	hospital, birth center	• may not accept high-risk patients • will transfer patient to OBGYN should complications occur • flexible in approach • provides care for newborn in hospital and afterward • may not have hospital privileges in some larger cities • may work in rotation • may be willing to consider home delivery
Certified Nurse-midwife	birth center home	• low-risk pregnancy and birth • may have hospital privileges • may do home delivery • cares for newborn • will be present for more of labor than most M.D.s • will generally do delivery of own patients • lowest fees

---

A woman who has a personal or family history of such problems should see a genetic counselor before becoming pregnant. Ask your physician to find one for you, since patients are usually seen by referral.

The most common reason to have an amniocentesis is to discover the presence of Downs syndrome, which occurs much more often when mothers are past the age of thirty-five or when there has been a history of Downs syndrome in the families of the prospective parents.

Until recently it appeared that Downs syndrome babies, sometimes referred to as Mongoloids because of the Oriental look of their eyelids, were ineducable. Parents of such children were often urged to put them into institutions. Now, however, interesting new evidence has appeared indicating that at least some of these children can be educated to lead virtually normal lives.

Prospective parents who are told that amniocentesis reveals Downs syndrome have a difficult choice to make. If they are young, have other children, or could not deal with the intense demands of caring for such a child, they may choose to terminate pregnancy. What if they are older parents, perhaps of uncertain fertility, who see this as their only chance to have a child? The new technology has first reduced and then increased the complexity of such a decision.

CHOOSING YOUR BABY'S DOCTOR

"I belonged to a large health plan designed to serve New York City unions," recalls one mother. "I had never met the pediatrician assigned to me, and she left on vacation after examining my newborn without telling the hospital who was covering for her. When problems developed, no one on the hospital staff would tell me what was going on. They said that only my own pediatrician could communicate with me. Since she could not be reached, I spent several days consumed with needless worry, wondering what was wrong with my baby. (It turned out the problem was minor.)

"Her careless attitude was the first sign of what became a very unsatisfactory relationship. Had I talked to her before delivery, I would have quickly discovered I did not trust her and would have asked to have another pediatrician assigned."

A nurse-midwife can only give care to the normal newborn. A family physician, as the name implies, gives total care. A pediatrician takes care of children from the moment of birth up to adolescence, and with special training, may continue to give care through the teen-age years. (For a discussion of how to select a pediatrician, turn to page 22.)

Be sure to identify a doctor for your new baby before you give birth. If serious problems should develop, you will have someone to turn to for information and for help in choosing subspecialists.

In addition, if you wish to breast-feed, you may need the doctor to leave orders directing the hospital staff to bring the baby to you frequently and to give no supplements in the nursery.

FINANCIAL ASPECTS OF CHILDBIRTH

Of course, the cost of giving birth to a baby is a small fraction of what you will spend on feeding, housing, clothing, educating, and entertaining a modern middle-class child. Nevertheless, childbirth can cost a nice chunk of money, especially if your insurance policy does not provide coverage.

Here are some choices or combinations of choices that can save you money—if you have a normal, uncomplicated pregnancy, labor, and delivery.

Find a hospital that encourages one-day stays.
Use a nurse-midwife.
Use a family practitioner who can also care for your baby.
Have your baby at a maternity center.

All the options above will cost less than the traditional combination of obstetrician plus three- or four-day hospital stay. For example, in one city the birth center cost $600 while a typical three-day hospital stay cost $1600.

Before making any decisions based on money, it is extremely important to get out a copy of your insurance policy, read the exact wording, and see how it applies to the kind of care you are considering.

For obstetrical coverage, there is often a waiting period (commonly eleven months) after the insurance policy goes into effect. Sometimes normal labor and delivery will not be covered and cesarean section will. Or there may be a limit to the total number of days of hospital care, including admission for false labor. The use of either a birth center or a midwife may not be covered.

HOW TO CHOOSE WHAT IS RIGHT FOR YOU

Based on present evidence, we believe that prepared childbirth, inclusion of the father when possible, minimum medical intervention, a relaxing and comfortable physical setting, and the use of pain medications only when women ask for them, are all desirable.

We are impressed with a number of scientific studies that have compared childbirth conducted along these lines with the standard "medicalized" treatment, with its bias toward intervention (drugs, routine electronic fetal monitoring, and forceps). These studies have shown that the former approach is better: mothers and babies are healthier, and the experience is far more satisfying for the family.

What we think is better may not be right for you. So much of the ease or difficulty of birth depends on how relaxed and safe the mother feels. You need to make your choices based not on what is currently the interesting or fashionable thing to do but on what makes you feel secure.

CHAPTER TEN

HOW TO
TAKE CARE
OF YOURSELF

Do you ignore most of your aches and pains or do you pick up the telephone and call the doctor at the first hint of a fever or twinge of a stomach ache? Or do you fall somewhere in between, in the worry zone? You want to ignore a symptom or treat it at home—but then you begin to wonder: am I missing the early signs, the important but subtle first symptom of something dreadful that the medical profession knows can only be treated if it is caught in time? "Why didn't you come to me sooner," says the doctor in this nagging fantasy. "If you had, I could have saved you."

We have all been sensitized by the overpromotion of screening tests, by a vast outpouring of articles on medical topics in newspapers and magazines, and by organizations like the American Cancer Society to look at symptoms as early warnings. To some extent this is good. There are some types of cancer that can be successfully treated if detected at an early stage.

Unfortunately, this attention to the early signs of disease has led people toward interpreting all kinds of temporary illness and discomfort as signs of the body's fragility. In fact, we have remarkable powers to repel disease and keep ourselves well.

We hope to reassure you that there are many problems you can quite safely treat yourself. We offer some guidelines for identifying what they are, how to take care of the most common, and when to call a physician. (Check the Bibliography for books exclusively devoted to this subject.)

Although most of the chapter addresses the subject of how to take care of yourself when you are sick, we have also included a section on preventing illness, with an emphasis on the practical things you can do to stay as healthy as possible to as old an age as possible.

HOW DO DOCTORS FEEL ABOUT SELF-CARE?

More and more doctors see the value in educating patients to understand and take care of their own medical problems, but we must warn you that a surprising number are violently opposed. In their view, only doctors can care for or cure any medical problem. In Chapter One, we noted that for thousands of years the medical profession, which did little to cure and much to harm, had to rely on mumbo jumbo to keep patients coming back. It was important to their livelihood to make sure their patients did not catch on.

Such opposition to educating people to care for themselves seems odd today. Patients know that doctors have the ability to cure serious disease. What makes this opposition even odder is that doctors, of all people, know that most illness is self-limiting: it goes away by itself.

Some critics of the medical profession blame financial self-interest for this attitude; according to their reading, doctors are afraid that people will learn so much about caring for themselves that medical incomes will suffer. We feel it is a rare doctor who is that selfish.

The medical attitude that we would blame is that Achilles' heel of the profession, the feeling that doctors know best. About everything! After all, most of the people with M.D. after their names got all A's in high school, mainly A's in college, spent seven or more additional years learning about things that are mysterious to most of the rest of the world, and have incredible power—both legally and in the eyes of those who walk into their offices. If you were one of those people, you might even think that you knew everything.

THE DOCTOR'S SECRET:
MOST THINGS GO AWAY BY THEMSELVES

The standard line here is, "Your cold will go away in seven days without treatment, whereas with treatment, it will last only a week." Colds are caused by viruses, as are many other common ailments, and there are no treatments for run-of-the-mill viral infections. If you have one—a cold, a stomach upset, or a flu—doctors can treat your symptoms and reassure you that your body will heal itself, but they cannot cure your disease. (Certain serious viral illness, including polio, measles, mumps, and German measles, can be prevented by immunization.)

For some people, this is all fine. Others are upset by the fact the doctor can't do something. The classic medical joke on the subject tells of the man who comes to the doctor's office with symptoms of a bad cold. The doctor does an examination, tells him that he has a bad cold, and recommends rest, fluids, and aspirin for his fever. The patient is upset and demands treatment. "O.K.," says the doctor, rolling up the window, even though it is a bitterly cold January day. "Take off your shirt and stand in front of this open window." The man is aghast. "But I'll get pneumonia," he objects. "Exactly," says the doctor. "That I can cure."

Most primary care physicians estimate that eighty-five to ninety percent of the problems they see would go away by themselves. In fact, sometimes doctors get excited when they have a patient with pneumonia or a bladder infection because they can actually cure these problems. Having spent all those years learning to treat meningitis, pulmonary edema, congestive heart failure, or severe dehydration in infants, where is the medical glamour in explaining to patients that their colds and flus and rashes will disappear by themselves?

Part of learning to care for yourself is discovering which types of ailment are of the disappearing kind. If you feel you have wasted a visit to the doctor when he or she says, "Your problem will go away by itself," consider whether you really want to have one of the problems a doctor can cure. Try to use this visit to learn as much as you can, so you will save yourself the time, money, and effort the next time.

Ask the doctor how to recognize this particular problem.
Ask whether there is any treatment for uncomfortable symptoms.
Ask whether there is any symptom you should watch for that would mean you had a more serious problem.

When your doctor learns that you take care of your own colds and minor ailments, he or she will respond more quickly when you are concerned that you may have a more serious problem.

IS YOUR UPPER RESPIRATORY INFECTION VIRAL OR BACTERIAL?

Since there is little a physician can do to treat a viral infection but much to treat one caused by bacteria, it is useful to have a way to decide which kind of problem you have.

Fever or a cough are symptoms of either; most other symptoms point to a viral infection, including:

· runny nose
· headache
· achiness
· dizziness
· hoarseness

The more of these symptoms you have, the more likely the infection is viral in origin.

SYMPTOMATIC TREATMENT IS UP TO YOU

Whether to take a drug or not is entirely your decision. Some people are philosophically opposed to taking drugs. They feel good about not taking anything. And as long as they are dealing only with symptoms, this is perfectly fine.

Feeling better can be very important, though. If you are miserably congested and need something so that you can go to work, or school, or otherwise cope with life, there are effective and safe over-the-counter drugs that will reduce or suppress symptoms.

Before you begin to play doctor, you should memorize the doctor's cardinal principle, "First, do no harm." Try to respect the fact that your body is doing what it can to overcome the infection.

For example, if fever is your main complaint, remember that this is one way your body has to kill off the invaders by making it too warm for them to grow and flourish. Only treat the fever if it's making you uncomfortable.

If you have a cough, it serves a purpose: to bring up irritating mucus and clear your lungs. This kind of productive cough is doing you good, and you don't want to suppress it. To help nature, you can drink fluids to liquefy secretions, or take an expectorant cough medication.

YOUR HOME PHARMACY

We are going to discuss the basics of a home medicine chest. For a more detailed discussion we recommend you consult either *The People's Pharmacy, Take Care of Yourself,* or *The Well Body Book.* (Check the Bibliography under Drugs and also under Emergencies.) For most situations, a few standbys will meet most of your needs. In homes with young children, all medications should be under lock and key at all times.

If you have a chronic ailment, there may be additional drugs you should keep on hand. Check with your doctor to find out what he or she recommends.

Unless you have a special problem, your home pharmacy should consist only of OTC drugs. You don't want to stock up on antibiotics, for example, unless you live on an isolated farm in the Australian outback or some version thereof, or have a recurrent problem that your doctor wants you to treat with antibiotics whenever certain symptoms appear. (Women with chronic urinary tract infections sometimes keep a supply of Bactrim or Septra on hand.)

There are three reasons you would not want to keep antibiotics around:

1. They become outdated and either lose their effectiveness or actually become toxic. (During the fifties, many wives of doctors developed an unusual kidney problem because their husbands

had them take old samples of tetracycline that were sitting around the house.)
2. If you have a disease serious enough to require antibiotics, you should be evaluated by your doctor.
3. There is no way of knowing ahead of time which antibiotic you are going to need.

What to Have On Hand
acetaminophen
Afrin® spray
aspirin
bacitracin ointment
Ben-Gay®
Chlor-Trimeton®
Dramamine®
Gelusil-M®, Maalox® No. 2 or Titralac®
hydrocortisone cream
ipecac
Kaopectate®
Lomotil® (requires a prescription)
Robitussin®
Robitussin-DM®
salt
Sudafed®
Tinactin® cream
vinegar

CHECKLIST OF PROBLEMS
AND HOW TO TREAT THEM

Colds
We think you ought to treat just the symptoms that are bothering you, so we do not recommend products that contain multiple ingredients. The symptoms of a cold are discussed individually, below.

Cough
If you are coughing up mucus, you are doing what nature intended to get rid of infection. Don't take a cough suppressant.

Whether or not a cough medicine that is classified as an expectorant will help is not entirely clear. A number of studies have shown that no product is effective as an expectorant—and that staying well hydrated (six to eight glasses of fluid a day) is the only effective treatment. But a cough may be so irritating—to have or to listen to—that you feel you must try *something*. Robitussin is inexpensive and safe to use.

If you want to suppress a dry cough during an important meeting, at the opera, or while you sleep, take a single dose of Robitussin-DM.

You don't need any other forms of Robitussin, because you can buy separately the extra ingredients contained in those combinations.

Congestion
The simplest and cheapest way to treat nasal congestion is with a saline solution. Dissolve ½ tsp. salt in 8 oz. of water. Use an eyedropper (available in the drugstore for a few cents) to place two drops in each nostril every two hours. The solution is completely harmless and can be used as often or as long as you like. This solution is available for more money as an OTC preparation called Ocean Mist®. If saline nose drops don't work, you can use OTC preparations such as Sudafed tablets for congestion in adults (the liquid form for young children) or Afrin nasal spray. (Use Afrin for three days *at the most* and then stop even if your nose still feels congested. Otherwise you will encounter that unpleasant loop known as "nasal spray rebound," in which the spray begins to cause the congestion.) Chlor-Trimeton 4 mg. tablets are useful for allergic symptoms or to take in combination with Sudafed if you find the Sudafed makes you feel too jumpy.

Skin Problems
Bacitracin ointment for minor skin infections, such as swollen pierced ear lobes or scrapes that are a little tender. Also useful for putting on gauze and taping over a scrape—the ointment will not only help prevent infection but will prevent the gauze from sticking to the scab when you remove it. Tinactin cream for athlete's foot and jock itch. Hydrocortisone cream (there are a number of brands) for poison ivy, itchy insect bites, moderately severe diaper rash, allergic skin problems.

Benzoyl peroxide, the active ingredient in a number of different preparations, is very effective against mild acne. If self-care measures are not adequate, see a physician; there are now extremely effective treatments available.

One of these measures, the use of antibiotics in low doses, is sometimes resisted by parents. If you are a parent in this situation, you need to weigh your concerns about the over-use of antibiotics against the feelings of unattractiveness and anxiety your teen-ager is feeling.

Diarrhea
Kaopectate or other antidiarrhea agents. Take only after you have had a number of loose stools. The purpose of the diarrhea is to rid your body of toxins. You should not take anything for a brief episode of diarrhea (a day or two) unless you are getting physically or emotionally

irritated. The drug really doesn't treat the problem, only hides it. Drink a lot of clear liquids, and consume potassium in the form of citrus or tomato juice, or banana, if you feel weak.

Nausea and Vomiting
Treated not by drugs but by taking nothing by mouth for several hours and then sipping small amounts of weak tea with sugar or flat soda. If no further vomiting occurs, increase amount of fluids and gradually introduce easy-to-digest solids (plain rice or dry toast and jam).

Heartburn
Antacids such as Maalox No. 2, Gelusil-M or Titralac (the last two taste better[1] than most antacids) for "heartburn" or other problems with digestion. If you need them more than occasionally, consult your doctor.

Recurrent UTIs
If you are a woman prone to urinary tract infections, you may decide it will give you peace of mind to have some Pyridium® (prescription required) on hand. This is specifically to soothe the pain of a bladder infection to and will help relieve symptoms while you arrange for a visit to your doctor.

Fevers
Aspirin, or acetaminophen. Fever too is a way for the body to fight infection. If you are miserable, by all means take something. Otherwise there is no need to.

Recent studies have shown a correlation between the onset of a serious pediatric problem called Reye's syndrome, and aspirin taken for flu or chicken pox. If you have been treating your child for one of these problems with aspirin, and he or she develops persistent vomiting, call your doctor immediately.

Pain
Aspirin if the pain is accompanied by inflammation (sore throat), and choice of aspirin or acetaminophen if it is not (headache). Salt water makes a good gargle for sore throats.

Headache
Most headaches will respond to acetaminophen. If you have a severe headache, you may need three regular or two extra-strength. For recurrent headaches, check with a physician to make sure this is not a symptom of a serious problem.

In almost all cases, your headaches will turn out to be the result of muscular tension or emotional problems. Migraine headaches may respond either to avoiding certain foods or to medication. If you suspect you have migraine, see a doctor for further help.

If your headache is accompanied by ringing in the ears or jaw pain, you may have TMJ (tempero-mandibular joint) syndrome, a problem misdiagnosed and mistreated by most physicians. If you feel this is a possibility, be sure to consult a physician or dentist familiar with the syndrome, and insist on conservative treatment only. Avoid surgery or expensive appliances. (Many people with this problem are helped by learning techniques to reduce muscular tension.)

You can learn to treat your own headaches with techniques such as biofeedback, meditation, imaging, or a combination; your physician may be able to refer you to someone to teach you these skills or you can call the Department of Psychology at the nearest university for names of qualified practitioners.

Muscle Aches
Ben-Gay, which contains methyl salicylate (the active agent in oil of wintergreen), is very effective for muscle aches and pains.

Menstrual Cramps
May respond to exercise and acetaminophen. Herbal teas, such as chamomile or red raspberry leaf are sometimes helpful. Some women find that a Vitamin B_6 supplement decreases premenstrual and menstrual distress. If these measures do not help, get a refillable prescription from your doctor for one of the newly developed antiprostaglandins, and be miserable no more.

Vaginitis
Plain white vinegar (two tablespoons to a quart of water) makes a good douche. If the infection persists, you will need to see a doctor.

Multiple Symptoms
One general principle to keep in mind if you suddenly come down with something: the more different parts of your body that have symptoms, the less likely that you have a very serious problem. This runs counter to what most patients believe, and they become more and more anxious as each new misery manifests itself. But this multiplicity of symptoms is almost always evidence that they have one of life's passing—and untreatable—viruses.

ADVICE TO TRAVELERS

1. If you have a chronic disease and are going to be away from home for a period of time, discuss the situation with your doctor, who will make sure you have an adequate supply of medication, and may be able to recommend a local physician to call if your condition deteriorates while you are away.

2. If you are planning a trip outside the country, consider joining one of the organizations that lists English-speaking (some are American-trained) physicians practicing in various foreign countries. (See Resource Directory for details.)

3. If you are traveling in the United States and develop a serious urgent problem, don't hesitate to call your primary care physician. Almost all doctors have studied or trained or worked in a number of cities and have networks of associates through which they can find you a physician appropriate for your problem.

4. Dramamine is effective and safe for motion sickness. If you have severe problems, talk to your doctor about prescribing Transderm-Scop®, an effective long-acting treatment, applied to the skin!

Ginger has recently been demonstrated to be effective for motion sickness. In a study at Brigham Young University, volunteers who took capsules of powdered ginger and then submitted themselves blindfolded to six minutes in a rotating chair reported less stomach upset than those who took either Dramamine or a placebo.[2]

5. If you are going on a trip to an underdeveloped country or unhygienic area, ask your doctor to prescribe paregoric or Lomotil. (Be careful with Lomotil. The pills are tiny, and toddlers can easily ingest a handful and die.) Pepto-Bismol® has been shown to be helpful in preventing travelers' diarrhea, but must be taken in such large quantities that it is impractical for most people. A recent study showed that a short course of Septra or Bactrim is helpful in treating this problem; so you may want to ask your physician for a prescription so you can take one of these drugs with you.[3]

6. Be sure your immunizations (polio, measles, tetanus and diphtheria) are up-to-date prior to any foreign travel. If you are planning to travel outside Western Europe, consult with your physician at least six weeks before you leave. Depending on your itinerary, you may need immunizations against such diseases as yellow fever, typhoid, or cholera, and possibly a treatment regimen to protect you against malaria. Because there may be a change in the legal requirements for entry or in the existing health problems of a given country, be sure your doctor checks with the most recent edition of *Health Information for International Travel,* published by the Centers for Disease Control, for the latest recommendations on malaria chemoprophylaxis and immunizations.

WHEN DO YOU NEED TO SEE A DOCTOR?

1. When you suspect that your problem is more serious than the routine ailments we have discussed or that you have read about in a good self-care book.
2. When you are getting worse, despite whatever you have done.
3. If your symptoms remain the same for a long period.

In reality, almost nothing stays the same: if it gets better, forget it; if it gets worse, make an appointment. One doctor says as much when he tells his patients who have minor self-limiting problems, "If it gets worse instead of better, give me a call." According to him, "In all the years I have said that, no one has ever called me back."

This approach may be detrimental to the doctor's pocketbook. Those doctors whose closing remark is "If it doesn't get better, I'd like to see you again," have several repeat visits from people with minor illnesses who don't realize that their problems need time to disappear.

To be fair, some of the reason for this may lie in the difference between what doctors mean by "better" and what their patients mean. "Better" to most people means completely well, perhaps a remnant of what we say to children: "Is it all better now?" When a doctor asks you if you are better, he or she is really asking, "Are you feeling better than before?" The best way to avoid this kind of confusion would be to ask how long your illness can be expected to last.

WHAT TO SAY WHEN YOU CALL

If you have been treating a problem at home and it is not improving, when you call your doctor be sure to mention what measures you have taken; otherwise, you may receive telephone advice recommending that you do what you have already done. Make sure you mention how long the symptoms have persisted. This may be an important clue to your diagnosis. Tell your whole story; for example:

> I have a bad cough for two weeks that isn't getting any better, and I'm worried about it. I have been drinking two quarts of fluids a day, taking plain Robitussin, and getting plenty of sleep.

If the problem stays the same but is not worsening, how quickly should you act? The answer is more a question of temperament than of absolute medical need, as long as you do not ignore a problem or deny you have it. We are not suggesting you spend weeks or months mulling over symptoms that need to be discussed with a physician. But a week is not going to matter much so long as your condition remains the same.

One of the diseases people fear most is cancer; we have all become aware of the need to recognize early warning signs so that something may be done before the malignancy has spread out of control. However, there is some room for you to use judgment even here. For example, a woman finds a lump in her breast a day before her period. She may choose to wait until her period is finished to call her doctor, knowing that lumps that disappear after menstruation are benign. Or she may be so anxious that she calls to make an immediate appointment.

Note: If she does call, the doctor will probably strongly recommend that she postpone her visit, since the first step in evaluating the lump will be to see if it is still there after her period.

Since breast cancer takes many years to develop, and since it is no longer considered good practice to proceed from frozen section to mastectomy while the patient is lying anesthetized on the table, the woman who waits a few days has the same chances for cure as the one who goes for a biopsy the next afternoon.

Suppose you have come back from a vacation in Asia feeling tired and have no appetite. It suddenly dawns on you that you may be walking around with a case of hepatitis. You may. You may not. Since there is no treatment for mild or moderate hepatitis, and since it has now been shown that there is no reason to rest more or eat a special diet, you can, if you wish, wait another few days to see if the problem persists. Another possibility would be to make an appointment for a week or so in the future. By then, if what you have is a stomach virus or other passing problem, you will be feeling better and can cancel the appointment.

Almost nothing will be so much worse in a week that you will have made a poor decision by waiting. In fact, the kinds of problems that cannot wait a week generally cannot wait a day—they are either true emergencies or very urgent—and if that is the case you will not feel like debating with yourself whether you really need to see a doctor. You will know you need one.

What we are emphasizing is that you have a choice. You should do what feels most reasonable and reassuring to you. If waiting makes sense, you have some leeway. If you are worried, don't let someone else or your own fear of being thought foolish prevent you from seeking medical help.

WHAT DO YOU NEED THE DOCTOR TO DO?

Ask yourself the following:

Do I need a diagnosis?
Do I need reassurance?
Do I need a prescription?

Diagnosis

Life sometimes presents us with an odd rash, a peculiar twinge, or a stomach upset that cannot be dignified with a precise name. For example, if you go to see your doctor with some combination of nausea, vomiting, diarrhea, stomach ache, or cramps you may be told that you have a case of gastroenteritis. This means that after duly considering your complaint, the doctor has been unable to determine the cause and is telling you in medicalese that you have exactly what you already know you have.

For minor problems like this, having a diagnosis is not especially important. That minor problem may temporarily cause you major misery, but it will go away by itself without permanent ill effects.

One good way to deal with minor problems is to have on hand a book like *Take Care of Yourself,* which contains what medical professionals call algorithms. An algorithm is a branching sequence of steps to follow that will lead you to a decision, in this case whether or not to call a doctor.

Books can give you guidelines, but they cannot diagnose your precise problem. Your own gut instinct is often your best guide. Doctors, by the way, learn to rely on their patients' instinctive feeling that something is wrong. If a parent says about a child, "She just doesn't look right," this is sometimes more meaningful than the presence of a fever or other symptom.

Reassurance

If you have any doubts at all, call your physician. Don't be afraid that you are "just being nervous." If you are, you will get the reassurance you need and at the same time begin the process of learning what you can safely treat on your own. This is an important part of what a primary care doctor can do for you.

What if you are a worrier by nature? Chances are you will call the doctor more often than the person who assumes that everything will turn out fine. Some worriers find that knowledge decreases their anxiety by giving them more control over their bodies. If you are in this category, you especially need a doctor who is both reassuring and willing to explain things to you.

Prescription

There are times when you know not only what your problem is but also how to treat it. If you need a prescription in order to treat it, you will have to talk to a doctor. You may, for instance, have recurrent cystitis, and you may be utterly and miserably familiar with the symptoms. You know that you need Gantrisin.

If you have a doctor who knows about your cystitis, he or she will probably phone in a prescription to your pharmacist. If you have a recurrent problem, you could ask your doctor to write the prescription so that it can be refilled several times.

If you don't have a personal physician to call and can't get an appointment with a new doctor right away, you can try drinking very large amounts of fluid and acidifying your urine by taking vitamin C. You can drink cranberry juice, which has a specific ingredient that fights infection. A hot bath may help relieve the pain. Otherwise, you will have to go to an emergency room.

For many problems, with the newly expanded range of over-the-counter drugs available, you may find that there is a product that will relieve your symptoms. Ask the pharmacist for advice; he or she will be sure to recommend you see a physician if your problem is more serious than you thought.

SELF-CARE FOR CHRONIC PROBLEMS

Often people with chronic medical problems want to do as much for themselves as possible. Office visits can become very expensive, and the feeling of being out of control can eat away at independence and self-esteem.

Much depends on your particular problem and how you feel about it. If you would like to be more involved in your own care, you must find a doctor with an open mind and an innovative approach. Just because a problem has always been treated during an office visit by the physician does not mean that this must be so forever.

People with seizure disorders, for example, can learn to be more responsible for adjusting their medication. People with colostomies, arthritis, asthma, hemophilia, and a number of other diseases that have been diagnosed and stabilized can all contribute a great deal to their own treatment.

We discuss below three very common chronic problems: hypertension (high blood pressure), allergies, and diabetes. These three examples, we hope, will give you an idea of what people can learn to do for themselves.

Hypertension
First, of course, you need a careful diagnosis. One abnormal reading at a supermarket or street fair does not mean you necessarily have a problem. You must have several readings taken at different times to confirm the diagnosis.

You will need your doctor to establish a treatment plan. You may be advised to cut down on salt and lose weight to try to lower your readings, both things that you must do yourself.

What if you do need drugs? Your blood pressure will need regular monitoring, twice a month at first and then every month or two for the rest of your life. There is no reason why you must see a doctor on this schedule unless you have other problems as well. You can ask your doctor to help you learn to use a sphygmomanometer, a device used to measure blood pressure. You can buy one at your local pharmacy, but be sure to get a recommendation on what brand to use. (See the Resource Directory for more information.)

Instead of making frequent office visits, you can simply take a reading at home and then call your doctor with the results. When you call, you discuss any side effects you are having to the medication, so the doctor can make appropriate adjustments. There is a further advantage in home monitoring for those people who, because they are made nervous by going to the doctor's office, experience a rise in blood pressure there.

We hope that eventually more people will become actively involved in controlling their own hypertension. Right now, of the ninety percent of people whose condition is easily treated, half fail to get regular checkups and to follow their prescribed diet and drug regimen. Many of this untreated group then go on to suffer from heart and kidney disease and strokes that could have been prevented. Perhaps, had they been more actively involved in their own care, they might have been spared the serious consequences of neglecting this chronic problem.

Allergies
Even if regular shots are needed, once the diagnosis is established and the treatment program worked out, care becomes fairly routine. If you are interested in learning how to give yourself injections (difficult for most people) or better yet, in having a family member learn how, there is no reason why you cannot have your allergist make up the allergen and let you give the shots at home. If you have any questions, you can always call.

You may have to look a while before finding a doctor who is willing to work with you and teach you, but there are some who are more flexible and innovative. If you want to do home treatment, this might become a basis for selecting your allergist.

Diabetes
This is another chronic disease that lends itself to home care, and there is some new technology to help. Glucometers give a more accurate reading of the amount of sugar present in the bloodstream and enable patients to keep the disease under better control. Some diabetic patients, particularly those who are extremely sensitive to small variations in insulin dosage, may want to find out more about the recently developed insulin pumps that make it possible to administer insulin much more precisely. If your doctor does not have information on these advances, you can ask to be referred to a center that specializes in the treatment of diabetes.

WHERE TO FIND SUPPORT FOR SELF-CARE

One good way to find out what you can do for yourself is to seek out an organization or center that specializes in helping people with your particular problem. Many hospitals or medical groups offer special services for people with a given disease. In addition, lay people with various medical problems have formed their own self-help groups to promote knowledge and self-acceptance among those who share a particular illness or disability. (See the Resource Directory for information on how to locate special groups.)

PREVENTION AND WELLNESS:
WHAT YOU CAN DO
AND WHAT YOUR DOCTOR CAN OFFER

This book is primarily about how to deal with illness, but we would like at least to mention some of the measures you can take to prevent disease and promote positive health. Some of them are solely up to you; others require the participation of your doctor.

THE TERMINOLOGY OF PREVENTION

The medical profession uses specific terms to describe different levels of prevention:

Primary Prevention
Intervention to prevent the development of a disease. Immunizations are an example of what doctors can do in the way of primary prevention. Stopping smoking, decreasing alcohol consumption, increasing exercise, wearing seatbelts in cars, and losing weight are things you can do in this area.

Secondary Prevention
Early intervention in a disease so that it does not cause worse problems. Examples are detecting and treating high blood pressure to prevent strokes, doing Pap smears to detect and treat early cell changes in the cervix before they become malignant. Your role is to make sure you have those tests and screening procedures that are reliable ways to find treatable diseases. (See Chapter Eleven p. 251.)

Tertiary Prevention
Efforts to maintain a maximum level of independence in the chronically ill by restraining the progress of a disease after it has manifested itself. Generally this involves ensuring that the patient takes medication properly or is able to cope with the demands of everyday life. Your role here would be to participate, to ask questions, and to bring up any problems you are having in following a given regimen.

While most doctors consider secondary and tertiary prevention to be matters well within their sphere, not many are active in doing primary prevention. Then, too, not all patients want their doctors to insist they give up smoking, drinking, or consuming large quantities of food.

Many, in fact, resent a doctor's attempts to raise primary prevention issues as an unwelcome intrusion on their personal territory.

Those doctors who care about primary prevention will look for areas of risk in your medical history and will teach you what you can do to minimize them. For example, if you have a family history of heart disease, your doctor may advise you to increase regular exercise, lose weight and change your dietary habits, or stop smoking.

WELLNESS

Health is not a medical school subject. Physicians as a group have little training in how to make healthy people even healthier. Lack of training in this area may not really be a deficiency, since learning how to treat and cure disease provides an almost overwhelming amount of material to master.

Problems arise when people ask doctors, who are supposed to know all the ins and outs of the human body, to advise them on topics such as exercise, vitamins, and sex. For example, a patient laboring under this delusion asks the doctor whether a vitamin supplement would be a good idea. "Nonsense," answers the typical doctor, "you get everything you need from your food."

Unless you have already discussed in detail your diet and your concerns about possible areas of poor nutrition, the doctor's response is meaningless. Most doctors have no background or interest in the role of diet and nutrition in promoting health.

There are some, though, who are exceptions to the general rule, and if wellness is an important issue for you, you may be able to find a physician who shares your interest. Some doctors have begun to study nontraditional treatments for disease as well as the promotion of well-being through diet, exercise, and stress reduction.

If you want to find out whether the doctor you are talking to is among them, begin by asking whether he or she has a general interest in nutrition or stress or exercise before you raise particular questions.

STRESS: WHAT IT IS, WHAT IT DOES TO YOU, WHAT YOU CAN DO ABOUT IT

Stress is the nonspecific response of the body to any demand for change or adjustment (adaptation). If an event in your life requires such an adjustment, whether the experience seems positive (getting married, moving to a beautiful new home) or negative (losing a job, confronting your boss), there will still be an effect on your body. Understanding that the way you lead your life influences your physical well-being will encourage you to make decisions that promote rather than harm your health.

Our central nervous system is designed to protect us, to signal the body that it may have to meet some danger. A pioneer in examining this brain-body communication, the famous physiologist Walter Cannon, used the term "fight or flight" to identify the way the human body responds to a challenge. (If we were intelligent rabbits, would we instead be discussing the "flight or freeze" syndrome or if oppossums, the "flight or play dead" syndrome?)

When faced with a stressor (the stress-provoking experience), a trigger signal from the brain sets in motion a chain of chemical responses. Hormonal messengers alerted by the brain begin to prepare the body for action, either running away or standing and fighting. Changes include:

· increased heart rate
· increased blood pressure
· more rapid breathing
· increased muscle tone
· perspiration
· dilation of the pupils
· diversion of blood from digestive tract to muscles

This aroused state will not subside until the reason for it has disappeared or until we no longer perceive ourselves as being threatened.

In our modern world, running and fighting are usually inappropriate responses to provocation. We are supposed to be rational. The "fight or flight" response, however, occurs in a part of our brain untouched by logical argument. For example, if your husband/wife/boss/teacher accuses you of having done something stupid, you may, if you become sufficiently aware, notice that your body is preparing itself to fight or flee.

You could bristle your eyebrows, growl deep in your throat, and shove a fist in the offender's snout—or alternatively, sprint for the door, and run off into the night. Either action (although we are not recommending them) would burn up the adrenaline pumping through your veins more rapidly than what most people do: stay and explain in a reasonable way that the fault was unintentional, that it was due to a misunderstanding, sloppy accounting, or the fact that your lecture notes were stolen. In fact, the phrase "stewing in one's own juices" is an almost literal description of the state of the body when someone has not resolved a stress situation.

Having looked at the above list of responses, you should not be surprised to learn that stress is implicated in a number of diseases including:

cardiovascular disorders
high blood pressure

psychological problems
chronic diarrhea
ulcers
sexual problems
colitis
fatigue

Hans Selye, a major thinker and researcher in this area, described the body's three-part reaction to a stressor as the General Adaptation Syndrome (GAS).[4]

1. The Alarm Stage, the body's immediate preparation for fight or flight
2. The Resistance Stage: once the stress is dealt with, the body's attempt to restore itself to its pre-Alarm equilibrium
3. The Exhaustion Stage: if stress is too prolonged and the body cannot repair itself, adaptive energy becomes depleted, disease sets in, even death can ensue

Do not conclude, however, that all stress is bad. Some level of change and challenge is necessary to mobilize our energies, whether we are going out to hunt for roots and berries or look for a job. The optimum level of stress varies with the individual. Some people do better in a more highly charged atmosphere; others have a need for more stability and repose. What is stressful for one person isn't necessarily stressful for another; much depends on your own life history, your individual response to a given situation, and how well you have learned to cope with stress.

COPING IS THE KEY

If our lives are too stressful, if we begin to experience feelings of exhaustion, stomach aches, headaches, or loss of sexual interest, what can we do to stop, undo the damage, avoid reaching Selye's Stage Three? Depending on what appeals to you, there are a number of things you can do to take care of yourself before these warning symptoms turn into actual disease.

Exercise
This is an excellent way to calm yourself down and release tension. Exercise prompts the release of brain chemicals called endorphins, which are responsible for calming, tranquilizing and producing a sense of well-being.

Meditation
There are many different meditation techniques (yoga, transcendental meditation, progressive body relaxation exercises, deep breathing and

breath-counting): any one of them can be useful in evoking the "relax-ation response." Meditation requires learning and practice, and it must be done on a daily basis. Researchers have found that people who practice it are able to decrease heart rate, blood pressure, and respiration and increase feelings of well-being.

Biofeedback
This is the technological way to relax, and it can be especially effective as a way of learning to reduce tension in specific areas of the body. The person being trained is connected to a monitor with electrodes, which report the electrical state of the muscles. This information is trans-formed into a visual wave signal on a monitor and into auditory beep tones. Using this technique, people have learned to control such body functions as blood pressure and skin temperature, which were once thought to be completely unconscious.

Relearning
Since the way that we perceive a situation can make it stressful or not, learning new ways to look at and deal with situations can reduce their stress content. People can be trained to break old "worry habits" and to practice "thought-stopping," a technique that allows them to ac-tually block disturbing thoughts. By developing new coping skills, such as changing irrational ideas or learning to become more assertive, we can change the way events affect us—and our health.

Therapy
Our emotional problems may cause us to react to certain situations with a high level of stress. For example, if you felt strongly disap-proved of as a child, your response to even a mild and appropriate crit-icism might set your stomach to churning. By uncovering and dealing with problems in therapy, you may reduce the physical as well as the emotional toll they take. (See Chapter Eight for more on therapy.)

HOLISTIC MEDICINE

Traditional medicine views the body as a complex machine that is from time to time invaded by disease. The metaphors for treatment are often militant. Doctor and Disease are the principal characters; the pa-tient becomes the battleground upon which the war is waged with "the weapons of science." We have had a "war on cancer." The equipment (books, medicines, surgical tools) at the doctor's disposal are thought of as an armamentarium (an armory).

Great medical advances have been made using this model. Killers like smallpox and diphtheria and pneumonia have been slain by medi-cine *militans.*

But, as efforts to treat the major chronic diseases have intensified, doctors have come to realize that they must take into account more than purely biological factors. Family situation, state of mind, the intensity of the will to live may have a profound influence on whether people will become ill and if they do, how well they will respond to treatment.

More and more doctors are reemphasizing a concept that goes back to Hippocrates: that they must treat the whole patient, not just a diseased organ. Those who practice the art as well as the science of medicine have always instinctively known this to be true. Now, as researchers have begun to demonstrate how chemicals produced by the brain can affect health and disease, the instinctively holistic doctors have some scientific confirmation to wave under the noses of their skeptical colleagues.

The holistic movement, as distinguished from a return to holism in medicine, attempts to draw on a wide range of nontraditional approaches to healing and to wellness. If you attended a conference of holistic practitioners, you might find internists, psychologists, art and dance therapists, gurus of various Eastern religions, iridologists, poets, watercolorists, and clowns; and you would be able to take courses in subjects ranging from the psychology of cancer and basic anatomy to Tantric tennis, Celtic art and Congolese dance.

Although the mainstream of medicine has yet to incorporate Celtic art and Tantric tennis, it has begun to absorb some valuable nontraditional (for Westerners) techniques of healing, such as the use of acupuncture, hypnosis, and meditation. Doctors may be doubters, but they are also practical. Demonstrate to them that if you twirl a needle in someone's foot, a pain will go away, and they begin to pay attention.

HOW TO APPROACH A
NONTRADITIONAL TREATMENT

If you are healthy and want to pursue greater health through pleasurable and life-affirming activities such as massage, dance, music, body awareness, art—whatever appeals to you—you don't need medical advice. You are in the realm where your own feelings are enough to guide you.

We hope, though, that if you became ill, you would not neglect what medicine *can* do for you and that you would approach with caution any procedure that is invasive or seems unbalanced or distorted.

The greater the risks of a treatment, the more you would want some scientific confirmation of its safety and effectiveness. For example, regular fasting sounds good to many people; it seems like a rite of purification. Yet although a day without food won't hurt anyone, prolonged or regular fasting can be dangerous. The body, deprived of nourishment, begins to break down fat tissues, releasing toxic substances known as ketones. You can poison rather than purify yourself in this way.

There are people who, while they mistrust what they see as the powerful and "antinatural" interventions of physicians, unquestionably allow alternative healers to perform dangerous procedures. The results may be fatal.

For example, there is a treatment some chiropractors perform, a kind of enema called a colonic irrigation. It has no medical value whatsoever but appeals to some minds as a kind of internal housecleaning. A recent study in *The New England Journal of Medicine*[5] reported an outbreak of amebiasis (a parasitic intestinal infection) in patients who were given colonic irrigations at a chiropractic clinic in Colorado. Ten of the thirty-six people with the disease had to have surgery; and six of the ten died.

In considering a nontraditional treatment for an illness, we would suggest that you proceed with the same caution you would apply to any medical recommendation and that you ask the same kinds of questions:

Do I have a diagnosed disease for which a successful *medical* treatment exists?

Must I forgo the successful medical treatment to pursue the nontraditional one? (Sometimes you can combine the two.)

What are the credentials of the person who is treating me?

How well documented are the results of the treatment this practitioner is advocating? Has there been any scientific study of its safety and efficacy?

What are the risks?

What are the benefits?

HOLISM AND RESPONSIBILITY

A dominant theme in the holistic movement is that people are responsible for their own health and disease. At least some of this emphasis on personal responsibility has arisen, we think, as a reaction to the ignorance and dependence historically fostered by the medical profession—and to some extent is a response to the medical consumerist movement.

There are great virtues in this approach. As we pointed out earlier, there is very little a doctor can do to make someone stop smoking, stop drinking too much, get enough sleep, eat properly, maintain correct weight, control blood pressure, and exercise. These are all things that you must decide to do for yourself and are the very things that will have the most impact on your future health.

When it comes to disease, the feeling of individual control that this attitude fosters is positive and helpful—for some people. It allows them to mobilize their energies and creativity to find a cure. Norman Cousins, who in his book *Anatomy of an Illness* describes how he found his own way of treating a serious ailment, is a good example of the kind of person who benefits by feeling responsible.

There are problems, however, with assigning total responsibility to the sick person. A moving article by Alice Stewart Trillin, subtitled "A Cancer Patient Talks to Doctors," speaks of the "talisman of the will," her phrase for the confidence people feel in their ability to heal themselves. She then goes on to ask what happens if the talisman fails.

> *As much as I rely on the talisman of the will, I know that believing in it too much can lead to another kind of deception. There has been a great deal written (mostly by psychiatrists) about why people get cancer and which personality types are most likely to get it. Susan Sontag has pointed out that this explanation of cancer parallels the explanations for tuberculosis that were popular before the discovery of the tubercle bacillus. But it is reassuring to think that people get cancer because of their personalities, because that implies that we have some control over whether we get it. (On the other hand, if people won't give up smoking to avoid cancer, I don't see how they can be expected to change their personalities on the basis of far less compelling evidence.) The trouble with this explanation of cancer is the trouble with any talisman: it is only useful when its charms are working. If I get sick, does that mean that my will to live isn't strong enough? Is being sick a moral and psychological failure? If I feel successful, as if I had slain a dragon, because I am well, should I feel guilty, as if I have failed, if I get sick?[6]*

For some of us, the feeling that we are so personally responsible leads to feelings of fear or guilt or helplessness that may interfere with treatment. Those people who benefit from a healing relationship, who see the physician as the source of help, may not do so well with an approach that seemingly dumps the burden of illness back in their own laps.

It is interesting to reflect on the physician's role in this belief system. While at first glance it might appear that the physician who embraces this philosophy has only the patient's interest at heart, it seems to us that this point of view does much to protect him or her from having to take any responsibility for the failure of the recommended treatment. Since the traditional physician also tends to blame the patient for a treatment failure—"You didn't follow my instructions" or "Your body didn't react properly to the drug"—we seem to have traveled a long way without getting anywhere.

Once again, we suggest you need some amount of self-knowledge to find the right medical "fit" between your own personality and the style and philosophy of the practitioner you choose. Taking care of yourself means remembering that your emotional needs are not something apart from your purely medical needs. Perhaps it is an insistence on mind/body unity that will be the greatest general contribution of the holistic movement.

CHAPTER ELEVEN

HOW TO BE
AN INFORMED
CONSUMER
AND WHY

Many of the articles or books written about this topic have an underlying assumption: you must learn as much as you can in order to protect yourself against incompetent and/or greedy doctors. But we are assuming that you are going to use only well-trained and well-intentioned ones. The purpose of this chapter is to help you protect yourself against the confusion and ignorance you may encounter even in good-to-excellent physicians.

There are otherwise knowledgeable physicians who simply do not understand, for example, that abnormal laboratory results are frequently meaningless; that making clinical decisions based entirely on their own experience can be dangerous; and that certain treatments or procedures are done because of ritual and tradition, not scientific evidence.

HOW DOCTORS GATHER INFORMATION

Most of us, including most physicians, base our judgments and decisions on what is known as "anecdotal evidence." That is, we recall an individual situation, remember how things worked out, and generalize from that. If, for example, you learn you have breast cancer, you may think of your aunt who had a radical mastectomy and is still alive twenty years later. You may want to have the same treatment, even though recent medical studies have shown less drastic procedures to be just as beneficial. Or you have an arthritic friend who says, "Nothing helped until I tried Drug X." Should you need treatment for arthritis, Drug X comes to mind and you ask for it, even though you do not know your friend's exact diagnosis. (Arthritis is a word that means different things to different people.)

Doctors are practical. They want to use what they have seen to be effective. So if they remember that certain patients did well after trying a given treatment, they may conclude that this is the best treatment for all patients with similar problems.

Anecdotal evidence has its points. It was, for a long time, the only scientific tool medicine possessed. It is firsthand, and it is observable. But it is limited by the smallness of the group of people one doctor treats and the doctor-observer may be biased. What appears to be cause and effect may really be only coincidental or a result of the "placebo effect."

An additional problem is the possibility of a "skewed sample" (the opposite of a random sample): a certain surgeon sees a number of patients other surgeons have failed to cure—the successful cases do not get referred—and based on this group of people, draws the gratifying but false conclusion that the operative procedure the other surgeons used is inferior to his or her own.

HOW MEDICAL STUDIES AFFECT YOUR CARE

Good doctors continue to educate themselves once they leave training. One of their basic sources of information is what they refer to as "the literature": that is, the medical journals and recent textbooks that contain the latest thinking on a given problem. At times, consulting the literature is a little like reading tea leaves: the angle from which you approach the problem and the exact choice of journal will significantly influence your conclusions. And, like tea leaves, the literature is occasionally just plain wrong.

One example of this occurred during the 1940s as researchers struggled to identify the cause of retrolental fibroplasia. It had become obvious that many early premature babies were afflicted with a particular kind of blindness. What was especially puzzling was the fact that the incidence was highest in certain medical centers, where the care was supposedly superior.

The literature offered a number of explanations and suggested close to fifty different treatment approaches. Eventually, the cause of blindness was correctly identified as the high level of oxygen being given routinely to these babies in the medical centers on the assumption that the more oxygen, the better.

A medical study, like any form of research, is bound by the constraints of the researchers' imaginations; if they do not suspect that high levels of oxygen cause blindness in newborns, they may study everything from salt in formula to fluorescent light bulbs, come up with only slightly suggestive statistical correlations, and go on blinding little babies.

Although the literature is fallible, it is right far more often than it is wrong. Your doctor should know what the most recent studies say about your disease and its treatment. Often before making a definite recommendation, a good doctor will tell you that he or she must read up on your case. Based on the latest studies, he or she will then advise you as to what seems to be the most effective treatment. If your doctor learns that there is a great deal of disagreement in "the literature," you would probably do best to choose the safest alternative.

If you are the sort of person who wants to play a part in decision-making, you need a doctor willing to share information with you. "Why do you think I should have this treatment?" you ask. Listen for an answer like the following: "A recent study in *The Journal of the American Medical Association* showed that ninety-two percent of people with your problem were helped by this drug."

WHY READ A MEDICAL STUDY?

We are all bombarded by medical information from many sources—newspapers, radio and TV, magazines. Some of it is sensational and not really valid; some is important. How do you sort out whether the latest diet or the newest treatment for cancer has some value? Is it really worth the effort?

In earlier times, there was no difference between medical knowledge and ignorance, except that ignorance might actually have been somewhat safer. The learned doctors of the Middle Ages and Renaissance bled their patients to death. Had you wished to become an informed consumer of, say, seventeenth-century health care, you would have learned that the medical consensus supported leeches as the best available treatment. Today, there is a much greater gap between ignorance and knowledge, and therefore, a much greater incentive to inform yourself.

People who feel most secure when they possess as much information as possible should consider reading the same medical studies their doctors read. We will explain how to go about doing this: what the essentials of a proper study are, how to have some sense of its validity, and how to ask your doctor questions based on your reading. In addition, we are going to explore, for your own protection, two questions that many doctors fail to consider: statistics and risk preference. First, how do those statistics, upon which all medical decisions are based, really work? Understanding how probable the possibilities are may save your money, your health, and your life. Second, how do you use those statistics to make a choice that fits in with your own needs?

HOW TO THINK ABOUT A MEDICAL STUDY

Whether you read the actual study in a medical journal or an account of it as reported in a newspaper or magazine, be alert to what characterizes a well-designed scientific study.

It must be reproducible. Independent researchers should be able to achieve the same results.

It should involve an experimental group and a control group. The control group receives no treatment, or standard treatment.

The two groups should be closely matched for factors such as age, sex, ethnic background, and previous health. Otherwise, differences in results may be a reflection of the inherent differences in the groups.

If possible, the subjects should not know which group they are in. The jargon used for that condition is "blind." Certain kinds of studies can be organized so that the researcher also does not know which group a given patient is in. Such studies are called double-blind and are generally considered the most definitive.

HOW TO KNOW IF THE STUDY SHOWS ANYTHING AT ALL

How many subjects were studied?

Were the groups really matched or was there something about the control group that was different from the experimental group?

How well was the placebo effect screened out of the results?

Was there a statistically significant difference between the control group and the experimental group in the outcome?

When researchers submit their findings to a medical journal, their results are looked at critically to find flaws. The loftier the reputation of the journal, the stiffer the criticism. One key question is whether the experiment really shows a "significant difference" between what happened to the experimental group and what happened to the control group.

SIGNIFICANCE VERSUS RANDOMNESS

"Significant difference" or "statistical significance" are key phrases used in medical studies. These phrases signify that we are not dealing with luck or chance.

If you call heads, flip a coin four or five times, and actually get heads four or five times in a row—you may begin to think that you have special powers or that the coin is weighted. You attach significance to what has happened. Eventually, though, as you continue to toss the coin you will get as many tails as you do heads. The coin toss is random, but you must do it a certain number of times to observe that this is so.

The same principle holds true of medical studies. If you cured four people of toothache by touching a needle to a caterpillar and then to the afflicted tooth (a treatment favored by the physician of King Edward II) you might conclude that you had hit on the perfect toothache remedy. If you tried your treatment on a much larger group, perhaps eliminating the placebo effect by dividing your subjects into two groups and offering the control group a needle untouched by caterpillar, you would find that your remedy was sadly lacking. (Since to our knowledge this experiment has never been done, we are perhaps being unscientific in guessing the outcome!)

If you are comparing two different treatments, how much of a difference in the results must the study demonstrate before you can conclude that the difference is real, not just the kind of "lucky streak" you might have with a coin toss? Unlike the coin toss, which can easily be repeated thousands and thousands of times, medical researchers have much greater difficulty in enrolling thousands of participants in a study. Still, a method had to be found to help decide whether the results of an experiment showed a real difference or were merely a random outcome.

In judging medical studies, physicians and researchers have decided to discuss how real they believe the results to be in terms of the mathematics of probability. Those studies in which the findings have a less than one-in-twenty chance of being random are considered to have real, or significant, results.

Look at a study in a medical journal and you will see those odds of one-in-twenty converted into the decimal .05. The researchers will state that their findings are "significant at the .05 level." Or you will read "$P < 0.05$," meaning "the probability of this being random is less than five in one hundred." Bear in mind that this decimal still means that there is a one-in-twenty chance that the conclusion is false—that after five heads in a row, the next flip will be tails after all.

A more definitive experiment would be "significant at the .02 level" (there is only a one-in-fifty chance that there is no real difference); better yet is the .01 level (one in a hundred). By the time you reach the .001 level (one in a thousand), you have about as definite an answer as you will ever get in medical science.

THE LIMITS OF MEDICAL STUDIES

Unlike the concrete and value-free laboratory experiments in chemistry and physics you may remember from your high school days, experiments on human beings are bound by medical ethics. Thus, the subjects must be told that they are part of an experiment. Because most human experiments are carried out on relatively small groups of participants, the results are often not as significant as studies that can employ very large numbers of subjects and be repeated endlessly. The larger the number of subjects, the more likely it is that a "real" difference will emerge if one treatment is actually superior.

And, too, once a treatment appears to be of value, it then becomes unethical to withhold it from those who might benefit. This is what has happened with electronic fetal monitoring (EFM). Because it seemed to offer great benefits in detecting fetal distress, it was widely introduced before careful studies were done of its effectiveness. As fetal monitoring has spread, the cesarean section rate has soared.

What is not entirely clear is whether EFM really does help prevent brain damage in newborns. The whole question could have been examined more easily before the technology became so widespread; it is now extremely difficult to study because of the ethical problem posed by withholding something that so many physicians feel is life-saving.

HOW TO FIND INFORMATION YOU CAN TRUST

These days the human body and its care, feeding, and preservation are a popular topic. Go to a bookstore and you will find shelves filled with books on every conceivable topic. There are books by physicians and nonphysicians. There are guides to self-care, diet, exercise, surgery, pregnancy, cancer, stress, etc. There are authoritative-looking tomes and jazzy paperbacks. Every women's magazine has at least one article on some aspect of health; many feature regular columns written by doctors. News magazines and newspapers report regularly on medical advances.

All information, however, is not equal. How do you decide that what you are reading is reliable? Following are some questions to ask about what you are reading or hearing:

Is this an original article or report, or an account of what some other source said?

If these are new findings, have they been published in a reputable medical journal?

Is it prepared by a physician or other health professional, a professional health writer, or a general magazine or newspaper reporter?

If written by a physician, what are his or her credentials?

Does the publication or TV show have a reputation for accuracy?

Are the facts presented supported by references to authoritative sources?

If personal opinions are presented, are they so identified?

Answering these questions may be rather a large order, but let's take them one at a time. If you are watching the news on TV and are told that "an exciting new cure for cancer has just been discovered," pay close attention to the source of the discovery. If you investigate further, you may find that the researchers themselves are making only modest claims. Television and radio news departments look for the angle that will grab your attention; the pros and cons and maybes and tentative conclusions that are part of medical research lack punch and will not make their way as readily into the newsroom as the "amazing new treatments" and "miraculous new advances."

Often the media will quote new findings that have just been presented at a major medical meeting but have yet to be published. If your doctor is not greatly impressed, it is because physicians know that it is much easier to present a paper at a medical conference than to get that same paper published in a major journal. The prestigious medical journals have a very intensive process of review and re-review, a process that involves their own staffs as well as outside experts. The organizers of most conferences are much more casual about choosing which papers will be presented.

So the newspaper article or TV news spot should state that the study has been published, name the journal, and give you some information as to what kind of study was conducted and by whom. The two journals that are most apt to be quoted these days are *The New England Journal of Medicine,* and *The Journal of the American Medical Association (JAMA).* Both sources are extremely reliable; your only concern about them would be whether they are being quoted accurately.

You might think about going to the library and reading the entire article from the journal itself. If you can't get through all the technical material, read the abstract at the very beginning, the introduction to the article, and the discussion at the end. The two journals mentioned above usually have several articles in each issue that are of interest to the sophisticated lay person, so you may want to look through the table of contents to see whether anything else attracts your attention.

At times, you will hear of a study published in a journal with a fine-sounding name, without realizing that the source is, in effect, the house organ of a given industry, whether it be dairy products, sugar, beef, or food additives. Considering the source, such findings must be considered suspect. The doctor who is conducting the study is being paid to do so by that industry, a practice that can lead to a less careful research (even if unintentional). One rarely sees this type of research prove anything that the industry in question does not wish to prove. Examine the masthead very carefully if you suspect the journal is of this type.

What about the professional's expertise in a given area? A specialist in medical reporting like Lawrence Altman, M.D., who writes for *The New York Times,* will present authoritative articles on medical advances. Both this writer and his sources are reliable. Unfortunately, you cannot safely assume that a writer with a medical degree is by definition well informed. Many have convinced magazines to print what turned out to be unsupported outlandish theories.

A well-researched article by a professional health writer is apt to be an excellent source of information. For example, Jane Brody, a health writer who also produces a column that appears regularly in *The New York Times,* will usually quote several authorities, cite their credentials, present the existing range of opinion on a given health topic, and draw a balanced conclusion.

Each year a number of books appear, many written by physicians, that claim to have the answer to the riddle of life or death or sometimes just fat. We would advise you to adopt an attitude of suspicion in direct proportion to the magnitude of the author's claims. If the author says that you can lose twenty pounds a week by eating grapefruit seeds, onion skins, and honey cake in rotation, you might wonder how long life can be sustained by such a diet and whether the weight loss will be permanent or transient.

A careful reading of such books will provide you with clues as to their worth. If the authors make unsupported claims (i.e., claims without references to reliable studies) or present statements as fact that appear to be merely personal opinion, you might well wonder about the validity of their conclusions.

There are personal books that are extremely valuable such as *Anatomy of an Illness,* a book we have already cited several times, in which Norman Cousins describes his successful attempts to cure himself of a life-threatening disease. Here, the author is quite explicit about the personal nature of the material. He clearly labels his own opinions as such; there is no hard sell.

The kind of book or article we are warning you about is the one that makes statements like, "The amazing truth is that you will never get cancer if you follow my system," or, "There is now a vast conspiracy to prevent the public from using this harmless and inexpensive substance to cure arthritis."

Another kind of article to be wary of often appears in magazines; it usually describes various medical advances as "the latest word." The advances are usually noted very briefly, and their source is not always mentioned. Since there are thousands of medical journals these days, almost anything is apt to be proposed as a possibility by one of them. Magazines like to pick up novel ideas that will interest their readers; most are not substantiated by careful investigation. The people in the forefront of discoveries tend to look at the positive side of what they are doing and leave it to others to find the flaws.

HOW DOCTORS RESPOND TO NEW INFORMATION

Most doctors do not respond the way you might like to new information. They do not usually say things like, "What an exciting approach. How enormously intelligent of you to find all this out." They are far more likely to say, "Are you going to believe everything you read?"

Doctors should listen to what you have to say with an open mind. They should not make you feel as though you were trespassing on hallowed ground when you reveal that you have read or heard of a medical study that may throw light on your situation. What you are encountering is a very human reaction, or overreaction, to the suspicion that you do not trust his or her professional judgment.

Medicine is still more of an art than a science; there are many situations where your physician must sift through a number of possibilities and conclude that one of them feels like the right diagnosis or treatment, hoping fervently that this assessment is really correct. If you display your own doubts to a doctor who is engaged in this sort of educated guesswork, you may touch a sensitive nerve.

If you have read carefully, if your source is a good one, and your concern significant, especially if you have been following the recommended treatment without success, you have every reason to expect your doctor to listen to what you have to say, if not with intense enthusiasm, at least with respect.

HOW TO PRESENT INFORMATION TO YOUR DOCTOR

You will be more apt to get an attentive hearing if you know and cite the original source of your information. If you are facing gallbladder surgery and read about a *New England Journal* study in your newspaper, mention to your doctor that you understand that *The New England Journal* has recently published a study on the necessity of gallbladder surgery. It is likely that he or she will take the time to discuss the issue in detail.

If, on the other hand, you remark that, "I read somewhere that doctors do not always agree on the necessity for gallbladder surgery," your doctor will not be especially interested.

If you are not sure of the source, or know that it is not highly regarded by most of the medical profession, you might do well to tread with caution. You might say something like, "I just read an article about a new method of treating kidney stones with herbal tea. Do you think there might be something worthwhile in that?" If you are tactful, your doctor will not feel you are questioning his or her judgment and will be more apt to listen to you carefully and give you an informed answer. A good doctor who is not familiar with the subject will probably ask for more information, such as a copy of the article or the original reference.

The kind of article that will probably be least likely to impress your doctor is a personal account written by someone who has found a cure through means not seen as effective by the medical community. Unless there is no alternative available to treat your problem, the chances are that your doctor will shrug off this type of information as essentially meaningless.

SHOULD YOU TRY A NEW DRUG
OR AN EXPERIMENTAL TREATMENT?

Being an informed consumer is obviously easier when a body of reliable information exists. If you have a medical problem for which the treatment is agreed upon by the medical community, you will have a much easier time asking questions and getting answers.

What do you do, though, if there is no established treatment for your problem or if you have a life-threatening disease for which there is no known cure? People with genital herpes, an extremely painful condition, are interested in any new development that promises relief or cure. Several drugs have been researched; one or two show promise. Should someone with herpes volunteer to be an experimental subject for the latest ray of hope, or wait to see if the proposed treatment really makes a difference? What about the person with incurable cancer who reads that a clinic in Mexico promises to cure his or her condition?

Before signing up for an experiment or asking for a newly released drug, you need to ask the following questions:

1. Do I have a serious or life-threatening medical problem?
2. Have the standard treatments failed?
3. What are the known or possible risks of the new treatment?
4. What are the proven benefits?

If you are truly at death's door and a researcher appears to have come up with something that might save you, you will probably want to try it. The risks of the treatment are outweighed by the probability of dying without it. But if, like the heroine of the old grade B (or possibly C) movie *Queen Wasp,* you are an aging beauty who tries a poorly tested treatment for eternal youth and turns into a version of the insect from which your cure was extracted, you would have been better off aging gracefully.

Who will answer your questions? Pioneers of a new approach are always extremely enthusiastic; they will tend to emphasize the successes and minimize the failures. Listen to what they say, but get another opinion on the subject from a physician who is not involved in the research or testing.

If you have a painful condition that is not life threatening, you have a more difficult decision to make. You will want to know at a minimum whatever the researchers have learned about potential risks and benefits. The problem lies in what they don't yet know. New drugs and treatments are first tested on animals, but no animal is exactly the same as a human being. Until a treatment is tested over time on large numbers of people—some adverse effects show up only after several years—no one can be sure of its safety. The more minor your problem, the more reluctant you should be to try a new drug or treatment.

INFORMED CONSENT

Except for critical emergencies, in which moments make a difference, a physician must obtain your written consent prior to performing a procedure that entails any risk. After a detailed discussion, the doctor will give you a form to sign that spells out what procedure will be done and the specific risks and consequences. This process of giving you all the information, the negative as well as the positive, is what makes your consent "informed."

> The parents of a college student drop her off at the school's health center because she has a urinary problem. When they get back to their hotel, there is a message awaiting them to call the hospital. It seems the physician had decided their daughter needed an intravenous pyelogram to determine if her infection were caused by an underlying abnormality of the urinary system. She had suffered an extremely rare, but not unheard of, reaction and died despite all medical efforts.

Could this death have been prevented? Perhaps by a patient alert to the significance of informed consent. Because it is known that there is a chance of dying from an IVP—however unlikely—patients have to sign to indicate that they understand the risks. But because the possibility is so remote, physicians almost never mention it. The preprinted form that the patient signs may have no reference to the possibility of death and may be written in difficult technical language.

If you are alert to the way the system works, you will be alerted by *the fact you have to sign a form.* This means that there is *some* risk, even if no one has discussed it, and the doctor or hospital wants legal protection. Tell the doctor that before signing you want to know exactly what the risks are; if told "none worth mentioning," then ask why you must give signed consent, something you don't have to do for procedures with literally no risk, like drawing blood.

If pressed, even a reluctant physician will acknowledge that there is a "one-in-a-million" chance of having a bad reaction; further questioning will elicit the information that this bad reaction is that your heart will stop beating. The doctor may add that equipment is available to treat that eventuality.

Pushing once more, you will learn that occasionally no treatment will work but that the risk of your dying from an IVP is less than the risk of dying in an auto accident on the way home after the procedure is done.

This may be true, but it is irrelevant. Only you should decide whether even that tiny risk is worth it, and you can't make the decision unless you know the risk exists.

There are a number of procedures besides IVPs (IUD insertions, spinal taps, arteriograms, kidney and liver biopsies are examples) that are presented as routine but that have rare yet serious risks.

Before signing anything, ask what is to be gained from the procedure and what are the risks of skipping it. Only with this information can you make a truly "informed" choice.

WHAT IS THE DIFFERENCE
BETWEEN A NEW TREATMENT
AND SOMETHING TRULY
EXPERIMENTAL?

Some drugs or procedures are truly experimental, ruled as such by the FDA, and can only be used legally by certain doctors. In such situations, you will usually have to sign an elaborate consent form that spells out the risks. Read it carefully, and discuss it with the doctor. If he or she says, "Oh, the risks have been exaggerated so that patients won't have a basis for suing if they do poorly," be suspicious. An ethical doctor will take every risk very seriously and show you what benefit you can expect that would make the risk worth taking.

A procedure or drug may not be officially experimental, but there may be only one or two doctors in your community who use it. For example, chymopapain injections have just been approved by the FDA for use in certain types of disc problems. Some orthopedists are very interested in this new approach; others are not. You may want to avoid surgery by trying the injections. The doctors who use them will be quite enthusiastic; the doctors who do not may be skeptical. Your best bet would be to discuss your questions with your primary care doctor and have him or her try to get as much information as possible for you.

WHAT IS A QUACK AND CAN YOU TELL?

History will separate the true medical advances from the false. The problem is that at any given time some things that history will vindicate are denounced by the establishment as being nonsense. We mentioned the now famous observations of Semmelweis in our chapter on childbirth. In his day, he was treated with contempt by colleagues who refused to consider that their unsanitary practices were the cause of childbed fever. All he suggested they do was to scrub their hands before examining patients, a remarkably inexpensive and noninvasive approach to preventing mortality.

We use the word quack to describe a medical charlatan; this may be an M.D. or a self-anointed "professional" who claims to have a medical cure and who knows how to turn people's desperate need for help into cash.

There are certain characteristics that are shared by almost all quacks:

They never publish their findings or theories in a reputable journal;
they rarely publish anything at all. Nevertheless, they claim their
treatment has miraculous results.

They claim there is a conspiracy to prevent the world from benefiting from the new treatment.

Their credentials are questionable.

They are usually loners, unaffiliated with reputable hospitals, professional organizations, or respected doctors.

You will not find references to their treatments in medical libraries.

They often recommend elaborate special diets and injections.

Their treatments require many visits or are otherwise expensive.

When you ask quacks why they have not shared the wonders of their new treatment, you will get an answer like, "My treatment is so revolutionary that it will put establishment doctors out of business, so they won't let me publish," or "Other doctors are working on this and they are preventing me from getting any credit." Or they may tell you that "I just want to cure people and don't want to take time away from that."

Next, their credentials are usually dubious. They may have an unusual degree. Mel Brooks gave us an example of this characteristic in one of his wonderful creations, a personage who introduced himself as Docker Haldanish and, when questioned on his pronunciation, revealed that his degree was not M.D. but Dcr.

The quack may have a degree that sounds better than a Dcr., perhaps a Doctor of Science from an obscure university. (According to *Health Quackery*—see Bibliography—Ernest Krebs, Jr., who with his father patented Laetrile, obtained an honorary D.Sc. from a small college in Oklahoma that is not accredited to grant such a degree.) Quite often the degree turns out to be of the mail-order variety.

If a quack claims to be an M.D., you will have an easier time checking his or her credentials (see Chapter Two). Often they turn out to have been graduated from schools you have never heard of. They will not be affiliated with a reputable hospital or be a member of a prestigious medical society.

Doctors are trained in groups from their very first weeks in medical school when they are divided into fours for their dissection training. They tend to be gregarious, going off in packs to conferences, meetings, and seminars, and joining organizations of like-minded physicians. Even those who are on the fringes and are experimenting in areas that their more traditional colleagues sniff at, like acupuncture, spinal manipulation, or hypnotherapy, will be involved with the Establishment Fringe. The doctor who uses acupuncture may be the only one in town who is doing it, but he or she will be involved with doctors elsewhere who are doing the same thing and is apt to be a member of an organization promulgating the new approach.

Quacks, on the other hand, are usually loners. Occasionally, several of them will practice together as partners, but they will not have any sort of network with other doctors.

Many quacks use a lot of hocus-pocus: elaborate tests, special diets, large doses of vitamins, minerals, drugs (especially injectable ones), special foods, various rituals. They will use terms of their own invention to describe the effects of their treatment, attributing the effectiveness to a mysterious-sounding force or effect of some sort.

Some of this may be difficult to sort out from the mumbo jumbo of establishment medicine, especially when you look at some of the concoctions the oncologists use these days, or the new technology available to any of the "ologists," for that matter. The difference is that you will be able to look up medical mumbo jumbo in a library. It will be familiar to other doctors, who may be able to translate it into English for you.

Ask a quack for further reading or supporting materials and you will get an anecdotal answer. "I've treated dozens of these patients with this approach, and all of them are alive today, thanks to me." They are not apt to quote controlled studies or published reports. They are generally grandiose (that is, even more grandiose than other doctors), talking about all the people whose lives they have saved. They will probably be able to refer you to several patients who will give testimonials.

The patient whom they claim to have cured of an incurable disease may have been misdiagnosed, may have been the one in twenty who was going to survive anyway (almost nothing is universally fatal), or may be in a temporary remission. The one thing to be said for quacks is that they are very effective in mobilizing the placebo effect, the powerful and very real ability of human beings to cure themselves through belief. If the medical establishment has no treatment to offer you, Dr. Quack may be worth the money.

But beyond the cost, there are some serious questions here, ones you will have to ask yourself, since the quacks are not given to self-doubt. One is, "Am I forgoing an established treatment of real value for something with no scientific merit?" For example, the treatment of childhood leukemia has improved dramatically; many children are now completely cured with chemotherapy. If your child is diagnosed as having leukemia, do you have the moral right to decide that you really prefer to try Laetrile, a substance that has been scientifically studied and found to be of no benefit?[1]

The other question is one of the stickier ones in medicine. Is any hope better than no hope? If you are dying of incurable cancer, should you try to come to terms with your condition or should you try every possible treatment up to the last moment? If you have provided for your family and can afford to try the treatment you want, and if you are not forgoing something with a good chance of success for something that is scientifically pretty shaky, there is no reason why you shouldn't do as you please. It is really a personal decision.

THE ISSUE OF UNCERTAINTY

One recurrent theme throughout this book is that there is much that is uncertain about medical diagnosis and treatment, to the despair of both doctors and patients. To attempt to cope with this uncertainty, many doctors resort to unnecessary lab tests and even to inappropriate treatments. Patients often try to evade the issue by seeking out a practitioner who will give them a guarantee, and this may be one of the strongest appeals of quacks.

This is most apt to occur when someone who has a serious disease learns that the established treatment has less than a hundred percent chance of saving his or her life; that is, the doctor is not promising that the disease will not win.

At this point, the sick person is sometimes tempted to abandon a trusted doctor (and the chance of receiving the best treatment available) to search for a practitioner who will promise a cure. We would recommend instead getting a second or third opinion or doing some reading.

It is frustrating and disappointing that doctors always seem to hedge their bets—but it may be because they are humble enough to understand the limits of their knowledge. Honest practitioners cannot guarantee life to anyone. They can only do their utmost to make the odds more favorable.

DO YOU NEED HEALTH CARE WHEN YOU'RE HEALTHY?

So far, we have discussed how to get health care when you are sick. (It really ought to be called sickness care.) Unless whatever is wrong with you is very minor and self-limiting, you will usually turn to a physician for help. When it comes to health care, as opposed to sickness care, it is really up to you to decide whether you want or need a "physical," how often you need one, and whether to avail yourself of various screening procedures from stool tests for blood, to Pap smears, to blood tests designed to detect carriers of Tay-Sachs disease.

WHAT SCREENING TESTS WILL DO

Since most health insurance pays rather skimpily for preventive care, you might want to find the least costly way to get screening tests. Most communities offer programs to detect some of the common treatable diseases. For example, your employer may offer hypertension screening; the local hospital or another health organization may sponsor a free screening program for glaucoma.

There is a lot of confusion in the area of screening. Patients often believe that a single x-ray or blood test will reveal whatever abnormalities lurk within the body. In fact, their doctors must specify which abnormalities are to be tested for. Doctors, too, are confused about the usefulness of screening tests and commonly order tests that not only have little chance of helping you but also may harm you by leading to recommendations for risky procedures that you don't need. Obviously you need to ask a few questions:

Will the test detect disease if I now have no symptoms?
What are the risks of the test?
How meaningful will the test results be?
Will this test lead to effective treatment if I have the disease?
Will an earlier diagnosis make a difference in the long run?
Is the possibility of finding a treatable abnormality worth the cost, inconvenience, or discomfort?

A screening test must be able to pick up disease in an asymptomatic person. An electocardiogram (EKG), commonly used as a routine screening test, often fails to do this. People can have a normal EKG one day, and die of a heart attack the next day.

The test should be safe. A cardiac stress test for someone with no symptoms cannot be justified, since people occasionally die as a result of such a test.

Screening tests should reliably identify people with medical problems. The SMA-12, a dozen blood chemistry tests that laboratories have lumped together in one package for reasons of economy, not necessarily because of their diagnostic usefulness, yield at least one false positive in almost fifty percent of cases.

Will a treatable disease be found? A CBC (complete blood count) is inexpensive and safe, but its primary purpose as a screening test is to detect asymptomatic anemia. There is no evidence that anyone is really better off being treated for asymptomatic anemia. (The test may possibly pick up early leukemia, but the odds of that happening are so remote, and the advantages of early treatment so minimal, that most authorities do not support that indication.)

To justify doing a screening test, your doctor should be able to show that treatment will be more effective if the diagnosis is made earlier. The American College of Radiology now no longer recommends a screening x-ray to detect lung cancer. By the time the disease can be diagnosed in this way, the cure rate is no higher than it is for symptomatic disease. Thus, the tests become a waste of money and an unnecessary exposure to radiation.

There is an additional wrinkle that many physicians do not understand: sometimes early diagnosis adds years to your *disease,* rather than years to your life. For example, suppose mammography reveals a tiny breast cancer, undetectable by physical examination, in a fifty-year-old woman. She has surgery and lives for fifteen years before dying of metastatic disease. If the average woman lives only ten years after detection of breast cancer, it appears that early diagnosis added five years to this woman's life.

But let us suppose that she had not had mammography, and that she discovered the cancer at fifty-five by physical examination of her breast. She has surgery and succumbs ten years later to the disease.

In the first case, she lived fifteen years after diagnosis, and in the second, only ten—but either way she died at age sixty-five. Many authorities on the subject are still not convinced of the benefits of early detection if it does not lead to an increase in actual life-span. Not only does the woman in our example fail to live longer with early detection, she spends five extra years as a cancer patient, with all the emotions and stresses her diagnosis and treatment cause.

WHAT DOES AN ABNORMAL
TEST RESULT REALLY MEAN?

There are two basic goals in developing a test. The developer of the test may make it highly *sensitive,* so that it will always be positive in the presence of a certain disease, or highly *specific,* so that it will only be positive if one given disease is present and no other. Ideally, all tests would have a specificity and sensitivity of 100 percent. But no one has been able to come up with such a test.

Every test has a "false positive" rate; that is, some number of people will have abnormal results even though there is absolutely nothing wrong with them. There is also a "false negative" rate to contend with: some people will have the disease in question, even though the lab test says they don't.

How would you design a lab test? Take tonometry, the test for glaucoma, as an example. You sit in front of a machine, put your chin on a metal bar, and hold your eye open and at the ready for an enormously startling puff of air. The puff test measures something called intraocular pressure. Up to a certain point the amount of pressure is normal; above that point, your eyes may be in trouble. The question is where to draw the line.

On a scale of 1 to 100, for example, you might find that people with readings of 20 or under are always normal and those who have readings over 24 always have early glaucoma. What do you make of readings of 21 to 24? Some people in this range will turn out to be abnormal, others perfectly normal.

If we set 20 as the upper limit of normal, we will make the test highly sensitive; that is, we will not miss a single case of glaucoma. But the specificity of the test will be terrible. Very few people in the "abnormal" range will actually have any disease. They will be subjected to the expense, discomfort, and anxiety of several unnecessary visits and further testing until their freedom from glaucoma is established.

On the other hand, if we set 24 as the upper limit of normal, everyone with an abnormal reading will have the disease. The test now becomes 100% specific. Unfortunately, by doing this we will be missing thousands of cases of early glaucoma. By moving up the number we have destroyed the sensitivity.

In the end, the line between normal and abnormal is a compromise. We choose a number between 21 and 24, so that the test will be reasonably specific and reasonably sensitive. Neither is 100% now.

To many people the statistical basis of modern medicine is upsetting. Why cannot ways be found to determine things with absolute precision? How do you know whether your abnormal result means you have the disease? (Most of us are so happy to get a "negative" result that we don't worry whether that also may be false.)

Doctors too have difficulty dealing with the concept of false positives. Part of their ignorance stems from the fact that, in general, statistics is underemphasized in medical education.

The authors of an article in *The New England Journal of Medicine*[2] decided to find out if doctors really knew what false positives meant. "We asked twenty house officers, twenty fourth-year medical students and twenty attending physicians ... at four Harvard Medical School teaching hospitals, the following question: "If a test to detect a disease whose prevalence is 1/1000 has a false positive rate of 5 percent, what is the chance that a person found to have a positive result actually has the disease, assuming that you know nothing about the person's symptoms or signs?"

Only eighteen percent of the subjects gave the correct answer: one in fifty. The most common answer to the question was that there was a ninety-five percent chance that the person had the disease.

The problem for you, the patient, is that a doctor who is unable to estimate the significance of your test results is apt to order further and more invasive tests. Let us suppose that you are feeling fine but have decided to have a routine physical. Your doctor orders some tests and one comes back abnormal. He or she does not focus on the fact that the machines that do these tests are programmed to define the five percent of results that are farthest from the average as abnormal. Your doctor repeats the test. Still abnormal. The next recommendation is to send you to the hospital for an expensive and invasive biopsy.

Now suppose that this particular disease occurs in 1 out of every 400 people, and you know that five percent of normal people will have an abnormal test result. Are you sick or are you well?

You can calculate that 20 people out of 400 will have a false positive, but only 1 in 400 will turn out to have the disease. So only 1 out of the 21 people (4.8%) who had an abnormal test will actually be sick. Although you are still not sure whether you are sick or well, you now know the odds substantially favor your being well. Because the biopsy is risky, you may decide to forgo it, unless your doctor can identify factors in your genetic makeup or health history that put you at higher risk for the disease this test would reveal.

There is a mathematical tool called Bayes' Theorem that takes into account the sensitivity and specificity of the particular test and the prevalence of the disease; that is, how commonly the disease is found in the population being studied. (The more common the disease, the greater the likelihood that a positive test result really shows the presence of that disease.)

After the numbers are plugged into the formula, Bayes' Theorem will yield the predictive value of a laboratory test—that is, the probability that your abnormal result really means something. Now you know more about the subject than most doctors.

Why do we say that? As we noted earlier in the book, doctors are trained on sick patients. When they order a blood test to detect cirrhosis of the liver for an alcoholic patient who is vomiting blood, it will usually come back positive, since almost every one of these patients will actually have cirrhosis. A high percentage of lab tests in the hospital are true positives.

Once the doctor goes into private practice and begins to use these same lab tests for screening people with no particular symptoms, most of the positives will be false. But because doctors have so often seen the people who do have the problem, they often lose track of the fact that the tests are not nearly as specific on "asymptomatic patients," a bit of medical lingo used to describe normal people.

Also, as we have mentioned, during their training doctors are constantly warned of the importance of making the correct diagnosis. An article in the highly regarded British journal *The Lancet*[3] points out that "A mistaken diagnosis is categorically condemned . . ." and then goes on to describe the pressures on the doctors in training to make the right diagnosis. "The basic message is that discipline and faithful adherence to the proper method and procedures cannot but lead to the right outcome." If things don't go well for the patient—or, in medicalese, if there is a "wrong outcome"—this is seen as "the inevitable result of omission and ignorance, which should be condemned." Little wonder, then, that doctors who are severely criticized for missing a diagnosis and who are more familiar with desperately sick patients than with healthy ones, generally order too many screening tests and have too much faith in their usefulness.

WHAT PHYSICALS WILL AND WON'T DO

There are a lot of misconceptions as to the real value of regular physical examinations for people who are not sick. To see if you share one or more, answer the following statements true or false:

> The doctor will be able to detect all illness by doing a physical examination.
> An annual physical can give me a clean bill of health for the year.
> The physical and tests are so thorough that I do not need to mention any embarrassing or scary symptoms I have had.
> Medicine has made so much progress that there are definitely some problems I should be checked for on a regular basis.
>
> [Only the last statement is true]

The value of physical exams and screening tests depends on your age, the state of your health, and the particular risk factors you have acquired or inherited. If you are a forty-five-year-old woman who smokes and drinks heavily, and whose mother and older sister have both had breast cancer, you will need more in the way of checkups and screening than will a twenty-year-old with a negative family history (medicalese for a family with no history of significant medical problems).

Regular physicals *cannot*
· prevent sudden death
· give you a clean bill of health from one year to the next
· reveal everything that may be wrong with you

They *can*
· establish a baseline of what is normal for you
· reveal the presence of certain diseases at an earlier stage
· help you and your doctor get to know one another
· give you a chance to ask questions that are troubling you
· give your doctor a chance to counsel you on behavior that is detrimental to your health, such as overeating or cigarette smoking
· give your doctor a chance to make sure your immunizations are up-to-date: (rubella for young women, tetanus/diphtheria every ten years for everybody, influenza for those over sixty-five or with serious chronic disease, and pneumovax and hepatitis B immunization for selected high-risk patients).

THE SIGNIFICANCE OF YOUR MEDICAL HISTORY

You may recall that at the beginning of the book we emphasized the enormous importance of the medical history. The forms you fill out that ask if you have ever had any number of diseases, broken bones, operations, hospitalizations, etc., and the questions the doctor asks you are part of history-taking. If you are careless or embarrassed about providing information, you may limit the ability of your doctor to diagnose or even suspect the presence of a problem, or to rule one out.

For example, discharge from the penis may be a symptom of gonorrhea. If a man mentions this, the doctor will do a smear. The presence of this disease would otherwise be missed.

Actually, as we mentioned earlier, physicians believe that they get as much as seventy percent of the information needed to make a diagnosis from the questions they ask you. People who assume that the physical exam will reveal whatever problems they may have are expecting their doctor to play veterinarian.

(For a discussion of habits detrimental to health and the role of stress in lowering resistance to disease, see Chapter Ten.)

HEALTH RISK APPRAISALS

Some physicians or health promotion programs use an interesting tool called a "Health Risk Appraisal." Your answers to a series of questions about health habits and family history are fed into a computer that then produces an individualized profile. These appraisals compare your "medical age" to your chronological one and also compare your statistical life expectancy to that of your peers. They then show you how by changing your health habits, you can add years to your life expectancy. For some people, this kind of analysis provides a strong motivation for change.

With this background information, let's discuss the issue of how often you should see a doctor when you are well. The following recommendations are based on: (1) an extensive study commissioned by the Canadian government to determine what problems really are worth screening for, and (2) the most recent guidelines issued by the American Cancer Society, plus a major study by two public health specialists published in *The New England Journal of Medicine.*[4]

Men Under Forty
If there is no personal or family history (parents, grandparents, and siblings) of any unusual medical problems and no particular risk factors based on ethnic origin, work history, etc., the only problem really worth testing for in someone who feels generally healthy is high blood pressure (hypertension). This should be done every year or two. Although a checkup is not medically necessary, this does not mean that there is no good reason to have one if you want one.

Talking about health concerns with a doctor is very reassuring to many people, and the sense of security they derive is possibly even therapeutic. In addition, there are a number of self-care issues that are important, including learning how to do a self-examination for testicular cancer and Hodgkin's disease as well as having the doctor review health habits, including smoking, drinking, use of drugs, use of seatbelts, and any risk factors pertaining to ethnic origins (sickle cell disease and G6PD deficiency for blacks, Tay-Sachs for Jews of Eastern European origin, certain anemias for those of Mediterranean ancestry).

Men Over Forty

Once a man reaches forty, he should be screened for blood in his stool on a regular basis, in the hope of detecting colorectal cancer at an early stage. (This is a simple test the patient can do at home.) Some authorities feel that, in addition to the test for blood, it is worth doing a sigmoidoscopic exam every few years. Because this procedure is very uncomfortable, some men avoid getting any sort of checkup.

If you are in this category, tell your doctor you do not want sigmoidoscopy unless you have symptoms, but make sure you get a blood pressure check and a test for blood in the stool.

What about all the other tests you or your acquaintances have been subjected to—electrocardiograms (EKGs), chest x-rays, the SMA-12 (a group of blood tests), urinalysis, complete blood count (CBC), spirometry (a test for lung function), and tonometry (a test for glaucoma). Do you need all of these?

Tonometry seems to be worthwhile and is in itself harmless, although we have already discussed the problem of false positives. It is particularly important for anyone with a family history of the problem. Many physicians do a blood test for serum lipids, believing that abnormal results, which indicate an increased risk of cardiovascular disease, may motivate patients to improve their health habits. The other tests on the list, according to almost all careful studies of the subject, are not worth much as screening tests for people with no symptoms.

Why are they done so often? Because, as we have pointed out, doctors are trained to diagnose sick people, not well people. They know, for example, that an EKG is an invaluable tool for diagnosing someone with heart problems but simply do not understand how little value it has for healthy people.

Women

Women should have all the screening tests recommended for men in their age group. In addition, authorities recommend that they have regular Pap tests. How often is regular?

Annual testing is no longer the rule for the women with no special risk factors. The American Cancer Society is now recommending that a woman have a Pap test two years in a row. If both these tests are negative, they feel that once every three years thereafter is sufficient.

The usefulness of going to a physician for regular breast exams is not as well established, although most doctors feel it is well worth it for women to examine their own breasts monthly and to see a physician if any change is noted. If you are a woman who examines her breasts carefully, you would probably not really benefit from a routine physician exam. If you don't do breast self-exams, it would be a good idea.

The use of mammography (a kind of x-ray) to screen women for possible breast cancer seems to be well established as being worth the risk of the extra radiation only for women over 50, or for those younger women whose mother and/or sister has had breast cancer. The new equipment delivers a low dose of radiation; if you are having this test for screening, insist that it be done by a machine that delivers less than one rad per breast.

Many doctors feel women over forty should have regular pelvic exams to screen for cancer of the ovary.

Children

There is general agreement that frequent examinations of infants and regular examinations of children are beneficial. In the first eighteen months, babies need five or six visits for their immunizations, so it is convenient to have an examination at the same time.

If your child's physician seems helpful and knowledgeable about development and behavior, be sure to schedule several visits just before and during the first year or two of school. New problems and concerns having to do with social and learning behavior at school may appear, or a previously unnoticed medical problem, such as a hearing loss, may be unmasked.

Adolescents

Medically, the only special screening test for this age group is for scoliosis (curvature of the spine), particularly prevalent in girls. The screening is simple and the problem can be treated effectively if it is caught early.

There is very little serious disease in this age group. The value of checkups lies in the reassurance they can provide; preteens and teenagers have a lot of concerns about their bodies, their height, weight, skin, sexual development. They may need to know that all is normal. A sympathetic physician who is experienced in caring for this age group may be able to play an important role as an authoritative adult they can trust, since they will begin to fight against having their parents play that role.

Commonly, they have trouble asking for help or advice on their own, but if they find themselves in a doctor's office for a checkup and a couple of open-ended questions are asked, they will often share their concerns quite readily. In this process, the doctor is actually screening for the greatest risks to this age group: suicide, accidents, substance abuse, unwanted pregnancy, and sexually transmitted diseases.

WHAT IF YOU WANT THE TESTS AND CHECKUPS?

Have them. If you feel more secure having had a blood test or two, there is no reason not to get them, so long as you understand the issue of false positives and the sometimes dangerous trail that leads from a meaningless statistical variation to a potentially risky diagnostic procedure.

The information in this chapter is intended to help you decide whether you are shortchanging yourself or endangering your life by not having annual checkups or numerous screening tests. There almost seems, at times, to be the implied promise that if you have such exams or tests, you will live forever, that you will never die of cancer, diabetes, heart disease, etc.

If you feel healthy, you probably are healthy and will most likely stay that way, especially if you have had the few tests recommended. If you do not feel healthy, see a physician, preferably a primary care physician you feel you can talk to comfortably.

CHAPTER TWELVE

HOW TO PAY
FOR WHAT
YOU NEED

Margot, a registered nurse, decided to be a full-time homemaker when she and her husband Bill moved to a new community. After all, with their first child on the way, she thought she would enjoy staying home for a while. She and Bill are pleased with the way things have worked out. His new job, unlike his old one, will not require very much travel. What seems like perfect planning is marred by one expensive oversight. It seems that Bill's health insurance will only cover deliveries that occur eleven months after the policy goes into effect.

Nowadays, relatively few of us pay directly for our large medical expenses. Insurance, Medicaid, and Medicare take care of the hospital bills and, depending on the plan, various other costs, such as some portion of doctors' fees, drugs, lab tests and psychotherapy. Members of health maintenance organizations pay almost nothing for medical care either in or out of the hospital, provided they follow certain guidelines.

There is a tendency to develop a false sense of security. Thinking that "the insurance will take care of it," some people have made expensive assumptions about just what their particular policies would do for them.

All policies are not the same. Some are generous, some stingy; and the benefits listed in the policy can be affected by the way in which the insurance company administers and interprets what seem to be simple provisions. For example, one northwestern insurance company issues a policy that states that care of sick newborns is covered. Parents who are told that their babies must be treated for jaundice quite reasonably assume that their insurance will pay. Not necessarily, according to the administrators, who have ruled that they will not pay unless the bilirubin reading (a measure of the severity of the jaundice) is twelve or over. Thus, if a physician feels that an infant with a reading of eleven must be treated, that treatment will not be covered.

DO YOU REALLY HAVE
A DECISION TO MAKE?

Should you spend time comparing the features of different policies—or can you skip that step and concentrate your energies on reading the policy you have? If you are single and if your company has one plan covering everyone, you have no decision to make. Similarly, if you are married, if your spouse is not employed, and if you can add your family to your present policy at little or no cost, then you obviously sign up for that policy.

You do have decisions to make if you must buy your own insurance (later in the chapter, we discuss the risks of choosing to have no insurance) or if your employer offers more than one type of insurance. The federal government, for instance, offers its employees several different plans. An increasing number of employers offer the opportunity to join a health maintenance organization (HMO) as an alternative to a traditional indemnity plan, which reimburses you for incurred medical costs.

If you have choices to make, you need to know which type of plan is the best deal.

Should you choose the policy that covers most of your expenses or should you take one with a high deductible?

If you and your spouse are working, should you both have coverage under each other's insurance?

Which plan should you choose for family coverage? If an HMO is being offered, should you join?

This chapter has a dual purpose: to give you the information you need to choose insurance and to help you make the best use of the policy you presently carry. Before you read on, think about your own attitudes. Do you feel secure only if you carry a lot of coverage? Do you approach the subject analytically, performing careful calculations to decide whether you will fare better financially by taking the money you would have mailed off to the insurance company and putting it in the bank? Will you conscientiously file claims as expenses arise, or are you so impatient with the paperwork involved that you simply pay small bills yourself? How you feel about insurance affects the way you use it—and its value to you.

WHY BOTHER TO READ YOUR POLICY?

Insurance prose is not exactly spellbinding, and the prospect of spending an evening with your policy may seem less than enticing. But before you decide to skip the whole thing, consider the following: a recent study by The National Center for Health Services Research found that most consumers are unaware of what their health insurance really covers. Seventy percent don't know whether they are covered for outpatient mental health services and eighty-three percent are mistaken about nursing home coverage. Similar confusion was found in a number of other areas.

Have you ever read your policy? Its exact wording, and the waiting periods and exclusions it specifies for certain types of problems, may make an enormous financial difference to you. If you know what is covered beforehand, you may be able to arrange your care to take advantage of these conditions, but it's too late to do anything once you have received treatment and put in your claim. You will be out the money if you find your insurance will not cover the bill. For instance, many policies specify a waiting period before certain procedures will be covered. If the couple in our example at the beginning of this chapter had read their policy and planned the pregnancy accordingly, they might have saved as much as $2,000.

Pay particular attention to the terms of coverage for the following areas:

1. psychotherapy
2. emergencies
3. setting in which care is covered
4. doctors

Therapy

If your policy covers therapy, read carefully the terms under which it will reimburse you. Is the coverage for psychotherapy restricted to psychiatrists and Ph.D. clinical psychologists? If so, and you were thinking about using the services of an Ed.D. psychologist who had been recommended to you, that choice might cost you $1,000 a year in coverage. Learning this after you have begun to establish a relationship with a therapist could be a real cause of conflict.

Emergencies

How does your policy cover emergencies? Will it pay only for treatment given in a hospital emergency room or will it also cover treatment given in a doctor's office? Better to know ahead of time rather than trying to fumble for the information while your child is bleeding from the scalp. Is there a time limit on such visits? If so, you may be better off seeking care earlier in the course of a problem rather than waiting and finding out that you haven't met the time requirements.

Setting

Certain procedures and treatments may be covered only if care is given in a hospital. Even though office surgery might be cheaper, you cannot safely assume that you will be reimbursed. (If you want out-patient surgery, you may be able to get the insurance company to agree to cover it if you discuss it with them beforehand.) On the other hand, some progressive companies cover certain procedures only if done on an out-patient basis.

Which Doctors?

Are you covered by a plan that pays "member doctors" in full and other doctors only in part? If so, you certainly want to know that before choosing a doctor. If you join an HMO, (discussed later in the next chapter), you must know exactly what the rules of the plan are prior to getting care; otherwise, you may not be covered at all.

FREE CARE FOR NONCOVERED PROBLEMS

If immunizations are not covered by your insurance, you may be able to get them free from a community health center. Free treatment is also often available from community health centers that specialize in treating sexually transmitted diseases.

A BRIEF GUIDE TO INSURANCE TERMINOLOGY

Whether you are about to buy health insurance or are trying to understand what kind of coverage you already have, you are really going to have to read the entire boring, probably confusing, policy from beginning to end. If your coverage is through your employer, the company's benefits or personnel department may be a useful source of explanations. If you are self-employed, an honest and knowledgeable agent or broker can be helpful—but there is no substitute for your own efforts. Depending on your situation, it may be very important to you to have certain expenses covered. Or there may come a time when you feel that the company is not living up to its contract.

In order to read policies, whether they are written in so-called plain English or not, you need to understand a few terms.

Deductible

The amount you yourself must pay before the insurance comes into effect. For example, if you have a plan with a $100 annual deductible and you see your doctor for an illness ($35 for the visit), with two follow-up visits ($25 each), you have spent a total of $85. You will receive no reimbursement because you did not exceed the deductible.

If later in the same year you have another illness, you will exceed the deductible and begin to benefit from your insurance. The deductible may be imposed on each person covered in the policy, or there may be a single sum for the whole family. If per person, there is usually a family limit so that a large family does not have exorbitant sums to pay before the insurance goes into effect.

Remember that only the cost of covered benefits can be used to meet the deductible. If, for example, your policy does not cover routine physical examinations, the $100 you just spent on one cannot be used to satisfy your deductible.

Most group policies have a feature called a "deductible carry-over," which may save you money. Check your policy (or talk to your benefits officer or agent) to see if you can apply expenses incurred in the previous year to satisfy the deductible in the present year.

Co-Payment

A co-payment is similar to a deductible but is only charged in certain defined situations. For example, your policy may state that you have a $25 co-payment for an emergency room visit. You would be responsible for the first $25 in charges, and your policy would cover the rest. Co-payments are commonly charged for maternity care.

Co-insurance

It is common for you to be required to pay a certain percentage of your bill; this is called co-insurance. The most common percentage is 20 percent: for example, if your surgeon's bill were $800, you would pay $160. There is usually, but not always, a ceiling, or "stop-loss," so that once you have paid $500 to $1,000 of your own money, the insurance pays 100 percent of additional charges (up to the UCR, defined below), until a set, high maximum is reached. Then coverage stops completely. It may be useful when buying insurance to think in terms of your total risk: add the deductible (e.g., $100) to the maximum co-insurance (e.g., 20 percent of $2,500, or $500), to get a total ($600, in this example). The only additional costs would be co-payments (usually small) and costs of non-covered services (usually elective), unless you were to exceed the limits of the policy.

This high maximum is a lifetime maximum amount for which the insurance company will reimburse you. Some policies have a feature called an "annual restoration provision," which reinstates a portion of the lifetime maximum on an annual basis.

UCR

The Usual, Customary, and Reasonable charges of the physician based on your community and the doctor's general pattern of fees is referred to by the letters "UCR." The insurance will base its payment on the UCR charge it has established. If you find that your doctor's bill is substantially greater than the UCR fee your insurance company quotes you, discuss this first with your doctor, who may lower the fee.

If the doctor does not lower the fee, call a couple of other physicians in your community in the same specialty to see if their fees are similar to what you were charged. If so, challenge your insurance company; their UCR schedule may not be up-to-date. If your doctor's fee is truly out of line, you can report this to the county medical society, which may take the matter up with your doctor.

Waiting Period

This is the period of time during which your policy will not cover a given problem. A waiting period is usually somewhere between six and twelve months. It may apply to certain defined problems or to any problem for which you have consulted a physician in the year prior to the one in which the policy takes effect.

Exclusions

These are problems your policy will not pay for at all. Common exclusions are cosmetic surgery and experimental treatments, but there may be other categories specific to the policy.

HOW TO READ A POLICY

Due to the historical development of health insurance, you are apt to be provided coverage by two or occasionally even three different entities. The components include:

1. Coverage for hospital bills, including emergency room visits (Blue Cross sells most of the hospitalization insurance in the United States).
2. Coverage of doctors' bills (Blue Shield commonly covers these).
3. A major medical plan (generally sold by an insurance company), which picks up most of what the other components of your insurance do not.

How does this work? Generally, the Blue Cross portion, for example, will cover all hospital costs (semiprivate room) in full. In some cases, costs will be covered in full for only the first 21 to 60 days and will then drop to less than full coverage. The Blue Shield component will pay up to a certain amount for a given procedure—let's say, $500 for an appendectomy. If the doctor's bill is $800, you will have to pay the extra $300—or will you? You won't if you have the kind of plan that identifies certain doctors who will accept the insurance payment as payment in full and you go to a participating doctor. You won't if you brought this issue up prior to surgery and your doctor agreed to accept the insurance fee as payment in full. You won't if you have a major medical plan that will pay for eighty percent of the "usual, customary, and reasonable" (UCR) charges.

If the UCR charge for that doctor in your community for that procedure is $650, then the major medical would pay 80 percent ($520) once you meet your deductible (generally $100 or so). Since the $520 will more than cover the $300 that the basic insurance did not, you will have to pay $100 only—unless you have already met the deductible, in which case the $800 will be covered in full.

Got that? If you need an extra reading or two to make sense out of this, we sympathize. It is a very elaborate system.

If you see here an opportunity to make a profit in what looks like confusion—after all, with the $500 from Blue Shield plus the $520 from major medical, minus the $100 deductible, you could pay the $800 and clear $120 (maybe do even better if you are also covered by your spouse's insurance)—think again. Insurance companies have worked out a system called "coordination of benefits" to make sure that if you have several different policies, you are "made whole" (you owe nothing) and also to prevent policy holders from actually turning a profit from their medical woes. Therefore, there is no plus in being "overinsured."

Hospital Coverage

Once you have determined whether you have one, two, or three different plans to review, the first category to look at is hospital coverage, because that is the big ticket item. Some policies cover all hospital costs for a certain number of days; others allow a certain amount toward the room charge, and a certain amount toward miscellaneous charges—lab, x-ray, pharmacy, etc. As a rule of thumb, the former are much to be preferred; hospital bills grow very rapidly, and $1,000 of miscellaneous charges can be eaten up in a day or two, especially if you have surgery or need an Intensive Care Unit. In addition, the daily room charges are $200 or more in most cities, so a policy that only pays up to $100 a day for room charges won't cover much.

If the hospital coverage looks inadequate, it may be made up for by a good major medical plan. Most major medical plans cover 80 percent of costs after a modest deductible is met, with a defined maximum out-of-pocket cost to you—perhaps $1,000. That would mean that once the bill reached $5,000 more than the basic coverage, you would be covered in full thereafter—generally up to a high limit ($50,000 to $250,000). If that maximum is less than $250,000, you may want to consider purchasing an excess-coverage liability policy. This type of policy picks up after your major medical ends. The premium for such a policy is very low, since the coverage is seldom needed. When it is, however, you can protect your financial future.

Physician Coverage

How does the policy treat doctors' fees? Are office visits covered, and if so, under what circumstances? Most policies cover visits only for illness, not for "routine care," which would include checkups, well-child visits (including immunizations), and gynecological exams (including Pap smears). There is now a trend toward more coverage for such visits, often with a limitation: one checkup a year, for example. Read the policy carefully. Some employers offer plans that give fuller coverage to employees than to dependents.

Many plans differentiate between accidents and illness, generally covering accidents more completely. For example, you may be covered for a visit to a hospital emergency room for an injury but not for an illness, unless the illness leads to hospitalization. Time frames may be defined. A visit to the ER for illness may only be covered if the visit occurs within 24 or 48 hours of the onset of the illness but not thereafter. Are there dollar limits placed on reimbursement for physician visits, and how do those limits compare with actual fees in your community? Again, if the major medical plan picks up where physician coverage leaves off, this may not matter.

Surgical Fees

What kind of schedule is used to cover surgical fees? Is surgery only covered in the hospital or also in an ambulatory surgery center? What about procedures performed in the surgeon's office? You can see that the type of coverage you have may define the way in which you receive medical care.

COVERAGE FOR OTHER PROBLEMS

Because policies differ most in the way coverage is given outside of general medical/surgical problems, you need to pay special attention to certain categories: eye exams, coverage for prescription drugs, psychotherapy, abortions, obstetrics, sterilization procedures.

Psychotherapy

The most complex and variable of these areas is usually psychotherapy; coverage is often provided for a certain percentage of the cost (commonly 50 percent) up to a maximum reimbursement per visit (perhaps $20 to $30) up to a maximum number of visits (52) or dollars ($1,000 to $1,500) per year. Check the definition of year. Is it calendar year, contract year, or consecutive twelve-month period? Later we'll discuss how to get the most from your insurance in this area.

In addition, the policy will often define what credentials the therapist must have in order for the coverage to be in effect. If therapy is a benefit, a psychiatrist would be covered. In most cases, a certified or licensed clinical psychologist would be too. Commonly, a certified social worker would also qualify. If you choose a therapist without these credentials, you will most often not be reimbursed.

Pregnancy

If you are planning to have a baby, read your policy carefully to see just what your coverage is. For example, there may be a waiting period, commonly eleven months after you have signed up, before the costs of a delivery are covered. In addition, many plans do not cover the costs of routine nursery care for your new baby: these can run $100 to $200 a day.

Exclusions

Examine, in particular, those categories for which the policy will not reimburse you.

1. *Cosmetic surgery* is almost always excluded, but how does the insurance company define it? If your ears stick out, you can be sure that the correction will not be covered, but what if your child is born with webbed fingers or other birth defects? Would correction be considered cosmetic?
2. *Dental work* is not usually covered, except perhaps for some accident-related problems; if you have dental insurance, this won't matter. Otherwise, the extent of dental coverage may be important. Some policies cover hospital costs associated with certain kinds of oral surgery that must be performed in the hospital—or occasionally even in the office.
3. Sometimes *unusual exclusions* are found (for example, orthognathic surgery—surgery of the jaw to correct your bite) that are not applicable to most people, but you may be the one person affected. There may also be limitations that would not occur to you; one policy we reviewed covered circumcision only in the newborn period, for example.

Changing Coverage

If you are changing jobs, make sure that you will have insurance during the transition. There is often a waiting period before health insurance from a new employer goes into effect, usually from one to three months. Sometimes it depends on which day of the month you start your new job. The insurance may start on the first of the month following your date of hire; if you start on the last day of the month, your coverage would start the next day, but if you started one day later, you would go a month without coverage.

Your insurance from your previous employer may still be in effect for a few weeks after you leave or you may be able to purchase a conversion policy to cover you for a month or two until the new coverage is in effect. You should look into this latter option if you are now going to be in the market for an individual plan. For someone with a serious or chronic medical problem, the conversion policy is often superior to what can be purchased as an individual.

A number of large insurance companies now offer temporary medical coverage (3 to 6 months), effective immediately but excluding preexisting conditions. Check with a reputable agent for more information on this kind of plan.

HOW MUCH INSURANCE WILL YOU NEED?

Once you understand your options and have examined what each policy you are considering will cost you and what each will cover, the next step is to think about your particular needs. To some extent, you can use your past medical experience to predict the future.

Past Problems
Think about the medical expenses you have incurred over the past few years. If you have a child subject to frequent asthma attacks, you can continue to expect related medical costs: doctors' visits, ER visits, possible hospitalization, perhaps allergy shots, certainly medications. If you or a family member has a very serious chronic disease such as lupus, cystic fibrosis, diabetes, or cancer, you know you are going to use doctors, hospitals, and drugs very extensively; and it will be worth it to you to have the most comprehensive coverage possible.

Be sure that any new policy you are considering does not put limitations on coverage for preexisting disease. Such limitations are routinely imposed when people apply for insurance on an individual basis, and, at times, even when they sign up through a group or employer. Be sure (on individual plans) that the policy cannot be canceled; otherwise, you will pay when you don't use it—and lose coverage just when you need it.

Your Particular Needs
Look for the particular features that really affect you. If you never bother with annual physicals, why pay extra money for a plan that covers them? If you have no children, and no immediate plans to produce any, there will be no advantage to you in having well-child care covered. If you are a single man, you don't need good obstetrics coverage. If you are a woman, coverage for Pap smears and abortions may be a very important feature.

Future Problems
Think about what kinds of expenses lie ahead. Have you been told you may need a hysterectomy in the future? Do you have a knee problem that may at some point result in surgery? Will you or someone in your

family need allergy testing and possibly desensitization therapy? Are you considering psychotherapy, or do you have a child with behavior problems that may lead to a recommendation for therapy or testing of some sort?

Take your genetic history into consideration. For example, if you or your children are at risk for an expensive problem such as sickle cell anemia, diabetes, or muscular dystrophy, you may feel safer carrying extra insurance.

Remember: your primary goal in buying insurance is to protect yourself against catastrophe; if you can save money on the premium by paying for preventive care yourself, you may end up better off financially. Some people put the money they have saved on premiums into a savings account and pay for non-covered items from those funds.

CHOOSING INSURANCE

The best and simplest way to decide which plan offers the best coverage for your particular situation is to do an actual comparison of benefits. Here's how:

1. Get out your checkbook or record of past medical expenses and list on paper all the medical expenses you have had in the past two years.
2. If you had an expensive, once-only problem (e.g., a hysterectomy for large fibroids), subtract those costs since that expense will not recur.
3. Divide by two to get a yearly average.
4. Then calculate any additional costs that you are able to predict: a new child, elective surgery. Add those costs to the calculation in step three. This will give you a guess at what your total medical expense will be for the next year.
5. Then, taking each item you have paid for, see how much of the cost each policy you are considering would cover.

For example, Don is a married man with two children. His employer is, for the first time, offering a family policy for $65 a month. This is "first-dollar coverage," meaning that there is no deductible that must be satisfied before the policy goes into effect. Until now, he has paid $40 a month for a major medical plan with a $1,000 deductible to cover his family. Should he switch to his employer's policy?

Let's use the method we just described to answer the question. We offer two different scenarios.

Example A
1. Expenses for the past two years were the following:

Don—hernia repair (out-patient)	$750
Pam—2 gynecology visits	100
Chip—(age 7) two checkups	80
repair of laceration	70
one ear infection	30
Jeremy—(age 4) two checkups	80
one visit for rash	30
Total	$1140

2. Subtract Don's hernia repair (unlikely to recur), leaving $390
3. Divide by two to get average of $195 per year
4. No anticipated extra expenses in coming year

Our analysis shows that Don is apt to lose money by taking the new policy. It will cost him $25 more per month, or $300 for the year; yet he expects to have only $195 per year in expenses. If the new plan featured a deductible instead of first-dollar coverage, there would be no reason even to consider it.

Now let's try a somewhat different set of assumptions.

Example B
1. Expenses are the same as example A, except that Chip has had four visits for ear infections. The total cost would now be $1230.
2. The one-time hernia repair, deducted from $1230, leaves $480
3. Average cost per year is $240
4. Chip's pediatrician believes he needs a referral to a specialist for a myringotomy. The first visit would cost $50, plus $40 for a hearing test. The myringotomy would cost $400 for the doctor's fee, $350 for the day surgery unit, and $150 for anesthesia. The anticipated extra expense in this case would be $990.

The average per year of $240 plus the extra $990 would now give this family a projected cost of $1230. Clearly, it would make sense to take the new insurance plan.

Before signing up, though, they would need to check carefully to make sure that there were no exclusions. If there were a six-month waiting period—a fairly common feature—and the pediatrician felt that treatment could not be deferred, the new insurance plan would do nothing for them, but the present major medical plan with the $1,000 deductible would give them some coverage because Chip would exceed the deductible.

Another useful, if somewhat grim, way to compare plans is to consider a serious medical problem that might befall you—a heart attack, cancer of the uterus, a serious auto accident: some problem involving large hospital bills, physicians' bills, and a number of follow-up visits.

Costs for Problem

1.	Hospital: 10 days at $600 per day	=	$6,000
	(The semiprivate room charge is usually only ⅓ of the total daily charge.)		
2.	Physicians' bills for hospital stay	=	1,500
3.	20 office visits at $35 each	=	700
4.	Medication	=	150
	Total cost of serious illness	=	$8,350

Now that you have the cost of your hypothetical problem, look at all the insurance plans you are considering to see how each would cover it.

Plan A: $500 deductible, with 100 percent coverage after that.

Total cost to you: $500

Plan B: $100 deductible, with 80 percent coverage of all expenses up to $5,000 and 100 percent coverage above $5,000.

Your portion is $100 + 20 percent of $5,000 = $1,000

Total cost to you: $1100

Plan C: Hospital: covered in full for 60 days
Physician: $100 deductible, then 80 percent of all expenses up to $2500 and 100 percent above $2500
Medications: $100 deductible, then covered in full
Your portion is: (Physical) $100 + 20 percent of $2200 = $540, and (medication) $100

Total cost to you: $640

For a serious illness or accident, Plan A would clearly provide the best coverage, even though there is a large deductible. If Plan A is less expensive than B or C, it would be the best choice for most families. It would provide them with "insurance," in the true sense of the word—protection against catastrophe. The money they would save on the premium could be used to offset expenses for routine care and minor problems.

THE RISKS OF BEING UNINSURED

Alison has been out of college for three years, leading an interesting life as a free-lance translator. She has traveled to London and Paris and is currently spending some time in New

York looking for her next assignment. She is also looking rather desperately for a way to buy health insurance to pay for the surgery she recently learned she must have. She is horrified by the rate she will have to pay as an individual—and even more upset by the limitations on payments the various companies impose as the result of her diagnosis.

Many people, especially young adults without families, postpone buying health insurance. If they have been generally healthy, they decide to save money by simply paying for doctors' visits out of pocket. They correctly estimate that the odds of having to go to the hospital are remote. The problem comes if they lose their bet.

Of course, when you buy insurance of any kind, you are really betting against yourself. With life insurance, for instance, you bet that you will die sooner than the insurance company thinks you will. If you are right, your family reaps the benefits of your good judgment. If you are wrong, you have the pleasure of living a long life, perhaps thinking that you spent a lot of money for peace of mind. With health insurance, if you "win" the bet, you will see your insurance paying some rather hefty bills.

You can count on a hospital costing you at least $500 a day for most problems, and that figure does not include doctors' fees. A five-day stay for an emergency cholecystectomy (removal of gallbladder), for example, could easily add up to $4,000. If you feel you cannot afford the cost of health insurance or do not want to spend the money, you need to have a back-up plan in case you become seriously and expensively sick.

At the very least, you should have insurance for medical catastrophe: expensive surgery or long-term illness.

IF YOU ARE SELF-EMPLOYED

Individual insurance policies can be extremely expensive. If you are young and healthy and must pay for your own insurance, look for a policy with a high deductible—$500, or $1,000, or even $2,500—to keep the premium payments as low as possible. This strategy will prevent you from being financially destroyed by a serious illness or accident and also protect you from being bled slowly by a substantial monthly premium.

> Often self-employed people are able to avoid the high cost of purchasing individual insurance by joining an organization or association. Your college alumni association, a professional association in your field, or a financial or consumer organization may offer group health insurance.

WHAT KIND OF PLAN TO AVOID

There is a kind of plan, generally promulgated by celebrities or offered through the mail by a bank card, which guarantees you cash for each day you spend in the hospital. It has nothing to offer in the way of coverage of your actual hospital bills, but it does pay money directly to you, a feature that evidently appeals to many people, since there seem to be a lot of these plans. The odds are stacked against making a profit from such a plan, or just coming out even. One plan, for example, would pay you $60 a day for each day you or your spouse spent in the hospital, at a cost to you of about $16 a month. (The exact cost varies with age.) Why is this such a bad deal?

Let's suppose that you and your spouse buy the coverage for a total cost of $192 a year. Because, on the average, each of you will spend at most one day a year in the hospital, you would collect about $120— substantially less if you live in cities that average only half a day per person per year, or if you are a member of an HMO, the average member of which spends only 0.4 days in the hospital each year. A clue to the scare tactics used to market such a plan is that it often pays double for cancer or a heart attack. There is no financial logic to this—you don't need twice as much money per day because you have cancer— but it is a sure attention-grabber.

WOULD YOU EVER NEED DOUBLE COVERAGE?

Usually, it is unnecessary for both you and your spouse to have family coverage. To decide, though, you need to work out what you would get for the money. Suppose your own employer pays for the family plan in full and your spouse's offers a family plan for $15 a month. Obviously, you will take up your employer's offer, enroll your family on your own plan and forgo the privilege of paying the extra $15 a month. What happens if one of you decides to go into therapy? Each plan may only cover $25 a visit, but the cost may be $70 a visit. If treatment should consist of one visit a week for nine months, you would get $900 more in reimbursement if you were covered by both plans, at a cost of $180 for the year.

If one of your employers offers the HMO option (discussed in the next chapter), you may decide to enroll your family. Some people continue their spouse's indemnity coverage for a while until they are sure of the quality of the HMO.

MEDICARE OPTIONS

Those of you who have Medicare know how many expenses still come out of your own pocket. If you are healthy, you may decide not to buy additional insurance since Medicare provides very good hospital coverage. If you have a chronic disease that requires regular visits to a physician and a lot of medications, you will probably save money by purchasing a "wraparound" plan from Blue Cross or by joining an HMO in your area, if it offers a special plan to Medicare beneficiaries. Read these policies carefully—many cover only 80 percent of what Medicare approves. Since Medicare commonly approves 80 percent of charges, coverage is only 64 percent!

In addition, beginning in 1983, employers with over twenty employees must offer active employees over the age of 65 their choice between Medicare and the company plan. Examine the alternatives carefully if you are in this category. You might even want to review them with the benefits department.

HOW TO GET THE MOST
OUT OF YOUR INSURANCE

By understanding how the deductibles and limitations work, you can make sure that you get maximum coverage for the care you need. For example, one policy that we reviewed paid up to $15 a visit for therapy sessions, with a limit of 50 visits per calendar year. If that were your policy and you decided to embark on a course of therapy, you would do well to start therapy in the summer. That way, you could have twice-a-week visits for the second half of the calendar year (50 visits), and the same for the first half of the next year (another 50 visits). If you started in January and were being seen twice a week, your coverage would have run out in July. Read your policy carefully, though; sometimes reimbursement is limited to one visit a week.

HOW TO SAVE MONEY
BY KEEPING AN EYE
ON THE CALENDAR

Stephen and Mary have a policy with a family deductible of $300 a calendar year. They and their three children had a predictable amount of routine care for which they received no reimbursement. Here is a record of the past year:

January 25	Anne's checkup	$35
	Martin's checkup	$35
February 3	Jean's checkup	$35
February 15	Mary's checkup with family physician (includes Pap)	$60
June 12	Martin's camp exam	$35
August 20	Anne's school exam	$35
October 11	Stephen's glaucoma and blood pressure check	$25
	Total for year	$295

The expenses are just below the deductible, so this family gets nothing from their insurance. But suppose they rearrange their schedule somewhat, with absolutely no loss of quality of care.

YEAR 1

January	Anne, Martin, Jean checkups	$105
	Mary's checkup	60
	Stephen's glaucoma and blood pressure check	25
June	children's checkups	105
December	children's checkups	105
	Mary's checkup	60
	Stephen's visit	25
	Total for year 1	$485

YEAR 2

June	children's checkups	$105
	Total for year 2	$105

The family has the same number of visits in a given 24-month period, but by adjusting these routine visits so that they fall within the policy limitations, they have exceeded their $300 deductible for year 1. They can use their insurance to cover the remaining $185. If their policy covers 80 percent of this, they will have saved $149.

Similarly, if medical expenses are running high one year, you might decide to get care you have been putting off but know you need so that you can exceed your deductible before the year ends. Perhaps you are due for a tetanus shot, one or more children are due for immunizations, or you have been putting off minor surgery that you know you must have.

If you have already met your deductible, schedule the visits during the same year. If you have been healthy all year, schedule the elective visits for early next year. If you are less fortunate in the coming year, at least your illness may be reimbursable. (Note: Many policies allow you to use the expenses incurred in the last three months of the year to meet the following year's deductible.)

Approach your insurance policy the way you do a tax return and use all the legal ways you can to save money by making the rules and regulations work to your advantage. Speaking of tax returns, medical expenses, as you probably know, are not deductible unless they exceed 5 percent of taxable income. If you have any chance of exceeding that 5 percent, it would be another reason to schedule as much necessary medical care as possible for one calendar year.

HOW TO MAKE SURE
THAT YOU ARE REIMBURSED

As usual, start by reading your policy carefully. If you have insurance provided by your employer, discuss your bills with the benefits office. Some people worry about confidentiality when dealing with company personnel; commonly they are concerned about issues involving sex (abortions, sexually transmitted disease), mental illness (hospitalization or even psychotherapy), and substance abuse (drugs, alcohol).

You have a clear right to have your medical information remain confidential: it is legally not to be viewed by anyone, including the company president. To reassure yourself on this point, raise your concerns with the personnel director *before* you have a confidential problem. Another alternative, available to many, is to join an HMO. Although it is offered by your employer, all medical records are maintained at the HMO, and your employer has no access.

There are two reasons to file your claim promptly: (1) most policies have a time limit on the filing of claims; (2) if any problems develop, the care will be recent enough that the trail is still warm. Most important, keep copies of everything. Otherwise you might waste weeks or months trying to obtain new copies of bills, or having your doctor fill out forms for the second time.

Find out how long a wait to expect before you are reimbursed, and if you are not, follow up promptly at the time specified. If you bother the benefits people prematurely, they may come to regard you as a pest and will not go out of their way to expedite your claim. If you follow their recommendations and are failing to collect, they are more apt to feel responsible for your problems and make extra efforts on your behalf.

Above all, before you go to the doctor's office, be sure you understand your coverage, especially for out-patient problems, and bring your insurance forms with you. You should discuss your coverage with your physician at the time of your visit. Why? The exact wording of the reason you saw the doctor may make a difference in whether your policy will pay or not. For example, many plans do not cover routine gynecological exams, but if the physician finds a minor abnormality and lists it as a diagnosis, your insurance will apply. Similarly, "removal of blackheads" would not be covered by most plans, whereas "acne surgery" (consisting of removal of blackheads) probably would be.

If you must pay for hospital expenses, examine the bill carefully and question anything you don't understand. You can call the hospital business office and go over each item in detail. It is not uncommon for hospitals to bill for tests and procedures the patient has never had.

If at all possible, get the hospital or doctor to bill the insurance company directly, thus sparing you expensive delays in collecting. Hospitals will generally do this for admissions but may not for emergency room visits. Doctors, on the other hand, are increasingly asking for payment at the time of service, except for surgery performed in the hospital. If you know the exact extent of your coverage as well as the process for reimbursement, you will have a better chance of convincing the doctor's office manager to bill your insurance company. Be sure to bring your claim form with you on your visit—that helps ensure your doctor will submit the form promptly, important if you are paying directly.

Even when the office agrees to bill your insurance company, you may continue to receive a monthly bill. From their point of view, the bill is still your responsibility, and they want to remind you of that fact. Ignore the bills for the first two months. If they have not been paid within 90 days or so, you should find out the reason for the delay and when the payment will be made. Then call the doctor's office and give the office manager that information. There is usually less reason to let a hospital know; they have probably already checked themselves.

WHO CAN HELP YOU
GET THE BILLS PAID?

If you are not reimbursed for what you believe to be a legitimate claim, you do not have to accept the insurance company's decision as final. Sources of help include your benefits officer or broker, your union, or your doctor. If you must deal with the insurance company directly, ask to speak to the claims manager and by-pass the service representative. Many insurance companies now have a toll-free number to their claims department. If all else fails you can write to the state insurance commission or hire an attorney.

CHAPTER THIRTEEN

PREPAID MEDICINE: THE HMO ALTERNATIVE

Prepaid plans offer some important advantages and some possible drawbacks to consumers. Because the authors have particular knowledge of and experience in this field, we feel especially qualified to help you decide whether HMO membership would suit you and what characteristics to look for before joining.

In some parts of the country, the abbreviation HMO is common; in other places, people are puzzled by those three letters, which stand for Health Maintenance Organization. Although prepaid medicine is not a new concept, many experts feel it now represents the only cost-effective way for the private sector to deliver high quality health care. Whether or not they are right, you the individual consumer are primarily concerned with finding the best possible medical care for yourself rather than the best answer to questions of public policy. This section will describe just what an HMO is and how to go about deciding whether to join one should the opportunity present itself.

For many people, an HMO is medical heaven. They no longer have to deal with choosing doctors and hospitals, filing claims, waiting to be reimbursed. There is a telephone number they may dial day or night for urgent problems. For some, the restrictions outweigh the advantages—for example, having to use only designated physicians. Although a large number of studies have shown that the *medical* quality of the care given by HMOs is equal to or better than that given in the traditional fee-for-service setting, there may be a wide variation in the personal concern with which plans treat their members.

The phrase "health maintenance organization" was coined in the early seventies by Paul Ellwood, a physician who had observed how effectively prepaid health plans could contain costs without sacrificing quality. Ellwood wanted to convince the federal government to encourage the growth of prepaid medicine as a way to put a brake on the exploding rate of increase of health care costs in the country. Prepayment had started in the West, with an experimental cooperative in Washington, with the Ross-Loos Plan in Los Angeles (now part of CIGNA Healthplan's national network), and with Dr. Sidney Garfield's idea to provide health care on a prepaid basis to several groups of workers, most notably those constructing the Grand Coulee Dam. This latter experiment became the present-day Kaiser-Permanente now serving over 4 million members in nine regions stretching from Hawaii to Connecticut.

A prepaid group practice is an organized system of health care delivery that combines the financing and provision of health care into one entity; subscribers pay their premiums to the plan and then receive all of their care from its physicians. This has several advantages to consumers; for one, after the premium is paid, there will be no further concerns about health care expenses. Prepaid plans provide their members with a comprehensive set of health care benefits, in exchange for the fixed monthly premium. Some HMOs ask their members to pay small co-payments of a few dollars for office visits. In addition, claim forms are eliminated; patients simply go to the appropriate physician and present their membership card. If hospital care is necessary, the prepaid plan arranges it and pays the bill. Finally, the problem of what kind of doctor to choose is eliminated. The HMO supplies both primary care physicians and specialists.

There are three basic ways in which a health maintenance organization may arrange to provide medical care.

Staff Model
In this type of prepaid plan, the physicians are employed directly by the HMO. They work together as a group and deliver care in one or more health care centers. Plan members select a personal physician from among the doctors on the staff. A small HMO will have full-time primary care physicians (family physicians, internists, pediatricians) and may also have obstetrician/gynecologists, but will contract with other specialists in the community to provide care for more unusual problems. As the membership grows, more specialists are needed on a full-time basis. The very largest plans employ a wide range of very specialized physicians such as neurosurgeons or pediatric cardiologists.

Group Model
This will look the same from the member's point of view, but the physicians are not directly employed; instead, they form a legally independent group that contracts with the plan to provide care to its members. The Permanente Medical Group is the best known group

model, and it contracts with the Kaiser Foundation Health Plan to provide care for its 4 million members.

IPA Model
The Individual Practice Association consists of individual physicians who agree to see patients in their own offices on a prepaid basis. Members who sign up for the plan are given a list of participating physicians from which to choose a primary care physician; this person will serve as their regular doctor and will arrange for any specialty care that is necessary. A variation of this model is the Network model, in which a number of physician groups, as opposed to individuals, contract with the plan. Members choose one of the groups for care and then pick a personal physician from within the group.

OTHER ADVANTAGES

The very process by which a high quality HMO contains costs proves to be financially, and even medically, beneficial to its members. Since the plan both provides the care and covers the cost, it will arrange for necessary care to be given in the most economical way without compromising quality. The more successful the plan is in containing costs, the lower the premium in the long run.

In staff and group model HMOs, members have the added advantage of being cared for by physicians who can freely consult one another. Good HMOs have formal programs to insure quality of care: several physicians and other health care professionals review charts, examine the use of lab and x-ray, look at hospital records, follow up on complaints, and generally make sure the care given is of high quality. Several years ago, Johns Hopkins University reviewed twenty-five studies that compared the quality of medicine in prepaid plans with that found in the community as a whole. Nineteen of the twenty-five studies concluded that care in prepaid plans was superior to what was available in the community; six found it to be as good. No study found it to be in any way inferior.[1]

HOW TO JOIN AN HMO

HMOs are generally offered by employers as an alternative to the indemnity insurance that otherwise covers employees. Your company will pay toward the plan whatever it would otherwise pay for the indemnity insurance. Some HMOs accept applications from individuals, generally limiting enrollment to those who can pass a health screening (a lengthy questionnaire and possibly a physical exam in addition).

There are federal and state laws that require employers, under certain circumstances, to offer the option of membership in HMOs. If there is an HMO in your city that you would like to join, discuss it with your benefits department. If you get no results, contact your local HMO for information on possible ways to persuade your employer to offer the plan.

If you live in or near a good-sized city, there is probably at least one HMO in your area. At the end of 1982, there were 269 HMOs in the country, serving most major metropolitan areas. Membership stood at about 12 million people and continues to increase rapidly.

SHOULD YOU JOIN?

We have already pointed out some of the general advantages of HMO membership, but since you will be considering a specific HMO, you will need guidelines for judging its quality and some way to decide whether you would be happy getting your care there. One credential you should look for is either federal (or state) "qualification." This means that the organization will have met certain standards of medical quality, range of benefits, and financial stability. By now, most reputable prepaid plans are either federally qualified, state qualified, or both.

What if a plan is not federally qualified? Ask whether it is a member of the Group Health Association of America (GHAA) (see Resource Directory); GHAA does an extensive site visit before accepting a plan as a full member in its organization. Group Health Cooperative of Puget Sound (GHC), for example, is a highly regarded plan that, although very active in GHAA, has never sought federal qualification. GHC evidently feels the reputation it has developed since its establishment in 1948 speaks for itself; its success—enrollment is now over 300,000—would seem to attest to that.

To get a firsthand impression of the kind of care you will get, talk to friends or co-workers who are already members. If they are enthusiastic, that is a good sign. If they are negative, find out why. Have they had a single bad experience or a number of complaints? Do they have the same expectations as you do? Talk to the company benefits office to find out how satisfied other employees have been or whether there have been consistent problems.

An HMO, because it is almost always offered as an alternative to other insurance, does not have a captive clientele. It must be able to please its customers or it will go out of business. Find out how many years the plan has been in existence. A new plan may or may not give excellent care, but an older one will have to be doing something right to have lasted. (Prepaid plans with a largely involuntary membership obviously cannot be judged on this basis.)

The key to the medical excellence and financial success of an HMO is the quality and commitment of the doctors. Find out their credentials from the HMO's marketing or customer relations department. Are they all fully trained (board eligible)? Are most of them board-certified? Where did they go to school and receive their training, and when? Although young doctors are up-to-date and can provide excellent care, it is desirable to have a sprinkling of older, more experienced physicians who can offer their wisdom to the group. High turnover indicates either that doctors are unhappy about their working conditions or that those who have been recruited are not well suited to the demands of prepaid group practice.

Find out what hospitals the HMO works with, and check out the reputation of those hospitals with friends or physicians whose judgment you trust. It will probably not be very helpful to ask those same physicians what they think of the HMO. Unless they are associated with it as consultants, they will probably be negative, since most doctors in private practice consider the HMO as a large competitor. If you can, read the May 1982 issue of *Consumer Reports;* it contains an extensive discussion of HMOs and how to evaluate them.[2]

Read the marketing literature carefully. HMO coverage is fairly standard and usually very comprehensive. What you need to pay particular attention to is the *way* you will get care. Do you choose your own primary care physician from among those who work for the plan or is one assigned to you? Is there a simple mechanism for complaints if the system is not working for you? Is one of the health care centers convenient to work or home? Are the hours the center is open convenient? Will you always have to miss work to see your doctor or are there extended hours to accommodate you? Are you willing to abide by the rules for getting care, such as always using HMO doctors and consultants?

Before you join an HMO, go on a tour of the health care center, preferably the one you will be using. Is it clean and well equipped? Does it seem to be an attractive, friendly place or does it have a depressing hospital-clinic atmosphere?

Does the person giving the tour understand the program thoroughly and explain things to your satisfaction? If the HMO does not make sure that the person who explains the plan to you is an expert, you might justifiably wonder how well trained the rest of the staff is.

Really excellent medical treatment depends on a concept called "continuity of care"—that is, that patients have an ongoing relationship with one physician who provides all of their primary care. The top HMOs take administrative measures to make this possible. One way to find out whether the HMO really believes that continuity is important is to ask what will happen if you call with an urgent problem that needs to be seen on that same day.

The HMO should have a system—usually involving a screening or triage nurse—to evaluate the urgency of your request. If you do need an appointment, you should generally be able to see your personal doctor; good administrators try to leave some unassigned time in the appointment schedules so that physicians can take care of their own patients with urgent problems.

One way to determine exactly how concerned the plan is with pleasing its customers is to find out how long patients can expect to spend in the waiting room. A given physician may fall behind because of emergencies, but the usual waiting time should be half an hour or less; anything more is unacceptable.

WILL AN HMO SAVE YOU MONEY?

In the previous chapter, we suggested you do some calculations to help you decide which health insurance policy to consider. You can use these same examples to calculate the savings associated with the HMO. If you come out ahead and the plan you are considering offers good health care, you should strongly consider joining. Since you sign up on an annual basis, you will have the option of switching back to conventional insurance at the end of the year if you are not satisfied.

Health maintenance organizations often have lower premiums and broader coverage than most indemnity insurance plans. This is because they can control wasteful and duplicative use of medical services far more efficiently than the fee-for-service sector, in particular by eliminating unnecessary hospital costs.

WHO SHOULD NOT JOIN AN HMO?

There are two questions to ask yourself in order to decide if you are someone who would not be a good candidate for membership:

Do I presently have a relationship with a doctor whom I like and trust?

Am I unwilling to let the HMO doctors make medical decisions for me?

If you answer yes to either one, you would probably not be happy as a member of an HMO.

If you have a primary care doctor whom you like and trust, you are already ahead of the game. Giving up a good medical relationship would not make sense for you unless you are having serious financial problems. Generally, losing such a relationship is not worth the dollars you will save.

If decision-making is an issue, the restrictions imposed by an HMO may be difficult for you to accept. You cannot self-refer to a specialist, and you cannot make a visit to an emergency room without prior approval unless you are critically ill. You will have to use specialists on the HMO's panel and the hospital the plan chooses.

You can certainly argue with your doctor or switch to one of the other HMO doctors, but if you would resent giving up the final say in these matters, you will constantly be fighting the fundamental principle of this type of organization.

WHAT TO EXPECT IF YOU JOIN

You will need to learn and follow the systems the plan uses. When you call for an appointment, you will be asked several questions to help determine how soon you should be seen and by whom. If your problem is not urgent, rather than scheduling an immediate appointment, a nurse may give you advice on how to deal with whatever is troubling you. In many cases, reassurance and telephone advice is helpful and saves you the nuisance of an unnecessary visit.

Don't let the system intimidate you. If you are either very worried or in pain and feel your problem really needs a doctor's attention, say so directly. If your problem really can wait, remember that the triage nurse is trying to make sure that people with more medically urgent problems will have necessary access to doctors. Someday you yourself may be in that situation.

If you are dissatisfied with the care you are getting, by all means let the appropriate administrator know. Most plans have a patient complaint system, sometimes even a special number to call. If you especially like something about the plan, a doctor, a health education program, a system that makes sure you are seen promptly—you might also write a note of praise. HMOs need to know what pleases their members as well as what displeases them.

Getting good care in an HMO is really no different from getting good care in other settings, and the same advice applies that we gave at some length in the beginning of this book: *establish a relationship with a primary care physician.* We suggest that the first thing you do when you join is schedule a routine visit for each member of your family.

If you need help in picking a doctor, you can call the member services department for advice. In addition to providing you with physician credentials, they will be able to match your preferences in style and personality. You may prefer going to an older or younger doctor or want someone who will be warm and outgoing as opposed to serious and scholarly. If you are not pleased with the first doctor you choose, you are free to change.

Once you have chosen and visited your HMO doctor, you will find that using the whole system becomes much simpler. For example, if you feel you need to be seen right away and your doctor agrees, he or she will instruct the appointments desk to book you. If you have a problem that clearly requires a referral to a consultant, your primary care doctor may send you to one directly without first insisting on doing a preliminary evaluation.

When you join, be sure you have read and understood the rules for getting care after hours or from non-HMO physicians. Except for a critical emergency (uncontrollable bleeding, unconsciousness, inability to breathe), a visit to the emergency room will not be covered unless you call the HMO and receive prior approval from one of the doctors.

An HMO must provide you with access to physicians on a twenty-four-hour basis. You will be given a number to call when the health care center is closed. Except in the very largest organizations, there is no one waiting by the office phone. Most plans use the same system that fee-for-service doctors use. A medical answering service will pick up the phone and will then contact the on-call doctor, who may either be at home asleep or possibly in the hospital with a sick patient. That physician will call back and, depending on your problem, give you phone advice, arrange to meet you for an evaluation, or authorize an ER visit.

How late should you telephone? You can call at any hour, but a good rule of thumb would be to call the HMO doctor only with the kind of serious problem that would prompt you to wake up a doctor in private practice.

IF YOU ARE OFFERED MORE THAN ONE HMO

You may have your choice of HMOs, and they may be of different types. If one of them is an Individual Practice Association (IPA), it will often sound appealing. There are usually hundreds of physicians to choose among. If you already have a doctor you like who is on the IPA list, this type of plan may work very well for you.

There are, however, some disadvantages to IPAs that may affect you in the long run. Because they are so decentralized, they may have difficulty controlling both costs and quality. In general, IPA physicians are less committed to making the plan work financially; the premium is bound to reflect this fact. It may start out the same but will almost certainly become higher than the premium charged by a staff or group model. In addition, the quality assurance program and credentialing process in an IPA are usually much less rigorous.

REFERENCES, BIBLIOGRAPHY, AND RESOURCES

his reference section is organized by chapter. All journal articles and books referred to in the text are listed under **References.** These are followed by an **Annotated Bibliography** of books for those who want to do further reading and a **Resource** section with names and addresses of organizations devoted to particular problems as well as especially useful reference works.

HOW TO FIND OUT
WHAT YOU WANT TO KNOW

Public Libraries
Whether you are looking for a book, an article, or the name and address of a self-help group, a good place to begin is your library, preferably at the branch that has the best reference section.

We would start by enlisting the help of one of the librarians on duty at the reference desk. Librarians are information specialists; if they don't have what you need, they know where to find it. If your library does not have a book or article you need, ask the librarian to request it through the inter-library loan system; many libraries now belong to larger information-sharing networks, and some have been specified as depositories for the reams of material turned out by the federal government.

Hospital Libraries
Most good-sized hospitals have comprehensive medical libraries. Some are now open to the public; if not, the medical librarian may be willing to help someone with a specific question.

Other Libraries
If you don't have any luck with a hospital library, there are other places to turn to. Libraries of nursing schools (both hospital and collegiate), county medical society libraries, and libraries of community colleges, especially those with a health sciences division, are all possibilities.

Ma Bell

Your telephone book is another good starting point. If you are looking for a government agency, check in the white pages under federal, state, city, and sometimes county headings. If you are trying to locate a private organization and cannot find it in the white pages, try the yellow pages under "Associations" or "Social Service Organizations."

Local Health Departments

The public health nurses who work for these agencies are excellent resources. They will be able to refer you to associations and self-help groups and will tell you where to find information on how to prevent various medical problems. Many of these departments offer classes and clinics. (Check your telephone directory under state, district, county, or city listings.)

Specialty Hospitals and Clinics

Places like birth centers, orthopedic hospitals, or cancer hospitals are good sources of information about organizations and programs related to their specialties. For example, if you want to find out if your community has a branch of La Leche or a certified nurse-midwife who does home deliveries, chances are the staff of a birth center will know; if you are looking for information on self-help groups for ostomy patients or for parents of children with leukemia, someone at a cancer hospital is apt to know what groups are active locally.

If you are calling a large institution, ask the switchboard operator to transfer you to the social service department. If no one there can help you, you may be transferred to educational services, to a clinical nurse specialist, or to the appropriate nursing unit.

Free or Low-Cost Health Information

If you want information on a specific topic such as nutrition, first-aid, or how to stop smoking, a wealth of material is available for little or no money.

One reference work you will find in many libraries is a book called *Help Yourself to Health* by Art Ulene (G.P. Putnam's Sons, 1980). It contains 3500 nationwide resources for a variety of health-related topics. The first section, organized by subject, lists brochures and leaflets. Each item is coded to a section in the second part where you will find the name and address of the organization that will supply the material.

The U.S. Government Printing Offices will send you a free catalog listing all the booklets the Federal government publishes. Write to:

U.S. Government Printing Office
Consumer Information Center
Public Documents Distribution Center
Pueblo, Colorado 81009

───────CHAPTER ONE───────

REFERENCES

1. Driver, Harold E., *Indians of North America* (2nd Edition). Chicago: The University of Chicago Press. (Paperback, 1969) pp. 508–510.

2. Thomas, Lewis, *The Youngest Science: Notes of a Medicine-Watcher.* New York: The Viking Press, 1983.

3. Osmond, Humphrey, "God and the Doctor." *The New England Journal of Medicine,* March 6, 1980, pp. 555–558.

4. Taylor, A.J.P., *Bismark: The Man & The Statesman.* New York: Random House, 1967.

5. Eichna, Ludwig W., M.D., "Medical-School Education, 1975–1979; A Student's Perspective." *The New England Journal of Medicine,* Sept. 25, 1980, pp. 727–734.

6. Parsons, Talcott, *The Social System.* Glencoe, Ill: The Free Press, 1951.

7. Osmond, Op. Cit.

8. McCue, Jack D., M.D., "The Effects of Stress on Physicians and Their Medical Practice." *The New England Journal of Medicine,* Feb. 25, 1982, pp. 458–463.

9. Cousins, Norman, *Anatomy of an Illness.* New York: W.W. Norton Co., Inc., 1979.

BIBLIOGRAPHY

Reiter, B.P., M.D., *The Saturday Night Knife and Gun Club.* New York: J.B. Lippincott Co., 1977

Vivid description of internship in a municipal hospital. Most physicians have spent part (sometimes all) of medical school, internship, and/or residency in such a hospital; this will give you perspective on that experience and how it may influence their attitudes toward you. A "Hill Street Blues" of medicine.

Shem, Samuel, M.D., *The House of God.* New York: Richard Marek, 1978; paperback edition, Dell Books, 1980.

An exaggerated—but only slightly—account of internship in a famous university teaching hospital. Very "black" humor, not to everyone's taste, but it may leave you surprised that your doctor communicates with you as well as he or she does after encountering the kinds of experiences and prevailing attitudes so well described in this book.

Miller, Jonathan, M.D., *The Body In Question*. New York: Random House, 1979; paperback edition, Random House, 1981

The book (and the TV show) contains fascinating and thoughtful examinations of the history and practice of medicine. The discussion of the history of the "healing relationship" is excellent.

Cassel, Eric, M.D., *The Healer's Art*. New York: Random House, 1979

An outstanding medical practitioner and an authority on physicians, patients, and their relationship discusses how he learned to heal as well as to cure and the importance of the healing relationship.

Thomas, Lewis, *The Youngest Science: Notes of a Medicine-Watcher*. New York: The Viking Press, 1983

Vivid personal picture of the progress of twentieth-century medicine in the United States, elegantly written by a physician who now heads a world-famous cancer institute.

Lear, Martha Weinman. *Heartsounds*. New York: Simon and Schuster, 1980. (See Bibliography for Chapter Five for description.)

———CHAPTER TWO———

REFERENCES

1. Belsky, Marvin S., M.D. and Gross, Leonard, *Beyond the Medical Mystique: How To Choose and Use Your Doctor*. New York: Arbor House, 1975.

2. Ibid.

BIBLIOGRAPHY

LeBaron, Charles, *Gentle Vengeance*. New York: Richard Marek, 1981; paperback edition, Penguin, 1982

Fascinating account of the author's first year at Harvard Medical School, giving insight into the process by which so many physicians are overtrained in "scientific" medicine at the expense of learning how to work with patients as people.

Belsky, Marvin S., M.D. and Gross, Leonard, *Beyond the Medical Mystique: How To Choose and Use Your Doctor*. New York: Arbor House, 1975; paperback edition, Arbor House, 1979

Excellent book on what to look for in a doctor and how to talk to a doctor. Useful discussion on how to cope with being in the hospital. If every patient could find a doctor who shared the author's point of view, his book and our book would be unnecessary.

RESOURCES

The American Medical Directory (28th Edition). Chicago: American Medical Association, 1983

To look up a doctor's credentials, start with this reference work; it is frequently updated, so try to use the latest edition. You will find all licensed physicians in the United States listed here, with address, medical school, primary and secondary specialty, and type of practice. Osteopaths who are members of the AMA are also listed here. Although you can consult this reference work to find out the area of a physician's special interest, you must use the reference listed below for information on board certification.

Directory of Medical Specialists (21st Edition). Chicago: A. N. Marquis Co., 1983–84 (updated every two years)

Lists only board-certified physicians by state and city or town. If you want a doctor who is fully credentialed in a given field, this is the place to look. In addition, extensive information is provided on each specialist's background, including hospital affiliations, faculty appointments, and membership in professional societies.

The Directory of Women Physicians. Published by the American Medical Association, 535 North Dearborn St.; Chicago, Illinois 60610

Similar to *The American Medical Directory.* Lists all women physicians in the United States, not only those who are AMA members.

To find a specialist in adolescent medicine or a clinic that cares for teenagers, contact:
Society for Adolescent Medicine
Box 3462
Granada Hills, California 91344
(Enclose stamped addressed envelope with your request.)

——————CHAPTER THREE——————

REFERENCES

1. Boulis, Z. F., et al., "Head Injuries in Children, Aetiology, Symptoms, Physical Findings and X-Ray Wastage." *British Journal of Radiology.* November, 1978, pp. 851–854.

2. Samuels, Mike, M.D. and Bennett, Hal, *The Well Body Book.* New York/Berkeley: Random House/Bookworks, 1973.

3. Oppenheim, Mike, M.D., "How To Get Your Money's Worth From Your Doctor." *Woman's Day,* March 3, 1981.

BIBLIOGRAPHY

Two useful books for anyone concerned about the necessity or risks of a given x-ray or test:

Laws, Priscilla W., Ph.D. and Ralph Nader's Public Citizen Health Research Group, *The X-ray Information Book.* New York: Farrar, Straus & Giroux, 1983

Fox, Marion Laffey, R.N., *A Patient's Guide to Medical Testing* (Professional Edition). Bowie, Maryland: Charles Press, 1979

Belsky, Marvin S., M.D. and Gross, Leonard. *Beyond the Medical Mystique: How To Choose And Use Your Doctor.* New York: Arbor House, 1975. (See Bibliography for Chapter Two for description)

Pantell, Robert H., M.D.; Fries, James F., M.D.; Vickery, Donald M., M.D., *Taking Care of Your Child.* Vickery, Donald M., M.D. and Fries, James F., M.D. *Take Care of Yourself.* Reading, Mass: Addison-Wesley Publishing Company, 1977. (See Bibliography for Chapter Ten for description)

————CHAPTER FOUR————

REFERENCES

1. McNeil, Pauker, et al., "On the Elicitation of Preferences For Alternative Therapies." *The New England Journal of Medicine,* May 27, 1982, pp. 1259–62.

2. Shapiro, M.; Muñoz, A., et al., "Risk factors for infection at the operative site after abdominal or vaginal hysterectomy." *The New England Journal of Medicine,* Dec. 30, 1982, pp. 1661–6.

3. Crile, George, Jr., M.D., *Surgery: Your Choices, Your Alternatives.* New York: Delacorte Press, 1978.

4. Brody, Jane, "How To Avoid Operations You Don't Need." *Woman's Day,* April 24, 1979.

5. Paradise, J. L., Bluestone, Charles D., et al., "History of Recurrent Sore Throat As An Indication For Tonsillectomy." *The New England Journal of Medicine,* Feb. 23, 1978, pp. 409–13.

6. U.S. Congress, House, Committee on Interstate and Foreign Commerce, "Getting Ready for National Health Insurance: Unnecessary Surgery." Hearings before the Subcommittee on Oversight and Investigation, U.S. Government Printing Office, 1975.

7. Scully, Diana, *Men Who Control Women's Health.* Boston: Houghton Mifflin Co., 1980, pp. 140–41.

8. See report by the U.S. Congress listed in reference 6.

9. Lavin, John H., "Same-Day Surgery: Why Everyone Is Learning to Love It." *Medical Economics,* June 7, 1982.

10. See the Lavin article listed in reference 9.

11. Detmer, Don E., M.D., "Ambulatory Surgery." *The New England Journal of Medicine,* Dec. 3, 1981, pp. 1406–09.

12. See the Lavin article listed in reference 9.

BIBLIOGRAPHY

Nolen, William A., M.D., *Surgeon Under the Knife.* New York: Coward, McCann and Geoghegan, 1976

A surgeon's account of his own coronary by-pass surgery. Good discussion of how he made the decision to have the surgery. Dr. Nolen's description of how he chose his surgeon and of his experiences in the hospital are illuminating, as is his discussion of risk/benefit decision-making.

Crile, George, Jr., M.D., *Surgery: Your Choices, Your Alternatives.* New York: Delacorte Press, 1978

An excellent book for anyone faced with possible surgery. This renowned surgeon has caused great controversy in the medical community for championing operations (especially for breast cancer) that are less radical than is standard in this country. In general, his recommendations are conservative; following them could save you from unnecessary surgery. We disagree, however, with his position on the need for hysterectomies and oopheorectomies in young women for cancer prevention.

Gots, Ronald, M.D. and Kaufman, Arthur, M.D., *The People's Hospital Book.* New York: Crown Publishers, 1978; paperback edition, Avon Books, 1981. (See Bibliography for Chapter Five for description)

RESOURCES

Second Opinion Surgery 800-638-6833 (in Maryland, 800-492-6603) is a toll-free number to dial for a list of physicians in your area qualified to give second opinions for a given problem.

Ambulatory Surgery:

Both the organizations below will supply you with a list of facilities they have approved:

Free-standing Ambulatory Surgical Association (FASA)
1040 East McDowell Road
Phoenix, Arizona 85006

Accreditation Association for Ambulatory Health Care, Inc.
4849 Golf Road
Skokie, Illinois 60077

Write to address below for information on ambulatory surgical facilities in your community. This organization will have information on hospital day surgery units as well as free-standing facilities:

Accreditation Council for Ambulatory Health Care
875 N. Michigan Avenue
Chicago, Illinois 60611

CHAPTER FIVE

REFERENCES

1. Risley, Mary, *The House of Healing: The Story of the Hospital.* Garden City, New York: Doubleday, 1961.

2. Cousins, Norman, *Anatomy of an Illness.* New York: W.W. Norton Co., Inc., 1979.

3. McNeer, J. Frederick, M.D.; Wagner, Galen S., M.D., et al., "Hospital Discharge One Week After Acute Myocardial Infarction." *New England Journal of Medicine,* February 2, 1978, pp. 229–232.

4. Mather, H.G.; Pearson, N.G., et al., "Acute Myocardial Infarction: Home and Hospital Treatment." *British Medical Journal,* Aug. 7, 1971, pp. 334–338.

5. Cassel, Eric, *The Healer's Art.* New York: Random House, 1979.

6. Thomas, Lewis, M.D., *The Youngest Science.* New York: Viking, 1983.

BIBLIOGRAPHY

General Interest and Insight
Lear, Martha Weinman. *Heartsounds.* New York: Simon and Schuster, 1980; paperback, 1981

Disturbing and moving account of a physician's battle with debilitating heart disease. Memorable descriptions of the best and worst of hospitals and physicians. The book dramatizes the kinds of problems patients and their families frequently encounter in hospitals.

Belsky, Marvin S., M.D. and Gross, Leonard. *Beyond the Medical Mystique: How To Choose and Use Your Doctor.* New York: Arbor House, 1975. (See Bibliography for Chapter Two for description)

Nolen, William A., M.D. *Surgeon Under the Knife.* New York: Coward, McCann and Geoghegan, 1976. (See Bibliography for Chapter Four for description)

Cousins, Norman. *Anatomy of an Illness.* New York: W.W. Norton Co., Inc., 1979. (See Bibliography for Chapter Ten for description)

How to Manage Your Hospital Stay
Gots, Ronald, M.D. and Kaufman, Arthur, M.D., *The People's Hospital Book.* New York: Avon Books, 1978; paperback edition, Avon, 1981

This excellent and comprehensive book, written from the physician's perspective, helps you choose a hospital and cope with the experience of being a patient there. It also contains useful discussions of emergency rooms, surgery, and anesthesia.

Its only flaw is the authors' over-riding enthusiasm for university hospitals. The statement in the Introduction that "ideally, your every problem, no matter how 'minor or routine,' should be managed in the world's greatest hospital," is just not true. For another point of view, read what Dr. William Nolen has to say about his personal experiences in Massachusetts General Hospital, in *Surgeon Under the Knife.*

Nierenberg, Judith and Janovic, Florence. *The Hospital Experience: A Complete Guide to Understanding and Participating in Your Own Care.* Indianapolis/New York: The Bobbs-Merrill Co., Inc., 1978

This is a thorough guide to hospital routines, particularly helpful in its descriptions of common tests, operations, and treatments. By translating medical jargon into plain English, this book enables patients to participate more easily in decision-making.

How To Stay Out
Breslow, Lori (ed.), *How to Get the Best Health Care for Your Money.* Emmaus, Pa.: Rodale Press, 1979

Alternatives to standard care and hospitalization are presented clearly, with both pros and cons discussed.

Murphy, Lois Barclay, *The Home Hospital.* New York: Basic Books, Inc., 1982

For a bedridden adult, a child with a chronic illness, a teen-ager recovering from an accident, the home may be far more supportive and comfortable than a hospital or nursing home. This book supplies the information you need to provide proper home care—whether its finding the right kind of bed, keeping adequate medical records, or enhancing the patient's will to live.

Patients' Rights
Annas, George J., *The Rights of Hospital Patients.* New York: Avon Books, 1975 (paperback)

This book, part of a series put out by the American Civil Liberties Union, is a classic. It covers the legal aspects of a hospital stay. Topics include informed consent, access to records, confidentiality, experimentation, and payment of hospital bills.

Huttmann, Barbara. *The Patient's Advocate.* New York: Viking Press, 1981

This books tells the lay person how to play the role of patient advocate if a friend or family member must be hospitalized. Huttmann, a nurse, has a real insider's view and can offer nitty-gritty information on hospital systems, terminology, and common hospital procedures. She also suggests some alternatives to hospitalization.

RESOURCES

Choosing a Hospital
Each year the American Hospital Association puts out a *Guide to the Health Care Field.* Here you will find a list of hospitals according to geographic location, addresses of state agencies, and sections on licensure, organizations, and nursing homes. The hospital listing is coded and provides a great deal of information about each hospital's size, specialties, affiliation, administrator's name, etc. The *Guide* is found in the larger medical libraries.

For specific information, arm yourself with a list of questions and call the administrator's office of the hospital you might want to use.

Sample Questions

1. How many beds?
2. What type of hospital is this? University affiliate, community or voluntary hospital, municipal hospital, or proprietary hospital? If proprietary, who owns it?
3. Is it accredited and by what organization?
4. What kinds of intensive care units does it have?
5. Is there a pediatric unit? An adolescent unit?
6. What kinds of special services such as rehabilitation or kidney dialysis does it offer?
7. How does it provide maternity care? (See Chapter Nine, pp. 202–204 for specific questions.)
8. What is the ratio of staff nurses, LPNs, and aides to patients?
9. How is nursing care organized? Is there primary or team nursing?

For information on hospitals (types, size, specialties) and nursing homes:
American Hospital Association
840 North Lake Shore Drive
Chicago, Illinois 60611

To find out whether a hospital is accredited:
Joint Commission on Accreditation of Hospitals
875 N. Michigan Avenue
Chicago Illinois 60611

Information on cancer centers and qualified cancer specialists:
The National Cancer Institute
Office of Cancer Communications
Building 31, Room 10 A 18
Bethesda, Maryland 20205

The American Cancer Society
777 Third Avenue
New York, New York 10017

To locate hospital and out-patient rehabilitation programs:
National Association of Rehabilitation Facilities
P.O. Box 17675
Washington, D.C. 20015

Central resource for hospice information:
The National Hospice Organization
11311 A Dolley Madison Boulevard
McLean, Virginia 22101

For information on PAS lengths of stay, write to:
Commission on Professional and Hospital Activities
Ann Arbor, Michigan

———————CHAPTER SIX———————

REFERENCES

1. *The Medical Letter,* January 21, 1983.

BIBLIOGRAPHY

(The first three titles are discussed in greater detail elsewhere. Each of these books, however, has a useful section on emergencies.)

Gots, Ronald and Kaufman, Arthur, *The People's Hospital Book.* New York: Crown Publishers, 1978; paperback edition, Avon Books, 1981

Has an excellent and comprehensive chapter on how to use hospital emergency rooms.

Vickery, Donald M., M.D. and Fries, James F., M.D., *Take Care of Yourself.* Reading, Mass.: Addison-Wesley Publishing Co., Inc., 1976.

Emergency department personnel will often recommend this book for its first-aid information. Especially useful are the decision-making charts that help you determine whether self-care will suffice or whether you must see a doctor.

Pantell, Robert H., M.D.; Fries, James F., M.D.; Vickery, Donald M., M.D., *Taking Care of Your Child.* Reading, Mass.: Addison-Wesley Publishing Co., Inc., 1977

The same format—with decision-making charts—as the book above, but specifically about children.

The American Medical Association's Handbook of First Aid and Emergency Care. New York: Random House, 1980

Many emergency manuals are so extensive that you would find it difficult to locate critical information quickly enough. This handbook, while being thorough, up-to-date and accurate, is also the most concise and easiest to use of any we have read.

Mack, John E., and Hickler, Holly, *Vivienne: The Life and Suicide of an Adolescent Girl.* Boston: Little Brown and Company, 1981; paperback edition, NAL Books 1982

Using material drawn from Vivienne's own writing, and with the cooperation of her parents, the authors have reproduced a book that portrays and examines one young person's struggle with despair. Reading this book is a difficult emotional experience, well worth undergoing for those who want to understand more about the way children and adolescents experience depression.

RESOURCES

How To Research Your Local Emergency Services
Places to call or write:
1. Hospital emergency department
2. Emergency Medical Services office
3. Fire department, police department
4. Private ambulance companies

The Hospitals
Call your local hospitals and ask for either the hospital Public Relations Department or the Emergency Department. If you are connected with the ER, ask to speak to the charge nurse. She or he will be able to answer your questions on the type of services provided and may also be able to give you an idea of how long patients can expect to wait.

The Emergency Medical Services (EMS) office
Most states have retained this network, which was originally established by the federal government. (To find out if there is an EMS office in your area, look in the telephone directory under the state listing for Social and Health Services, write to the state Department of Health, or contact your local fire or police department.)

Where an EMS organization exists, it is responsible for training emergency medical technicians and paramedics and providing them with continuing education. EMS staff are apt to be objective about emergency services.

If there is no EMS office in your state or area, you might be able to gather information from your local fire department or a private ambulance company. You may find someone who is willing to talk to you about which ERs are considered best and which offer specialized services.

First Aid Classes and CPR Instruction
Instruction may be provided through one or more agencies in your community. Try the following:

The American Red Cross
The American Heart Association
Your local fire department
The YMCA or YWCA

Poison Control Centers
A nationwide system has been established to provide emergency information. The number of your nearest Poison Control Center will be listed in the front of your telephone directory. If you can't find the number, ask the information operator or call a hospital emergency room.

Some national addresses that may be helpful:

The American Heart Association
Inquiry Section
44 East 23rd Street
New York, New York 10010
or
7320 Greenville Avenue
Dallas, Texas 75231

American National Red Cross
17th and D Street, NW
Washington, D.C. 20006

National Poison Center Network
Children's Hospital of Pittsburgh
125 DeSoto Street
Pittsburgh, Pennsylvania 15213

Emergency Identification
People whose chronic diseases (such as diabetes, heart disease, or epilepsy) may lead to an emergency situation often wear a bracelet or necklace in-

scribed with the name of their disease, plus a telephone number to call for more medical information. Some carry a card in their wallet. There are several organizations that supply this kind of identification; two are listed below.

For wallet emergency information:
Evergreen Safety Council
822 John Street
Seattle, Washington 98109

This organization will supply you with a wallet-sized plastic card that contains your information on microfilm plus a magnifying lens to read it. You can even have them include an EKG tracing if you wish. Write for details and charges.

For medical identification necklaces or bracelets:
Medic Alert Foundation
P.O. Box 1009
Turlock, California 95381

CHAPTER SEVEN

REFERENCES

1. Moertel, C. G., et al., "A Comparative Evaluation of Marketed Analgesic Drugs." *The New England Journal of Medicine,* April 13, 1972, pp. 813–815.

2. Geddes, A.M., "A Framework for prescribing." *The Lancet,* Sept. 4, 1982.

3. *The Medical Letter, Inc.,* 56 Harrison St., New Rochelle, New York 10801.

BIBLIOGRAPHY

Long, James W., M.D., *The Essential Guide to Prescription Drugs,* (Third Edition). New York: Harper & Row, 1982

Superb book listing precautions, side effects, risks, advisability of use during pregnancy, and a number of other factors for over 1450 drugs. Extremely well organized and clear. A must for anyone on medication for a chronic problem, and at $9.95 for 935 pages, a bargain for anyone who wants to be well informed about drugs.

The Physicians' Desk Reference (PDR)
(Published yearly by the Medical Economics Company in Oradell, New Jersey. They also publish *The Physicians' Desk Reference for Nonprescription Drugs.*)

A potential gold mine if you don't fall down the shaft. Helpful for someone who wants to know every possible side effect or interaction of a drug, or what precautions to take. Useful section in the front that enables you to identify unknown pills by their appearance.

The material in the *PDR* is provided by the drug companies, and one of their goals is to supply information on every conceivable risk, no matter how obscure, to protect themselves from legal action. The danger of reading the *PDR* is that you may become so upset by the long lists of risks and side effects you might decide not to take a drug you really need.

Wolfe, Sidney M., M.D.; Coley, Christopher M.; and the Health Research Group, *Pills That Don't Work.* New York: Farrar, Straus & Giroux, 1981; paperback edition, Warner Books, 1982

Useful discussion of most effective treatment of a number of common problems, plus compendium of 607 drugs or drug combinations found to be ineffective. If your physician prescribes any of these drugs, discuss this book's findings with him or her to see if the decision seems justified in your case.

Graedon, Joe, *The People's Pharmacy.* New York: St. Martin's Press, 1976; paperback edition, Avon, 1977

Written in a casual, almost flippant style, this book contains a good discussion about the risks of drugs in general as well as valuable information on specific drugs to take and to avoid. Many useful and inexpensive self-care tips, too. Somewhat rambling—one section entitled "Colds and Vitamin C" wanders off into a very interesting discussion of the potential for aspirin to prevent heart attacks—but worth sticking with.

The Medicine Show. Mt. Vernon, New York: Consumer's Union (Fifth Edition), 1980. (See Bibliography for Chapter Ten for description.)

RESOURCES

Sample Drug Profile

Name, Address, Date of Birth

Chronic Illnesses

1. _____ 4. _____

2. _____ 5. _____

3. _____ 6. _____

Drug Allergies

_____

Allergies

_____

Drugs Taken (include non-prescription drugs and vitamins)

Name of Drug   Type   Strength   Amount per Day   Dates   Reactions   Physician

_____

_____

_____

Pregnant   yes/no
Nursing mother   yes/no
_____

————————CHAPTER EIGHT————————

REFERENCES

1. Weissman, M. M. and Myers, J. K., "Affective disorders in a U.S. urban community." *Archives of General Psychiatry,* 1978, pp. 1304–10.

——Woodruff, R. A., Goodwin, D. W., Grize, S. B., *Psychiatric Diagnosis,* New York: Oxford University Press, 1974.

2. Gordon, Barbara, *I'm Dancing As Fast As I Can.* New York: Harper and Row, 1979.

BIBLIOGRAPHY

Mishara, Brian L., Ph.D. and Patterson, Robert D., M.D., *Consumer's Handbook of Mental Health.* New York: Times Books, 1977; paperback edition, NAL, 1979

A thoughtful and thorough discussion of all aspects of treatment. Includes information on evaluating therapy, patients' rights and responsibilities, hospitalization, causes of mental health problems, fees, insurance, and financial help.

Kovel, Joel, *A Complete Guide to Therapy: From Psychotherapy to Behavior Modification.* New York: Pantheon Books, 1976; paperback edition, Pantheon, 1977

A detailed guide through the maze of different types of psychotherapy by a psychiatrist who has written extensively in this area.

Chesler, Phyllis, *Women and Madness.* New York: Doubleday & Co., Inc., 1972; paperback edition, Avon, 1973

A fascinating and well-documented examination of women's mental health problems, how they are defined by society and dealt with by therapists. Chesler, a psychologist who specializes in working with women, points out how behavior may be interpreted differently depending on whether it is exhibited by a man or a woman.

Women and Psychotherapy. Prepared by the Task Force on Consumer Issues in Psychotherapy of the Association for Women in Psychology, 2nd Division of the Psychology of Women of the American Psychological Association (1981)

(available for $3.75 plus $1.00 postage from the Federation of Organizations for Professional Women, 2000 P Street, NW; Suite 403; Washington, D.C. 20036)

Although it is especially relevant to women, this would be an excellent general guide for men too. Topics covered include: whether to seek therapy, how to choose a therapist, the use of psychoactive drugs, racism and therapy, feminist therapy, and how to deal with grievances.

Napier, Augustus Y., Ph.D., with Carl Whitaker, M. D., *The Family Crucible.* New York: Harper & Row, 1978; paperback edition, Bantam Books, 1980

Describes the practice and goals of family therapy, but is as gripping as a novel. According to *The New York Times Book Review,* "The real payoff of the book . . . is the perspective you will gain on your own behavior and its causes, and on the ways you can nurture and liberate yourself."

RESOURCES

To locate names of mental health organizations in your telephone directory, look in the white pages under the name of your state or in the yellow pages under the headings **Psychologist, Social Worker,** or **Psychiatrist.**

To check credentials of clinical psychologists write to:
The American Psychological Association
1200 17th Street, N.W.
Washington, D.C. 20036

To check credentials of social workers, use the following reference work:
The N.A.S.W. Clinical Register

To check credentials of pastoral counselors write to:
The American Association of Pastoral Counselors
3 West 29th Street
New York, New York 10010

To check credentials of sex therapists write to:
The American Association of Sex Educators,
Counselors and Therapists (AASECT)
600 Maryland Avenue, S.W.
Washington, D.C. 20024

This organization certifies sex therapists and can provide you with a list of qualified people in your part of the country.

To learn more about self-help groups in your community, write to:
The National Self-Help Clearing House
Graduate Center of the City University of New York
33 West 42nd Street
New York, New York 10036

Self-help groups consist of people with a similar problem who have banded together to offer support and share experience. There are groups for every kind of problem: alcoholism, stuttering, schizophrenia, chronic disease. Some groups are for those who are suffering from a problem; others are for their families.

Rights of hospitalized mental patients:
Patient Bill of Rights
U.S. Department of Health and Human Services
Federal Register, October 3, 1979

For names of biofeedback practitioners in your area:
The Biofeedback Society of America
c/o Francine Butler, Ph.D.
4301 Owens Street
Wheat Ridge, CO 80033

———CHAPTER NINE———

REFERENCES

1. Scully, Diana, *Men Who Control Women's Health.* Boston: Houghton Mifflin Co., 1980.

2. Wennberg, J: Report read before the Annual Meeting of the American Public Health Association, Los Angeles, October 1978.

3. Haverkamp, Albert D., M.D., et al., "A controlled trial of the differential effects of intrapartum fetal monitoring." *American Journal of Obstetrics and Gynecology,* June 15, 1979.

4. Caldeyro-Barcia, Roberto, M.D., "The Influence of Maternal Position on Time of Spontaneous Rupture of the Membranes." *Birth and the Family Journal,* Spring 1979.

5. Anderson, Sandra F., R.N., "Childbirth as a Pathological Process." *The American Journal of Maternal Child Nursing,* July/Aug. 1977.

6. Caldeyro-Barcia, Roberto, M.D., "The Influence of Maternal Bearing-Down Efforts During Second Stage on Fetal Well-Being." *Birth and the Family Journal,* Spring 1979.

7. Morgan, Barbara M.; Bulpitt, Christopher, J., et al., "Analgesia and Satisfaction in Childbirth." *The Lancet,* Oct. 9, 1982.

8. Sosa, Roberto; Kennell, John, et al., "Effect of a Supportive Companion on Perinatal Problems . . ." *The New England Journal of Medicine,* Sept. 11, 1980, pp. 597–600.

9. Burnett, Claude A., III, M.D., M.P.H.; and Jones, James A., M.P.H., et al., "Home Delivery and Neonatal Mortality in North Carolina." *JAMA,* Dec. 18, 1980, pp. 2741–45.

BIBLIOGRAPHY

Arms, Suzanne, *Immaculate Deception.* Boston: Houghton Mifflin Co., 1975; paperback edition, Bantam, 1977

This controversial book is an eloquent plea for a more natural birth experience. The author discusses the role of midwives, contrasts the European approach to birth with the more impersonal American system, and raises important questions about the safety and necessity of common obstetrical practices.

Bean, Constance, *Methods of Childbirth* (Revised Edition). Garden City, New York: Doubleday and Co., Inc., 1982

A good general book, clearly written and easy to read. It provides information on alternative methods of childbirth with the aim of helping prospective parents achieve the kind of birth experience they want.

Feldman, Silvia, *Choices in Childbirth.* New York: Bantam Books, 1980

A thorough and objective guide to childbirth alternatives, containing information on birth assistants (midwives and physicians), settings, and the different types of prepared-childbirth education available. This book also discusses the postpartum period and suggests sources of community support after the baby is born. Resources for new and expectant parents are well covered.

Hazell, Lester D., *Commonsense Childbirth.* New York: Tower Publications, Inc., 1969; paperback edition, Berkeley, 1976

Here is a book that has been around for a long time for good reason. Still current, it is highly readable and frequently recommended in childbirth education circles. Contains down-to-earth advice on pregnancy, labor and delivery, and breastfeeding. Appendices include answers to frequently asked questions, a synopsis of labor and delivery, and a brief discussion of what to do in an emergency childbirth (if you have to deliver the baby yourself).

Parfitt, Rebecca Rowe, *The Birth Primer*. New York: New American Library, 1980

This book is devoted to labor and delivery, both traditional and non-traditional. Unusually clear descriptions of the birth process and a complete discussion of methods of natural childbirth, as well as explanations and excellent illustrations of procedures and drugs common to hospital births. Childbirth education resources and lengthy annotated bibliography.

Walton, Vicki E., *Have It Your Way*. New York: Bantam Books, 1978

If you intend to give birth in a hospital, this is a particularly good guide to obtaining the type of hospital birth experience you want. Discusses pregnancy, labor and delivery, medication, newborn physiology, breastfeeding, and postpartum adjustment.

RESOURCES

It is easy enough to find out what types of maternity services the hospitals in your community offer by picking up the telephone, but discovering alternatives to hospital delivery and hospital-sponsored childbirth education, may take a bit of research.

If there is a free-standing birth center in your town, the staff there will usually know what options are available. Nurse-midwives often work both at birth centers and hospitals, and may also assist at home births.

Other local sources of information are women's health clinics or women's resource groups, which may be affiliated with a college or university or an organization like the YWCA.

For information on family-centered maternity care:
International Childbirth Education Association
    P.O. Box 20048
    Minneapolis, Minnesota 55420

(Ask for the name and address of your state coordinator. He or she is the person who can help you locate physicians, nurse-midwives, childbirth groups, and instructors in your area.)

For information on the Cybele Cluster System:
    The Cybele Society
    414 Peyton Building
    Spokane, Washington 99201

For information on free-standing birth centers, write to:
Maternity Center Association
48 E. 92nd Street
New York, New York 10028

If you want to find a Lamaze instructor:
American Society for Psychoprophylaxis in Obstetrics (ASPO)
1411 K Street NW
Suite 200
Washington, D.C. 20005

If you are interested in the Bradley method of prepared childbirth:
American Academy of Husband-Coached Childbirth (AAHCC)
P.O. Box 5224
Sherman Oaks, California 91413

To find out more about home births:
Home Oriented Maternity Experience (H.O.M.E.)
511 New York Avenue
Takoma Park, Washington, D.C. 20012

For information on breast-feeding:
La Leche League International
9616 Minneapolis Avenue
Franklin Park, Illinois 60131

If you're having more than one:
National Organization of Mothers of Twins Clubs, Inc.
5402 Amberwood Lane
Rockville, Maryland 20853

————————CHAPTER TEN————————

REFERENCES

1. Klein, Kenneth, M. D.; Liberman, David, M. D., "A Good Little Antacid." *The New England Journal of Medicine,* June 17, 1982, p. 1429.

2. Mowrey, D. B., Ph.D. and Clayson, D. E., Ph.D., "Motion Sickness, Ginger and Psycho Physics." *The Lancet,* March 20, 1982.

3. Dupont, H. L.; Reves, R. R., et al., "Treatment of travelers' diarrhea with trimethoprim/sulfamethoxazole and with trimethoprim alone." *The New England Journal of Medicine,* September 30, 1982, pp. 841–44.

4. Selye, Hans, *The Stress of Life* (Revised Edition). New York: McGraw-Hill Book Co., 1978.

5. Istre, Gregory R., M.D.; Kreiss, Kathleen, M.D., et al., "An Outbreak of Amebiasis Spread by Colonic Irrigation." *The New England Journal of Medicine,* Aug. 5, 1982.

6. Trillin, Alice, "Of Dragons and Garden Peas." *The New England Journal of Medicine,* March 19, 1981, pp. 699–701.

BIBLIOGRAPHY

Self-Care and Prevention
The Medicine Show. Mt. Vernon, New York: Consumer's Union (Fifth Edition), 1980

Published by the editors of *Consumer Reports,* a very helpful guide to effective over-the-counter drug use. Can save you from wasting money on unnecessary drugs or physician visits, by teaching you when OTC treatment would suffice.

Vickery, Donald M., M.D. and Fries, James F., M.D., *Take Care of Yourself.* Reading, Mass.: Addison-Wesley Publishing Company, 1976; paperback edition, 1981

For many sophisticated health care consumers, this might be the most valuable book in their home health library. In addition to meticulous explanations of how to manage 93 common problems, there are excellent discussions of the home pharmacy, choosing a doctor or a hospital, preventive care, and medical fraud.

Especially useful to those who stay cool, calm, and logical when they are sick. Step-by-step "decision charts" help you decide when to see an M.D. right away, when to call for an appointment, or when to use home treatment. In an effort to make sure you do not overlook a serious problem, the authors have a tendency to slightly over-recommend that you see a physician.

Pantell, Robert H., M.D.; Fries, James F., M.D.; Vickery, Donald M., M.D., *Taking Care of Your Child.* Reading, Mass.: Addison-Wesley Publishing Co., Inc., 1977

Even better than its companion; there are 142 introductory pages (compared with 88). Useful discussions about prenatal care, the newborn period, growth and development of children and adolescents; sound information in areas such as school problems and sexuality. Excellent home safety check list.

Ferguson, Tom, M.D. (ed.), *Medical Self-Care.* New York: Summit Books, 1980

This is a wide-ranging reference-cum-workbook written from a medical perspective for non-medical people. Contains a guide to health tools and equipment.

Sehnert, Keith W., M.D. and Eisenberg, Howard, *The Family Medical Handbook.* New York: Grosset and Dunlap, 1975

A "how-to" approach to a variety of common medical conditions. Includes a brief section on self-examination.

Behrstock, Barry, M.D., and Trubo, Richard. *The Parent's When-Not-To-Worry Book.* New York: Harper & Row, 1981

Very practical book debunking hundreds of myths that, in the author's words, "You've learned from your parents, friends—and even doctors."

Cousins, Norman, *Anatomy of an Illness,* New York: W.W. Norton, Co., Inc., 1979

Remarkable story by a man who took the treatment for an "incurable" disease into his own hands. Dramatic example of the potential for mobilizing the body's ability to heal itself. Also contains memorable descriptions of other creative approaches to healing.

Kunz, Jeffrey R. M., M.D., (ed.), *The American Medical Association Family Medical Guide.* New York: Random House, 1982

In its own words, "The Family Medical Guide shows how your body is structured, how it functions, and what you must do to keep it healthy. It answers your questions about all the most common diseases and their symptoms." Useful self-diagnosis charts. If you feel reassured to have an "encyclopedia" of medicine around the house, you can't do better than this book.

Graedon, Joe, *The People's Pharmacy.* New York: St. Martin's Press, 1976 (See Bibliography for Chapter Seven for description.)

Books Combining Medical Self-Care and Wellness
Samuels, Mike, M.D. and Bennett, Hal, *The Well-Body Book.* New York: Random House, 1973

Ranges from traditional medical advice to alternative approaches to healing. Includes information on how to do a complete physical examination. Contains interesting chapter on how to create and use an imaginary doctor.

Tager, Mark, M.D. and Jennings, Charles, *Whole Person Health Care.* Portland, Oregon: Victoria House, Inc., 1979

Incorporates medical and alternative healing methods. Stresses personal responsibility for health in a common-sense way. This book is especially useful for people who live in the Northwest because it includes a "Northwest Health Care Directory."

The Boston Women's Health Collective, *Our Bodies, Ourselves* (Revised Edition). New York: Simon and Schuster, 1979

Holistic in approach, this book deals with the social, emotional, and physiological aspects of being a woman. Topics include female anatomy and physiology, sexuality and love relationships, birth control, abortion, parenthood, diet and exercise, menopause and use of the health care system as well as alternatives to it.

Bell, Ruth and members of the Boston Women's Health Collective, *Changing Bodies, Changing Lives*. New York: Random House, 1980

Similar to *Our Bodies, Ourselves* in approach but written for teen-agers.

Wellness and Alternative Healing Methods
Pelletier, Kenneth R., *Mind As Healer, Mind As Slayer*. New York: Dell Publishing Co., 1977

The author shows you how stress can produce real physical illness and suggests relaxation methods that help to prevent the build-up of stress to levels high enough to cause undesirable effects on your body.

Fisher, Donald D., M.D., *I Know You Hurt, But There's Nothing to Bandage*. Beaverton, Oregon: Touchstone Press 1978

Easy-to-read and conversational in style, this book focuses on the health problems people cause themselves.

Popenoe, Chris, *Wellness*. Washington, D.C.: YES! Inc., 1977; paperback edition, Random House, 1977

A non-medical approach to the subject of wellness.

Ryan, Regina and Travis, John W., *Wellness Workbook*. Berkeley: Ten Speed Press, 1981

Similar to *Medical Self-Care* but with more of an emphasis on alternative methods for promoting wellness, this book emphasizes the necessity of learning about and accepting oneself. Workbook style. Includes extensive wellness exam and a number of alternative methods for promoting health.

Benson, Herbert, M.D., and Klipper, Miriam, *The Relaxation Response*. New York: William Morrow and Company, Inc., 1975; paperback edition, Avon, 1976

In this examination of the ways in which relaxation can influence health, the author draws on recent scientific studies as well as traditional Eastern wisdom.

RESOURCES

With the growing interest in health, a number of community organizations have begun to sponsor health-education workshops, classes, and telephone hot-lines to provide information on a wide range of topics. Call any of the following to find out whether they are offering courses in what you need.

United Way
Hospitals
Health departments
Colleges and universities
Health Maintenance Organizations

Home care for high blood pressure (hypertension): If you have hypertension and want to do home blood pressure checks, read *The People's Pharmacy,* pp. 254–256, for a detailed discussion of which equipment to buy. (See Bibliography for Chapter Seven.)

Healthy People: The Surgeon General's Report on Health Promotion and Disease Prevention, 1979
(U.S. Department of Health and Human Services)
For sale by the Superintendent of Documents
U.S. Government Printing Office
(Stock #017-001-00416-2)
Washington, D.C. 20402

A valuable resource for names and addresses of preventive health services. Among the listings in the back of this book are organizations dealing with family planning, mental health, maternal and child health, immunizations, sexually transmitted diseases, hypertension, occupational safety, nutrition, substance abuse, stress control, and physical fitness.

Association for Holistic Health
P.O. Box 9532
San Diego, California 92109

Write to them for information on doctors or clinics oriented to a holistic approach.

The National Self-Help Clearing House
Graduate Center of the City University of New York
33 West 42nd Street
New York, New York 10036

Write to this organization to find a self-help group for a given problem.

For travelers:
    Intermedic
    777 Third Avenue
    New York, New York 10017

Lists English-speaking doctors in foreign countries who have the equivalent of U.S. board certification.

International Association for Medical Assistance
    to Travelers (IAMAT)
    350 Fifth Avenue, Rm 5620
    New York, New York 10001

Names of English-speaking doctors in 400 foreign cities.

——————CHAPTER ELEVEN——————

REFERENCES

1. Moertel, Charles G., M.D.; Fleming, Thomas R., Ph.D.; et al., "A Clinical Trial of Amygdalin (Laetrile) in the Treatment of Human Cancer." *The New England Journal of Medicine,* Jan. 28, 1982, pp. 201–206.

—— Relman, Arnold S., M.D., "Closing the Books on Laetrile." (same issue) p. 207.

2. Casscells, Ward, B.S., et al., "Interpretation By Physicians of Clinical Laboratory Results." *The New England Journal of Medicine,* November 2, 1978, pp. 999–1000

3. Benbassat, J., and Cohen, R., "Clinical Instruction And Cognitive Development of Medical Students." *The Lancet,* January 9, 1982, pp. 95–97.

4. The Canadian Task Force, Walter J. Spitzer, M.D., (chairman), "The Periodic Health Examination." *The Canadian Medical Association Journal,* Nov. 3, 1979, pp. 1193–1254.

—— Breslow, Lester, M.D., and Somers, Anne R., "The Lifetime Health-Monitoring Program." *The New England Journal of Medicine,* Mar. 17, 1977, pp. 601–608.

BIBLIOGRAPHY

Berkow, Robert, M.D. (ed.), *The Merck Manual* (Fourteenth Edition). Rahway, New Jersey: Merck Sharp and Dohme, 1982 .

Packed with medical information and updated frequently, this is a handbook written for members of the medical profession. A very helpful book for some lay people, the worst possible one for those prone to "medical student's disease" (i.e., imagining you have every disease you read about).

For most people, this reference book would have its greatest use once a diagnosis has been made or proposed, and it would be a valuable resource for someone close to a sick person who wants to know more about treatment and prognosis (probable outcome).

Health Quackery. (By the editors of Consumer Report Books). New York: Holt Rhinehart and Winston, 1980; paperback edition, 1981

Good discussion of traps for the unwary consumer who has to deal with arthritis, suspected hypoglycemia, or obesity, plus informative chapters on Laetrile, chiropractic, nutrition, and vitamin E therapy. Very sound in its criticisms; perhaps too readily accepting of the viewpoints of Establishment Medicine.

Johnson, G. Timothy, M.D., and Goldfinger, Stephen E., M.D., (eds.), *The Harvard Medical School Health Letter Book.* Cambridge, Massachusetts: Harvard University Press, 1981; paperback edition, Warner Books, 1982

Synthesis of information presented in the *Harvard Medical School Health Letter* from 1975–1981. Expert discussions of the latest viewpoints on topics ranging from allergies, baldness and cataracts to weight loss, x-rays, and zinc. For people who are happiest when they are as up-to-date as possible, this book, along with a subscription to the *Health Letter,* is indispensable.

Check this book before you undergo surgery or accept treatment for a serious problem; if what you read differs from your physician's recommendations, bring the book with you on your next visit and ask why.

Brody, Jane E., *Jane Brody's The New York Times Guide to Personal Health.* New York: Times Books, 1982

More than 700 pages packed with information in the form of concise discussions of a wide range of topics. This book is an "editing, updating and collating" of more than five years of Ms. Brody's carefully researched and thorough columns. There are suggestions for further reading and resource listings, charts, and illustrations.

Dorland's Medical Dictionary (Shorter Edition). Philadelphia: The Saunders Press, 1980

To assist you in your medical reading, you may want or need a copy of this abridged dictionary, intended for lay people as well as medical professionals.

"Those Costly Annual Physicals." *Consumer Reports,* October 1980, pp. 601–606

An excellent and reliable guide to the screening tests you do—and don't—need.

The Physicians' Desk Reference (PDR).
(Published yearly by the Medical Economics Company in Oradell, New Jersey.)
(See Bibliography for Chapter Seven for description.)

RESOURCES

Harvard Medical School Health Letter
79 Garden Street
Cambridge, Massachusetts 02138

The periodical from which the *Harvard Medical School Health Letter Book* was compiled. Thoughtful, careful and up-to-date, this publication is aimed at the sophisticated lay reader. Write for a free sample issue or to ask if there are back issues covering a specific topic of interest. ($15/year for 12 issues—lower price on bulk orders of 50 or more)

For consumer-oriented health information:
Center for Medical Consumers and Health Care
Information, Inc.
237 Thompson Street
New York, New York 10012

This organization puts out a useful and well-researched bulletin called "Health Facts." You may either become a subscriber or write for a listing of topics and order only those issues that particularly interest you.

National Health Information Clearinghouse
Office of Disease Prevention and Health Promotion
Public Health Service
U.S. Department of Health and Human Services
P.O. Box 1133
Washington, D.C. 20013-1133

Write to this address and tell them what you want to know. A staff member will locate the organization that can best provide you with the information and will have someone from that organization get in touch with you.

For large quantities of free or low-cost information, write for a catalog of what is available.
U.S. Government Printing Office
Consumer Information Center
Public Documents Distribution Center
Pueblo, Colorado 81009

——CHAPTER TWELVE——

BIBLIOGRAPHY

Harrington, Geri, *The Medicare Answer Book*. New York: Harper and Row, 1982

Filled with useful information on Medicare benefits, care that will not be covered, how to file a claim, how to disagree with Medicare and win.

RESOURCES

The American Council of Life Insurance (CLI) and Health Insurance Association of America (HIAA) has a toll-free daytime hot-line. Call 1-800-423-8000 with questions on products, services, and companies. Will *not* settle individual complaints.

——CHAPTER THIRTEEN——

REFERENCES

1. "HMO Quality of Care Found Superior to Other Systems." *Group Health News,* July, 1979.

2. "The HMO Approach to Health Care: Are Health Maintenance Organizations Finally Taking Hold?" *Consumer Reports,* May, 1982.

RESOURCES

Office of Health Maintenance Organizations (OHMO)
Department of Health and Human Services
12420 Parklawn Drive
Rockville, Maryland 20857
(The toll-free number is 800-638-6686)

OHMO can provide you with information on location of HMOs, costs, and services.

Group Health Association of America, Inc. (GHAA)
624 Ninth Street, NW
Suite 700
Washington, D.C. 20001

GHAA publishes a newsletter for member organizations and has up-to-date information on plans, programs, and costs.

Index

medical studies, 238–242
  evaluation of, 239–240
  importance of, 239
  limits of, 241–242
  patient care affected by,
    238–239
  significance vs. randomness in,
    240–241
Medicare, 86, 275–276
medicine:
  as art vs. science, 244–245
  holistic, 233–234, 235–236
  human part of, 9–10
  militant metaphors in, 233
meditation, stress and, 232–233
Memorial Sloan-Kettering Hospital, 97
men:
  health care profession and,
    23–24, 77
  health risk appraisals for,
    257–258
meningomyelocele, 211
menopause, fibroid tumors and,
  78
menstrual problems, 23, 25
  self-treatment for, 222
mental health, see psychotherapy
Men Who Control Women's
  Health (Scully), 77, 189
methyl salicylate, 222
Middle Ages, hospitals in, 83–
  84
midwives:
  certified nurse-, 210
  lay, 210
migraine headaches, 222
minor emergency rooms, 119
Monistat, 158–159
Monroe, Marilyn, 151
morphine, 140
Mount Sinai Hospital, 32
moving, choosing doctors after,
  33–34
mumps, 216
muscle aches, self-treatment for,
  222
muscular dystrophy, 92, 211
myocardial infarction, 55, 89
myomectomy, 67, 78

National Center for Health Services Research, 263
nausea, self-treatment for, 221
Nembutal, 150
nephrologists, 20
Netherlands, home births in, 207
New England Journal of Medicine,
  3, 5, 8–9, 61, 68, 76, 81, 197,
  235, 243, 254, 257
New York Times, The, 243
Nolan, William, 97
nosebleeds, 130
nosocomial infections, 87
nurses, 104–107
  for childbirth, 206–207, 210
  private duty, 92, 110–112
  psychiatric, 168, 170
  types of, listed, 106
  visiting, 81

obstetrics (OBGYN), 209
  board status in, 30
Ocean Mist, 220
One Flew Over the Cuckoo's Nest
  (Kesey), 185
oophorectomies, 24, 78–79, 80
open-heart surgery, 66, 67
Oppenheim, Mike, 56
Ortho-Novum, 158–159
orthopedic surgery, elective, 67,
  79, 80
Osmond, Humphrey, 3–4, 7
osteopaths, 25, 26
out-patient surgery, 80–82, 90–91

pain:
  as natural defense, 151
  self-treatment for, 221
pain killers, 150, 151
Pap smears, 78, 251, 258
paracervical block, 199
parathyroid, 55
Parents Without Partners, 182
Parsons, Talcott, 6
pastoral counselors, 98
patients:
  connotation of, 6
  dependency of, 12